Prakash's

Atlas of
Orthopaedic
Surgical
Exposures

The journey is as important as the destination.

Easiest way in and easiest way out, and get the best view; that's what should be our mantra for orthopaedic exposures.

L Prakash

Prakash's

Atlas of
Orthopaedic
Surgical
Exposures

Written and Illustrated by

L Prakash
MS (Orth), MCh (Orth) (Liverpool)

Institute for Special Orthopaedics
Chennai, Tamil Nadu

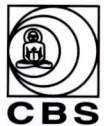

CBS

CBS Publishers & Distributors Pvt Ltd

New Delhi • Bengaluru • Chennai • Kochi • Kolkata • Mumbai
Hyderabad • Nagpur • Patna • Pune • Vijayawada

Prakash's

Atlas of
Orthopaedic Surgical Exposures

ISBN: 978-93-86310-73-6

Copyright © Author and Publisher

First Edition: 2017

Published by Satish Kumar Jain and produced by Varun Jain for

CBS Publishers & Distributors Pvt Ltd

4819/XI Prahlad Street, 24 Ansari Road, Daryaganj, New Delhi 110 002, India.
Ph: 23289259, 23266861, 23266867 Website: www.cbspd.com
Fax: 011-23243014 e-mail: delhi@cbspd.com; cbspubs@airtelmail.in.
Corporate Office: 204 FIE, Industrial Area, Patparganj, Delhi 110 092
Ph: 4934 4934 Fax: 4934 4935 e-mail: publishing@cbspd.com; publicity@cbspd.com

Branches

- **Bengaluru:** Seema House 2975, 17th Cross, K.R. Road, Banasankari 2nd Stage, Bengaluru 560 070, Karnataka
  Ph: +91-80-26771678/79 Fax: +91-80-26771680 e-mail: bangalore@cbspd.com
- **Chennai:** 7, Subbaraya Street, Shenoy Nagar, Chennai 600 030, Tamil Nadu
  Ph: +91-44-26680620, 26681266 Fax: +91-44-42032115 e-mail: chennai@cbspd.com
- **Kochi:** Ashana House, No. 39/1904, AM Thomas Road, Valanjambalam, Ernakulam 682 016, Kochi, Kerala
  Ph: +91-484-4059061-65 Fax: +91-484-4059065 e-mail: kochi@cbspd.com
- **Kolkata:** 6/B, Ground Floor, Rameswar Shaw Road, Kolkata-700 014, West Bengal
  Ph: +91-33-22891126, 22891127, 22891128 e-mail: kolkata@cbspd.com
- **Mumbai:** 83-C, Dr E Moses Road, Worli, Mumbai-400018, Maharashtra
  Ph: +91-22-24902340/41 Fax: +91-22-24902342 e-mail: mumbai@cbspd.com

Representatives

- **Hyderabad** 0-9885175004 • **Nagpur** 0-9021734563 • **Patna** 0-9334159340
- **Pune** 0-9623451994 • **Vijayawada** 0-9000660880

Printed at Rashtriya Printers, Dilshad Garden, Delhi, India

Foreword

Thirty-six years back, when my plastic surgeon friend explained to me that skin too had vascular dermatomes; and plastic surgical flaps are designed accordingly, I understood that anatomy existed beyond Henry Gray; we all knew so well.

This year too; when I saw the beautiful painstaking watercolour paintings including drawings of KRAISSL'S lines from the book *Atlas of Orthopaedic Surgical Exposures* by Dr L Prakash, my old schoolmate from Gwalior, I suddenly enriched my knowledge.

Realisation dawned on me that a time has come to revise our existing teachings as every orthopaedic colleague to whom I sent that picture and the PDF was impressed and astonished.

Now I realise that the knife too has to relearn its set of rules. Written lucidly in short and simple sentences, and illustrated with pictures emulating F. Netter, with a few words and many pictures, this *Atlas* was a pleasure to read, and I spent five fast hours reading it from cover to cover. I am astonished at the amount of work Dr L Prakash has single-handedly put in this book. He has written the text, made the drawings, painted the water colours, and even edited, formatted and made the layout on his fancy new Apple computer.

Hats off to Dr L Prakash for making both the audio and video versions of the book, and I had an immense pleasure in listening to the book on my car stereo during a long drive. It makes revision so easy.

Though I have twenty more things to learn from the orthopaedic legend Dr L Prakash, I begin first with exposures, before I begin to wade through the chest of his treasure trove of knowledge.

I wish that all Tyros and Maven in orthopaedics get an opportunity to read this book and benefit from it. This will take us closer to our ultimate goal towards better patient outcome, leading to wide smiled beaming relatives.

My beste ønsker… (best wishes) to Dr L Prakash for his new book, which I am certain will not only benefit the trainee and beginner, but also the middle to senior level surgeons like me, who would take this opportunity to brush up on their knowledge of orthopaedic exposures.

Arvind Jain Diwaker
Paediatric Orthopaedic Consultant
Lalitpur, India | Oslo, Norway

Preface

Most books on orthopaedic exposures are heavy on words and low on pictures. In addition, reading them feels like a chore and is seldom a pleasure. Many years back I decided to write a book with nice colour illustrations and crisp short text that could actually teach the operating surgeon how to reach a specific bone or joint.

This is not a book of operative orthopaedics. This is just a book that teaches you exposures. During my training days, whenever I read these books I was always fascinated by the history behind each approach and decided to incorporate the same in this book.

Unlike my earlier orthopaedic books, there is not much original in this book because I have borrowed heavily from the literature both the descriptions and the illustrations. The descriptions, however, I have simplified and the pictures I have redrawn and water coloured myself.

Though I have described most of the common and a few uncommon exposures, the book is by no means exhaustive enough to include all the exposures available in the literature.

However, I am certain that the incisions and exposures described in the book will certainly be adequate in most situations that an average orthopaedic surgeon faces during day-to-day practice.

The book is accompanied by two audio book CDs, that you can listen on long drives as you visualise the surgery. An additional atlas of cadaveric pictures is planned in the near future. I hope the readers enjoys reading the book as much as I enjoyed writing and illustrating it.

L Prakash

Acknowledgments

$\mathbf{M}$y parents Mr TS Lakshmanan, and Radha Lakshman. I owe my existence to them.

Dr TS Ramaswamy and Dr Pramila Ramaswamy, who made my live worth living, and because of whom I'm now a medical teacher and scientist.

Dr Mayil, my best friend, and more importantly my foul-weather friend.

TG Seshadri, my medical assistant, who learnt photography, designed a sterilizable camera sleeve, and who scrubbed up in every case, to take the brilliant close up photos and the excellent videos in the is book.

Jagga, my biomedical engineer, Puliarasi my orthopaedic nurse, and Babu my Man Friday who help me to stretch my day beyond 24 hours.

Mr LR Ashok, my editor, who has rendered the book flawless as far as the language and grammar is concerned.

My patients who placed their trust in me from the time I began implanting locally forged and machined implants 25 years ago.

L Prakash

Contents

Rules of Exposing Bones and Joints

1. The shortest and cleanest route from skin to the bone or joint is used.
2. As far as possible, the plane of approach is through intermuscular fascia.
3. Skin is incised parallel to the tension creases of Langer, or lines of Kraissl, Cox or Borges. This is not a hard and fast rule, and incisions can angle, deviate or even go at right angles to the creases, should the exposure require it.
4. Subcutaneous fat is cut in the same line as the skin.
5. The deep fascia is cut in the line of approach.

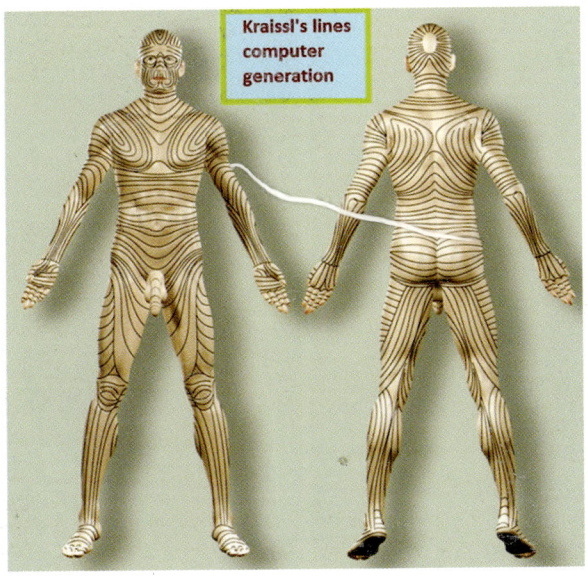

Kraissl's lines computer generation

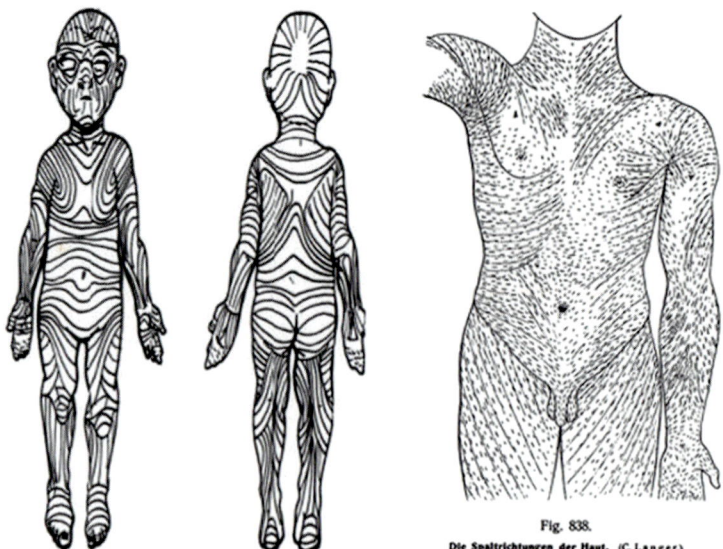

Fig. 838.

Die Spaltrichtungen der Haut. (C. Langer.)

6. Muscles should be split between fibres, or separated by blunt dissection. It is prohibited to make transverse cuts in the muscle belly.

7. Tendons should be retracted out of the way. When this does not allow a sufficient exposure, they can be divided by a Z plasty for later reattachment.

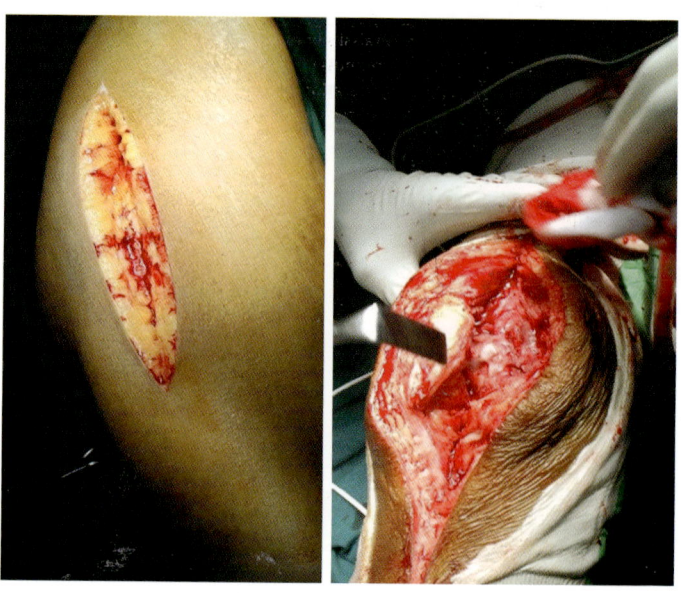

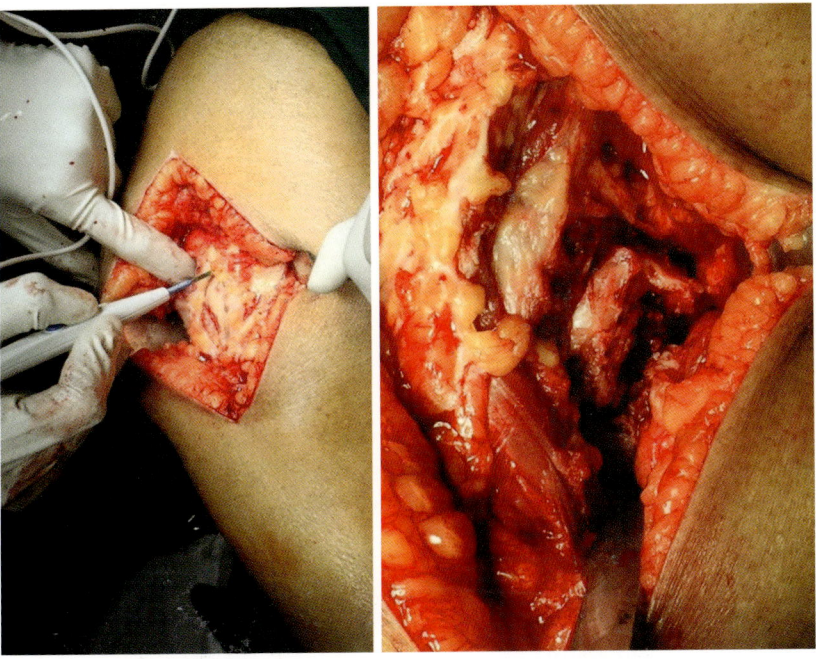

The above photographs show the exposure to the hip joint.

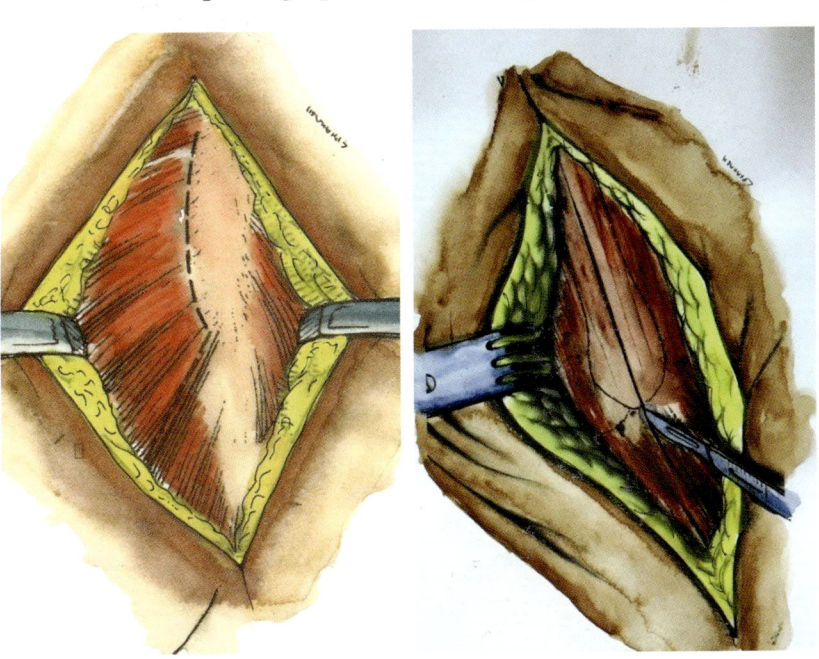

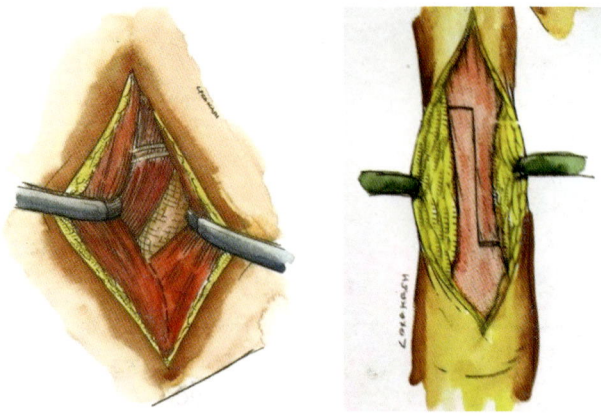

8. When tendons are cut, they should always be split in the direction of the fibres. Occasionally, a Z plasty might be required for a wider exposure.

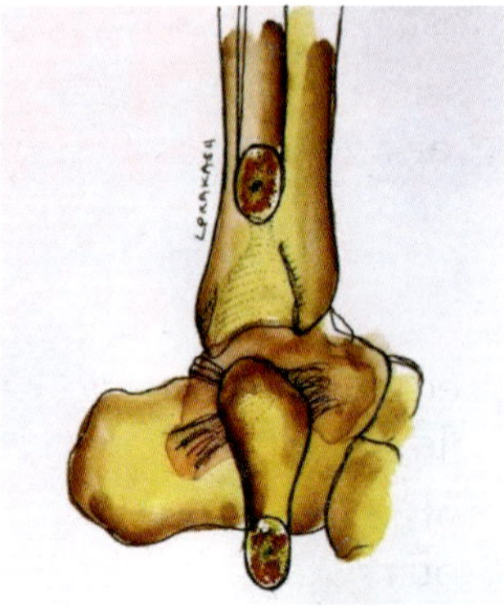

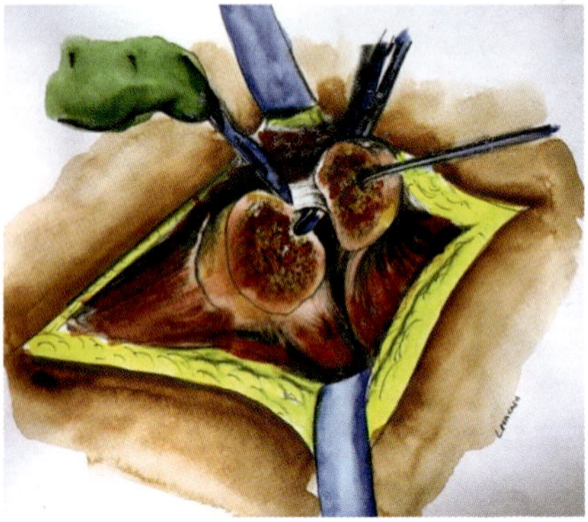

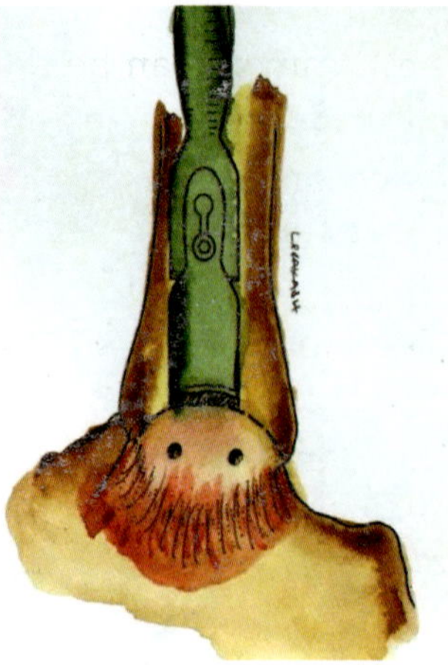

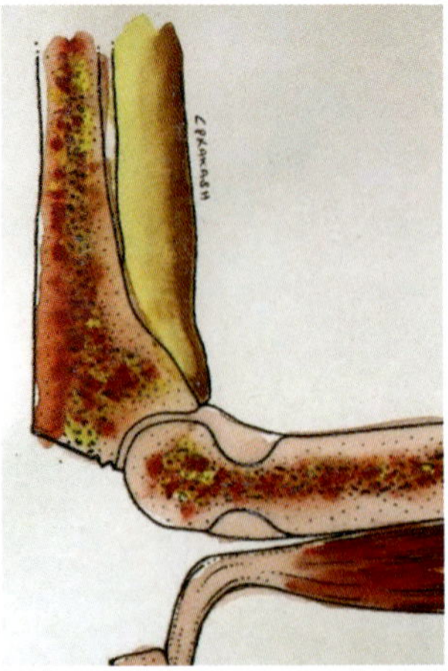

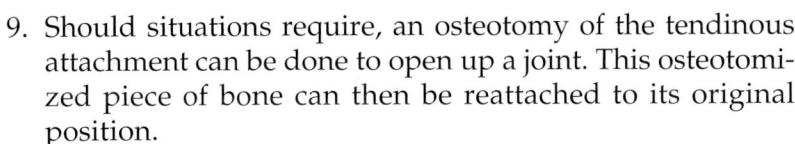

9. Should situations require, an osteotomy of the tendinous attachment can be done to open up a joint. This osteotomized piece of bone can then be reattached to its original position.

10. Small arteries, veins and nerves can be sacrificed. Medium-sized arteries and veins, if they fall in line of incision, are caught, cut ligated or coagulated. Large vessels are carefully identified and retracted out of the way.

11. As far as nerves are concerned, they should never be cut or even stretched. By very careful dissection, the nerve is mobilized and retracted in the direction of least tension.

12. The joint capsule can be cut in any direction, as the exposure warrants.

13. Periosteum is cut along the long axis of the bone and elevated off the bone using a periosteal elevator.

14. Anatomical closure in layers is essential for a functional and cosmetic postoperative result and the rules of closure are given below.

Rules of Surgical Closure

1. The joint capsule need not be sutured in an adult. If needed, it can be sutured by thin absorbable interrupted sutures.

2. All bony detachments and osteotomies are accurately repositioned and fixed with cancellous screws, tension band wiring or cerclage wiring.

3. In case of the trochanter, its attachment can be distalized to improve the abductor lever arm mechanism.

4. Accurate reattachment of osteotomized bone and rigid fixation are the most important steps in transosseous approaches.

5. Periosteum usually does not need to be sutured; it falls back in place.

6. Any detachment of a muscle or tendon from the bone for exposure should be performed leaving adequate bits for reattachment, and these are sutured under tension. This can be assisted by moving the limb in the appropriate direction to relax the tense structures while suturing.

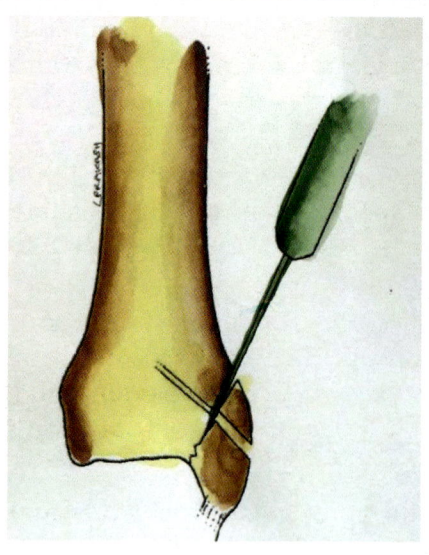

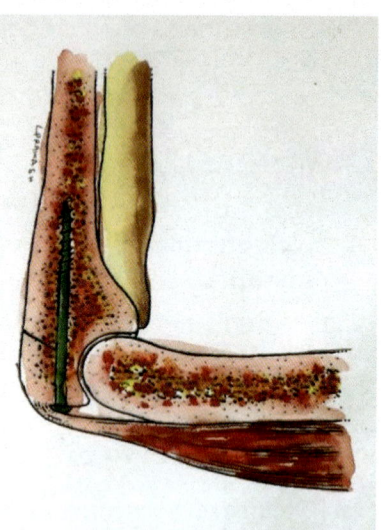

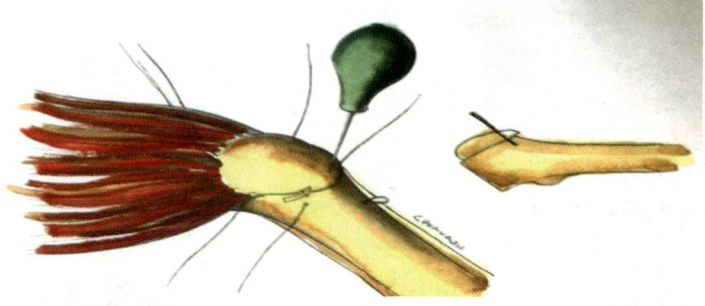

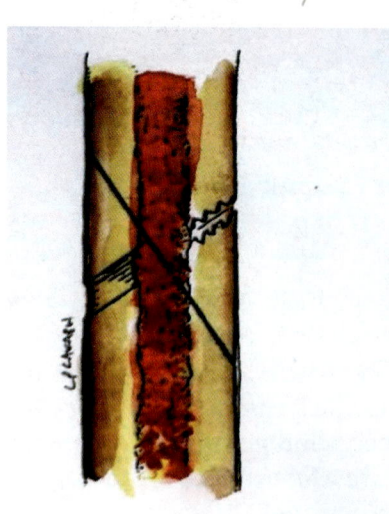

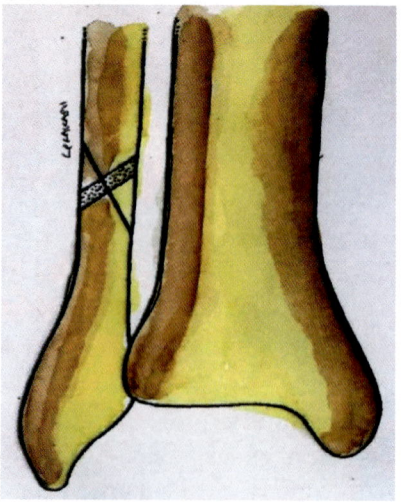

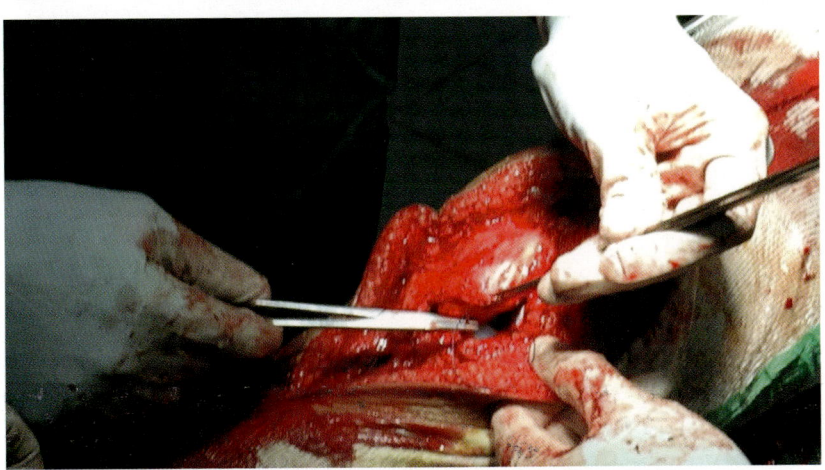

7. Split muscles don't need suturing; rather, transverse stitches strangulate the linear muscle bundles. Just relaxing the limb allows the split muscle to fall into place.

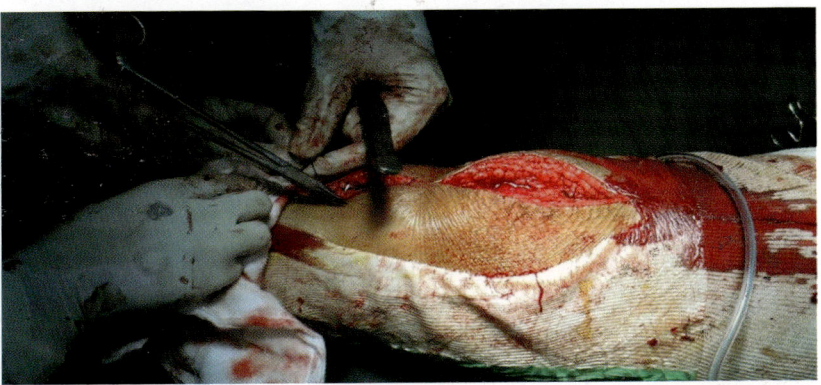

8. Deep fascia is stitched in the line of incision by synthetic absorbable sutures (continuous or interrupted) depending on the surgeon's choice.

9. A good approximation of subcutaneous fat is achieved by absorbable sutures. This should leave the skin edges close without eversion.

10. Though skin staplers are widely used, they are not recommended for joint replacement surgeries, because of higher risk of superficial and deep infections. I personally recommend and use one zero or two zero monofilament nylon.

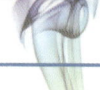

11. Use of postoperative drains and the duration of their presence is dependent on the part operated, intra- and post-operative bleeding and continuance of drain into the system. It is usually not recommended to keep drains for longer than four days.

12. Though some surgeons routinely open the dressings and inspect the wound a few days postoperatively, the author personally never opens the wounds once sealed in the theatre until two weeks, when the time is ripe for stitch removal.

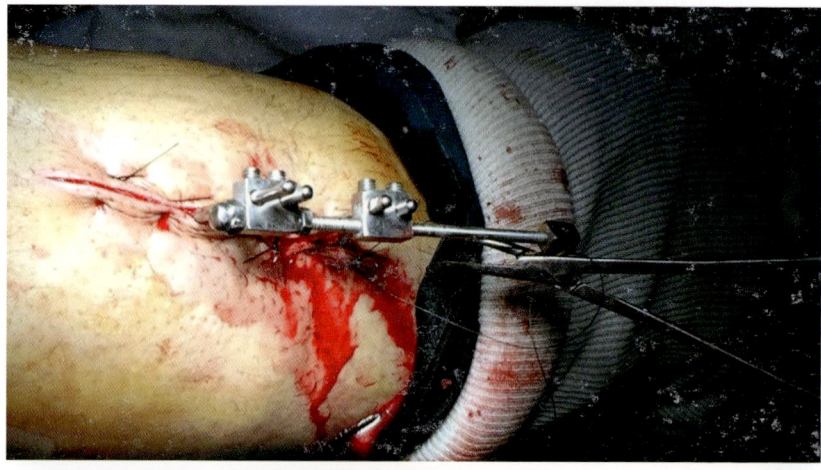

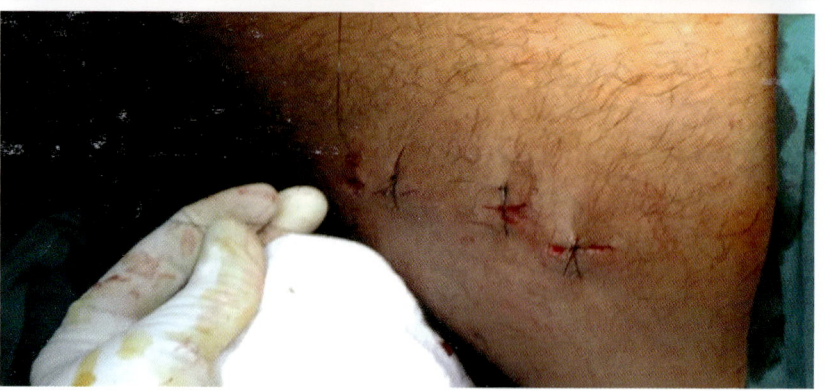

2

The Hip Joint

Bony Landmarks and Surface Anatomy

The following bony landmarks are easily identifiable:

- Symphysis pubis
- Anterosuperior iliac spine and iliac crest
- Posterosuperior iliac spine
- Greater trochanter
- Ischial tuberosity
- Pubic tubercle

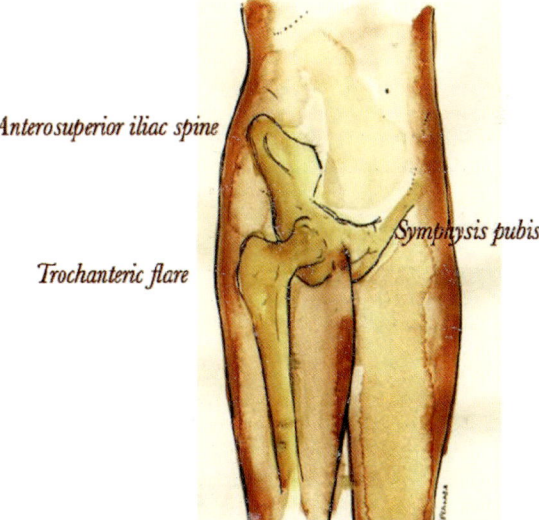

Anterosuperior iliac spine

Symphysis pubis

Trochanteric flare

Surface landmarks of the hip joint

9

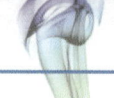

Vital Structures Around the Hip

Six arteries, four nerves, two veins and two cutaneous nerves are the important structures about which the surgeon has to be very careful! These are:

- Femoral artery, medial circumflex artery, lateral circumflex artery, obturator, superior gluteal and inferior gluteal arteries.
- Sciatic, femoral, superior gluteal and obturator are the deep nerves, while lateral and posterior cutaneous nerves are superficial.
- Femoral and long saphenous are the larger veins.

The three drawings below show the anterior, posterior and sectional anatomy of the hip.

The line between the pubic tubercle to the anterosuperior iliac spine is the groin crease. Over its midpoint lie the femoral neurovascular structures.

At the midpoint of a line between greater trochanter and ischial tuberosity lies the sciatic nerve.

The femoral and superior gluteal nerves are under risk with anterior approaches, while sciatic nerve should be identified and protected in posterior approaches. Likewise, obturator nerve is at risk with medial approaches.

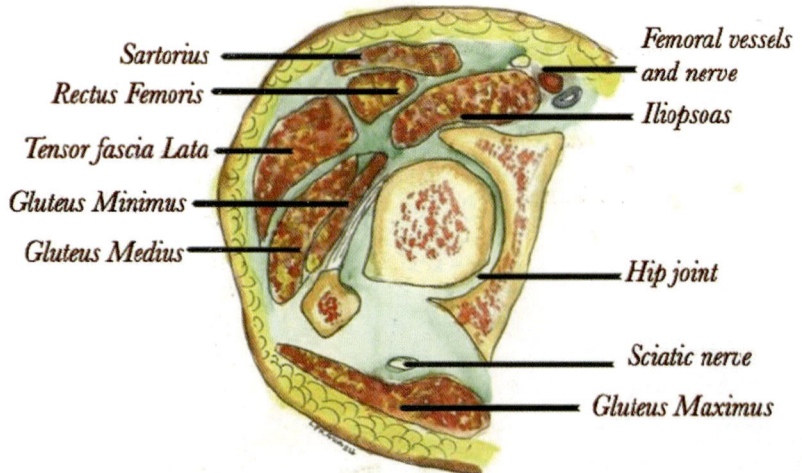

Sartorius
Rectus Femoris
Tensor fascia Lata
Gluteus Minimus
Gluteus Medius

Femoral vessels and nerve
Iliopsoas

Hip joint

Sciatic nerve
Gluteus Maximus

Anatomical planes for hip approach

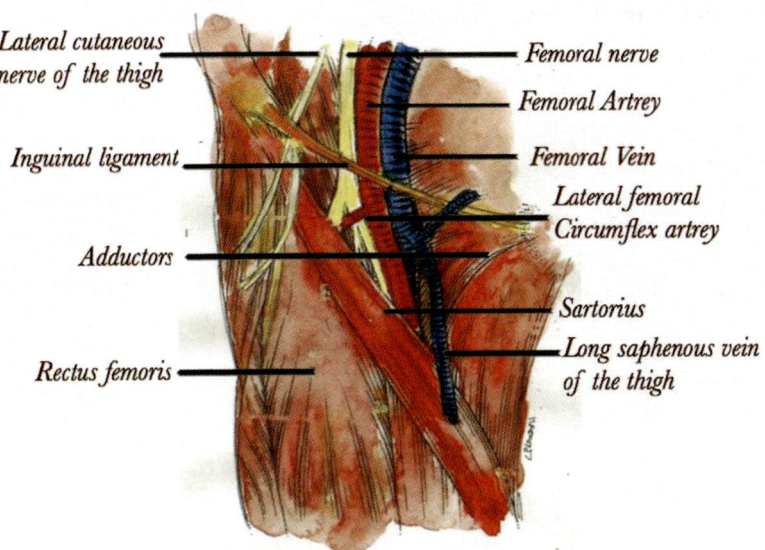

Lateral cutaneous nerve of the thigh

Inguinal ligament

Adductors

Rectus femoris

Femoral nerve

Femoral Artrey

Femoral Vein

Lateral femoral Circumflex artrey

Sartorius

Long saphenous vein of the thigh

Structures on the anterior side

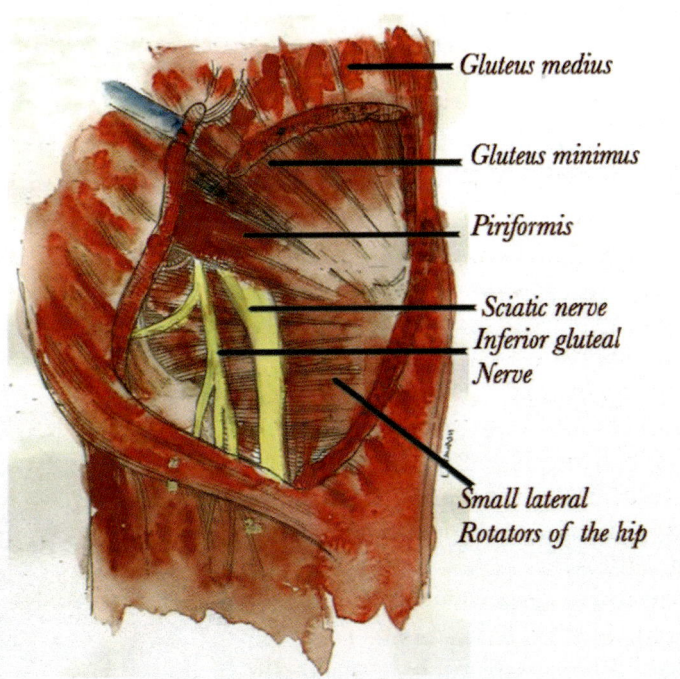

Gluteus medius

Gluteus minimus

Piriformis

Sciatic nerve
Inferior gluteal Nerve

Small lateral Rotators of the hip

Structures posteriorly

Classification of Approaches

Anterior

- Smith-Petersen
- Short anterior Bikini
- Ilioinguinal

Extensive (anterior lateral and posterior)

- Extended Smith-Peterson
- Judet and Letournel
- Ruedi transtrochanteric.

Lateral

- Modified Watson Jones
- Hardinge
- Transtrochanteric Charnley
- Lateral transgluteal

Posterior

- Posterolateral
- Southern

Medial

- Ludloff

Smith-Petersen's Approach to the Hip

History

Marius Nygaard Smith-Petersen (1886-1953), a pioneer hip surgeon, described this approach in 1917. He began his orthopaedic career under EG Brackett, prior to which he worked in physiology and neurosurgery. Dr Smith-Petersen started private practice in Boston, Massachusetts in 1923. He served as Assistant Instructor in Orthopaedic Surgery at Harvard Medical School from 1920–1930, as Instructor in Orthopaedic Surgery at Harvard Medical School from 1930–1946, as Clinical Professor of Orthopaedic Surgery at Harvard Medical School

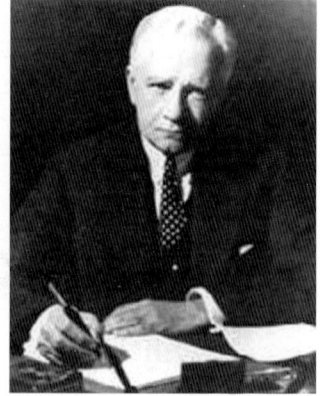

from 1935–1946, as Chief of Orthopaedic Service at Massachusetts General Hospital from 1929–1946 and as consultant to The Surgeon General from 1942–1945. He was internationally known for the development of the Smith-Petersen nail and hip nailing techniques and for hip-mold arthoplasty. Awarded the Grand Cross of the Order of St. Olav by the King of Norway, he was a brilliant surgeon and a gifted professor.

Plane
Between tensor fascia lata and gluteus medius posteriorly; and sartorius and rectus femoris anteriorly.

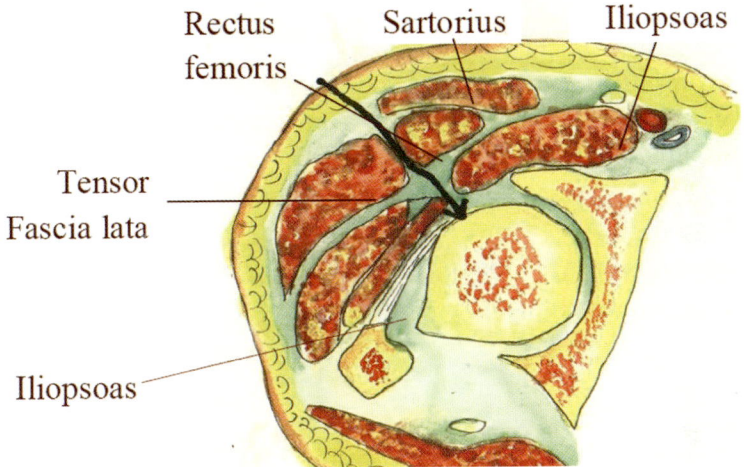

Access provided
- Inner and outer table of ileum
- Anterior and superior acetabulum
- Femoral head and neck
- Proximal femoral shaft

Dislocation
The hip joint is dislocated anteriorly.

Position and draping
- Supine with sand bag under the hip.
- Leg is draped free.
- Drape passes around upper thigh to expose anterosuperior iliac spine to gluteal tubercle.

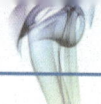

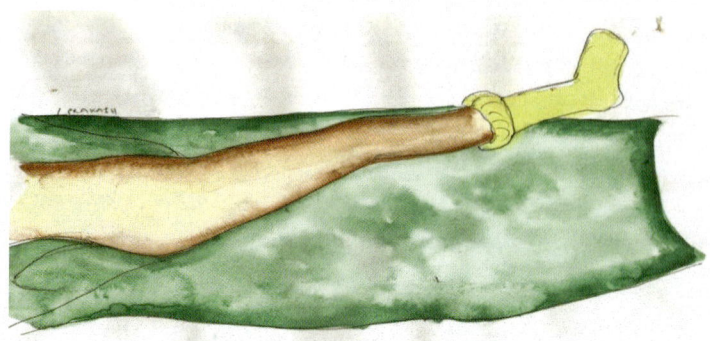

Incision

- Midpoint of the incision is anterosuperior iliac spine.
- This is extended superiorly along the iliac crest and inferiorly as a straight line leading towards lateral patellar border.
- Depending on the exposure needs, the skin incision can be extended upwards or downwards.

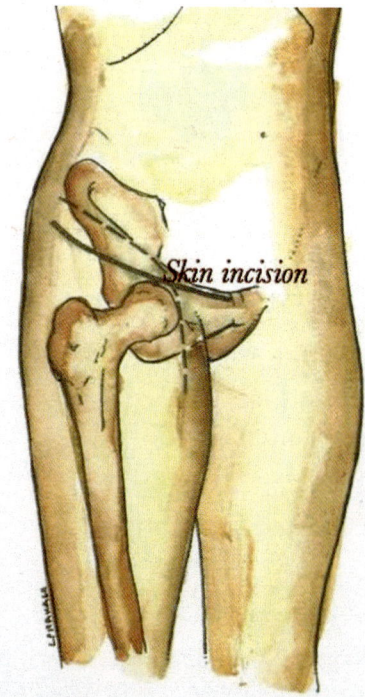

Skin incision

Smith-Petersen's approach

Dissections

- After skin and subcutaneous fat are cut, deep fascia over antero-superior iliac spine and that over anterior thigh is incised.
- A longitudinal incision is made over tensor fascia lata and the cleavage between it and sartorius is developed.

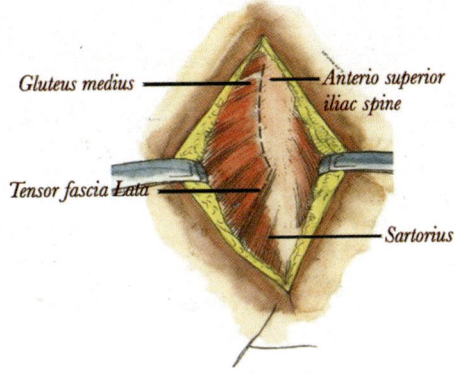

Anterior iliofemoral approach

- This is deepened, rectus femoris is identified and the plane between gluteus medius and rectus femoris is opened up.
- The ascending branch of lateral circumflex vessels is now located and ligated, to allow dissection to be carried above to ASIS.
- Deep to the lateral edge of rectus femoris, the hip capsule is visualized. Detaching the reflected head of rectus femoris increases the degree of exposure of superior acetabulum.

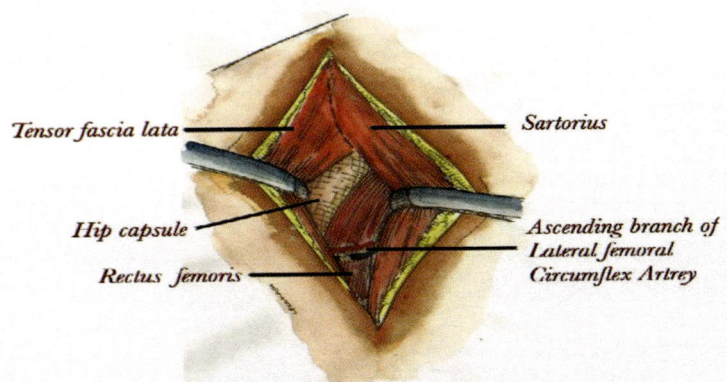

Anterior iliofemoral approach

- Muscles over lateral pelvic wall are subperiosteally stripped as far posteriorly as required, and one can go right up to the sciatic notch.
- Increased exposure can be obtained by detaching the attachment of rectus femoris from the anteroinferior iliac spine.

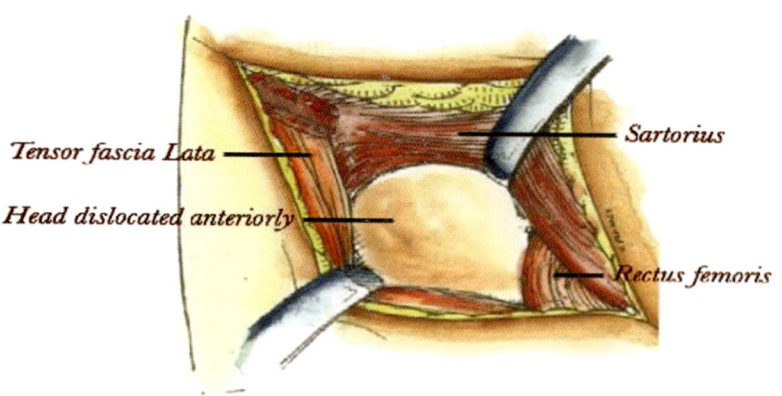

Tensor fascia Lata ——

Head dislocated anteriorly ——

—— *Sartorius*

—— *Rectus femoris*

Femoral head is dislocated by internally rotating the limb

- Adduction and external rotation of the hip stretches the hip capsule which is cut with a T shaped incision.
- Gluteus medius can be stripped off the lateral pelvic wall for additional exposure.
- External rotation and adduction will dislocate the hip after capsular incision.

Indications
- Paediatric hip exposures
- Congenital dislocation of the hip where both femoral and acetabular surgeries can be combined
- Pelvic osteotomies
- Traumatic anterior dislocation, and acetabular injuries involving anterior column of pelvis
- Arthrodesis or total hip replacement in selected cases
- Tumours of the anterior hip

Advantages
- Excellent proximal femoral and anterior acetabular exposure.
- Gluteal release in high riding hips, especially CDH.

- Posterior blood supply to head of femur is preserved.
- Bone grafts can be simultaneously and easily removed.

Disadvantages
- Restricted femoral medullary exposure.
- Detachment of glutei and TFL necessitates prolonged protection.
- Lateral femoral cutaneous nerve injury is common.

The Short Anterior Bikini Approach

History
Edgar Somarville described this approach in 1953. He was an outstanding figure of the generation that developed paediatric orthopaedic surgery in the UK in the postwar years. Somerville first made his name as co-author (with Girdlestone) of the second edition of the book 'Tuberculosis of Bones and Joints' (1952).

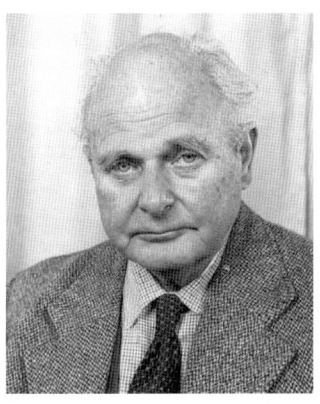

The children he treated were examined personally once a year in Oxford at clinics which soon became study sessions on skeletal development.

Miniaturized radiographs, meticulously mounted on a large cardboard sheet, told the story of each child's hip. Like frames from a slow-motion cinematograph, the yearly films were used to teach the importance of the fourth dimension (time) in paediatric surgery.

Plane
Between tensor fascia lata and gluteus medius medially; and Sartorius and rectus femoris laterally.

Access provided
Limited direct access to the hip joint alone.

Dislocation
The hip joint can be technically dislocated anteriorly, but a complete dislocation to the extent of viewing of the acetabulum is difficult with this approach.

Position and draping
- Supine with sandbag under the hip.

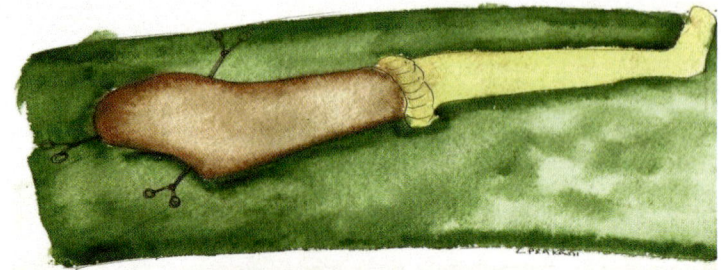

- Leg is draped free.
- Drape passes around upper thigh to expose anterosuperior iliac spine to gluteal tubercle.

Incision
Short oblique incision 4 cm below ASIS.

Dissections
- After skin and subcutaneous fat are cut, deep fascia over antero-superior iliac spine and that over anterior thigh is incised.
- The incision between TFL and sartorius is developed. Branches of lateral circumflex vessels are ligated. Rectus femoris is elevated to expose the anterior capsule.

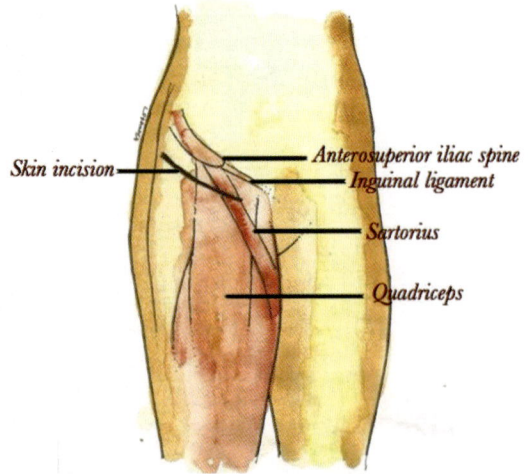

Skin incision —————————— Anterosuperior iliac spine
—————————— Inguinal ligament

—————————— Sartorius

—————————— Quadriceps

Short anterior approach to the hip

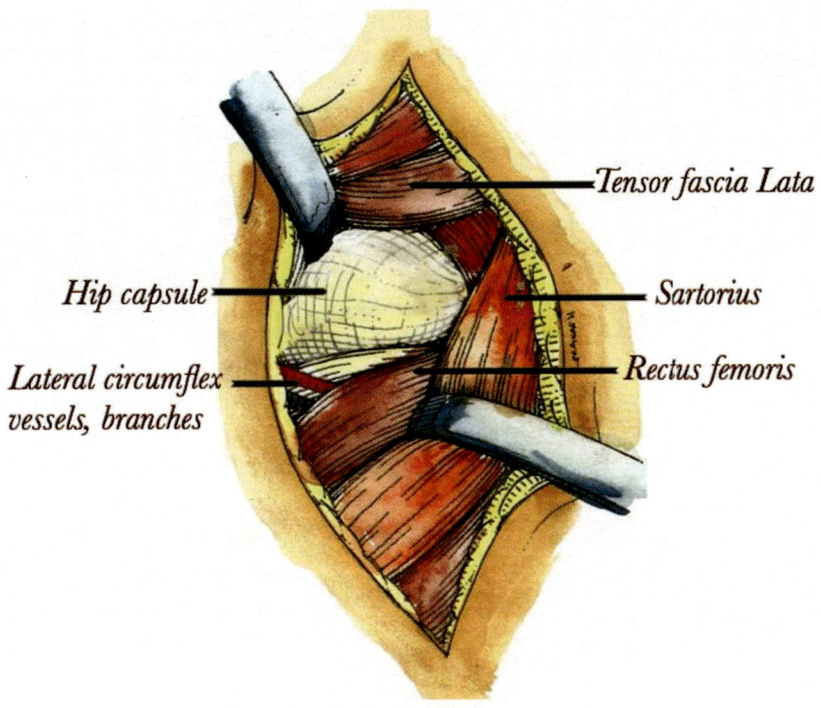

Tensor fascia Lata

Hip capsule

Sartorius

Lateral circumflex vessels, branches

Rectus femoris

Short anterior approach to the hip

- Inferior blunt dissection allows access to iliopsoas tendon and lesser trochanter.

Indications
- Access to anterior hip capsule, without detachment of hip abductors.
- Psoas tenotomy and anterior capsular releases.
- Biopsy and septic arthritis.

Advantages
- Small scar, cosmetic incision.
- Reduced morbidity due to preservation of gluteal origin.

Disadvantages
- Limited exposure.
- Difficult to dislocate hip.

Ilioinguinal Approach

History

Henri Judet described this approach in 1964.

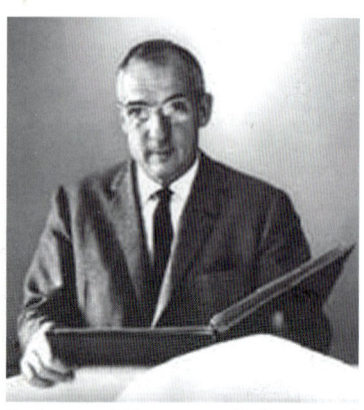

Judet was one of the first to practice orthopaedics exclusively in France. His reputation was authoritative at the time. He devoted considerable time on research and developed numerous surgical techniques for congenital hip dislocation, clubfeet, and other birth defects. His sons John and Robert started their clinic "Jouvenet" which became a Mecca of orthopaedic surgery. It was located at 6 Square Jouvenet in Paris' 16th arrondissement.

Plane

• Between iliopsoas and the pelvic wall

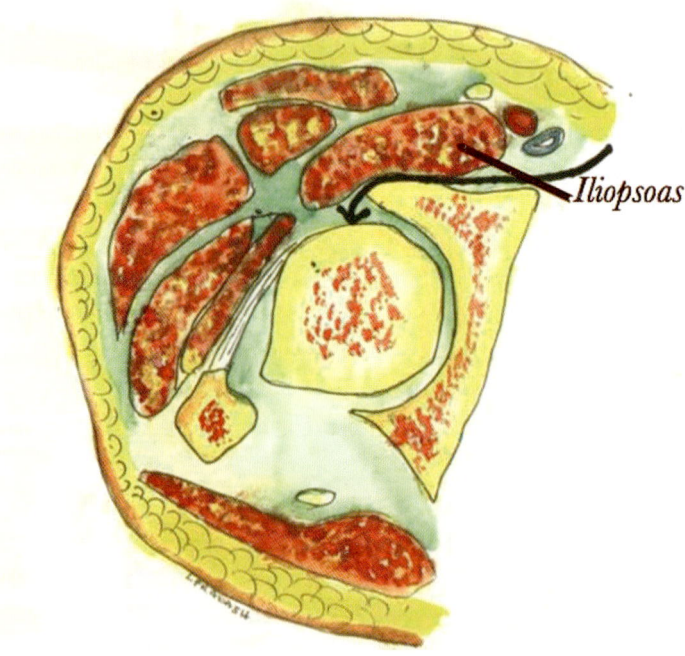

Anterior ilioinguinal approach

Access provided

A decent and extensive acetabular exposure giving access to:

- Interior of hemipelvis
- Iliac crest
- Exterior of pelvic crest
- Sciatic notch inferomedially
- Symphysis pubis anteriorly
- Ala of sacrum posteriorly

Dislocation

Hip can be dislocated superiorly, anteriorly or posteriorly depending on the requirements of the area of acetabulum to be exposed.

Position and draping

Supine with sandbag under buttock.

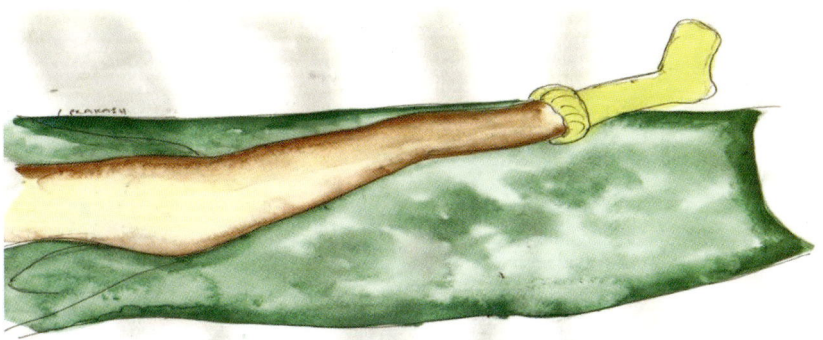

Incision

Long incision from posterior iliac crest to symphysis pubis, which is curved distally.

Iliac crest is exposed and structures can be stripped off the pelvis both from outer and inner tables.

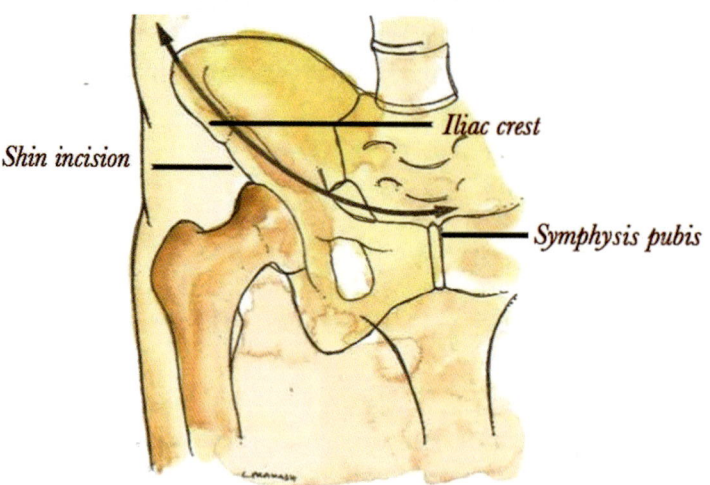

Ilioinguinal approach

Dissections

On the inner side, abdominal muscles are either gently erased off the iliac crest, or the anterior third of the iliac crest is osteotomized and then snapped inwards, breaking the inner table and allowing a subperiosteal dissection of the iliacus muscle.

This stripping can be carried as far back as the sacroiliac joint, if required.

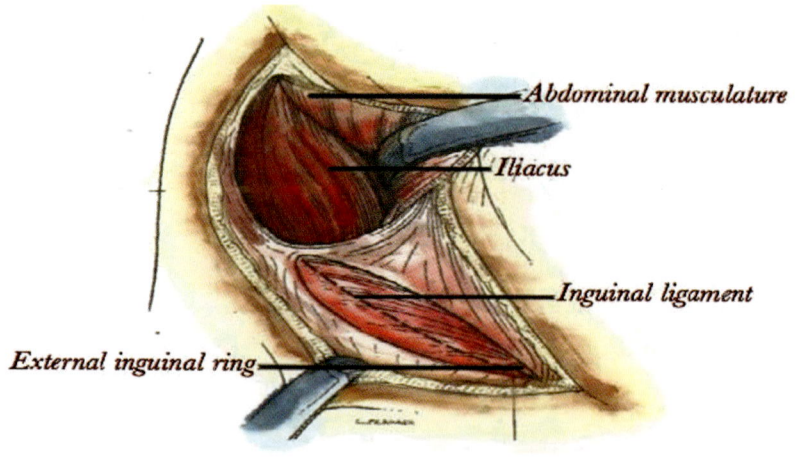

Ilioinguinal approach to the hip

The aponeurosis of external oblique is divided from ASIS along the iliac crest. The lateral cutaneous nerve of the thigh is now identified and protected.

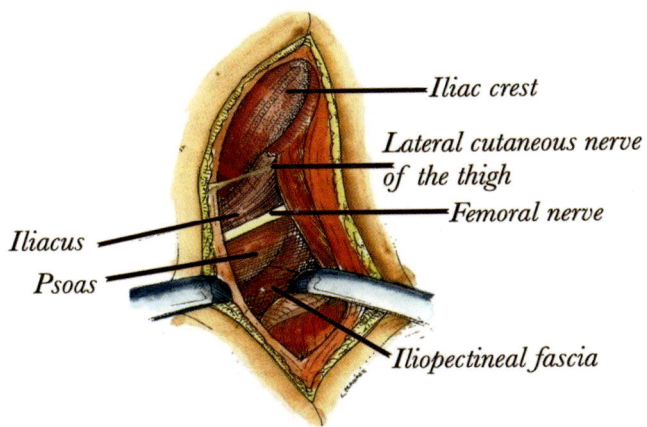

At this stage, starting from the conjoint tendon, the inguinal ligament is detached from its origins, leaving a dense fibrous strip for reattachment.

The iliopsoas muscle mass and femoral nerve come into view. The iliopectineal head is identified and detached from pelvis, allowing mobilization of iliopsoas muscle mass along with the femoral nerve.

By passing a loupe of soft tape or rubber catheter, these can be retracted in either direction.

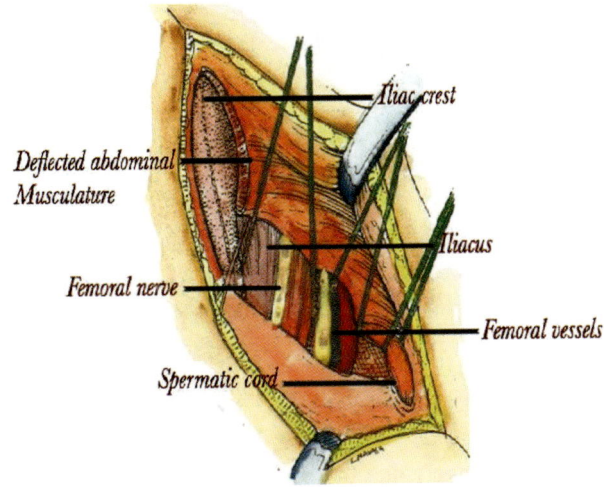

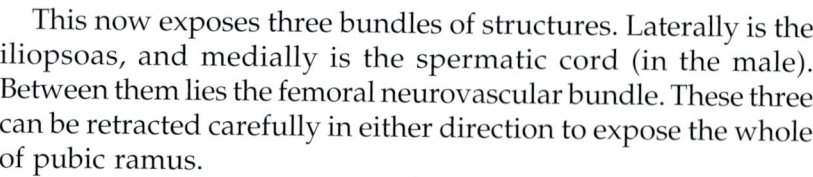

This now exposes three bundles of structures. Laterally is the iliopsoas, and medially is the spermatic cord (in the male). Between them lies the femoral neurovascular bundle. These three can be retracted carefully in either direction to expose the whole of pubic ramus.

The incision can be carried across the midline should there be a need to expose the contralateral pubis, and the whole anterior brim of the pelvis can be exposed by this approach.

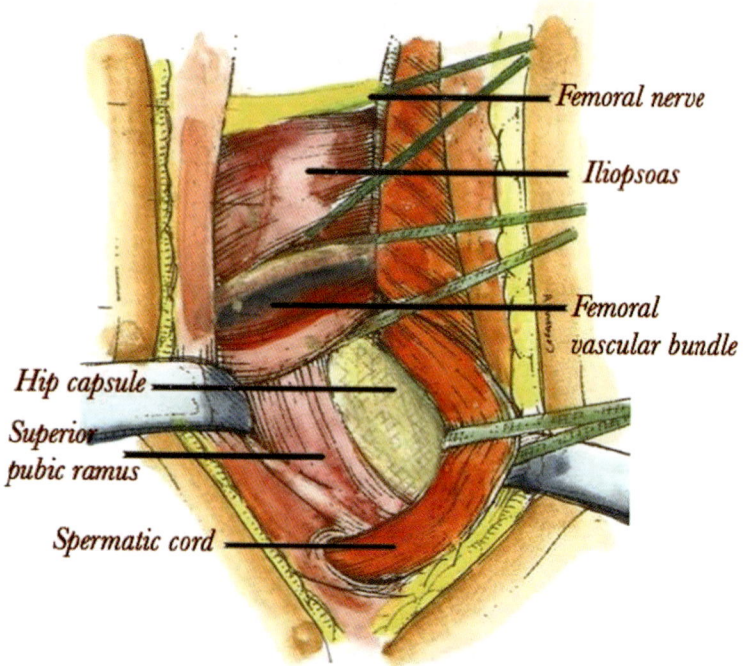

Femoral nerve

Iliopsoas

Femoral vascular bundle

Hip capsule

Superior pubic ramus

Spermatic cord

Indications
- Pelvic fractures, except those involving sacrum.
- Fractures of the anterior column.
- Superior pubic ramus fractures.
- Floating symphysis pubis or disruption of symphysis pubis.

Advantages
- Good field of exposure from one side to the other, especially in anterior column fractures.
- Good clean cosmetic scar.

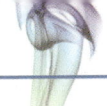

Disadvantages

- Difficult and technically demanding operation.
- Lateral cutaneous nerve is in danger and irritating complications occur if it is cut.
- External iliac and femoral vessels have to be carefully protected.

Ruedi Approach

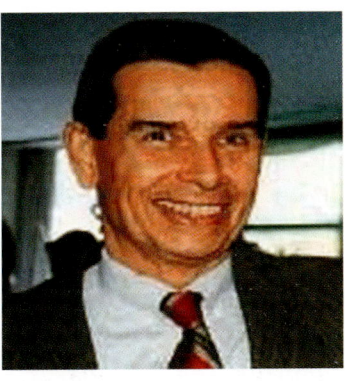

Surgeons confronted with acute trauma are frequently under great pressure to act quickly. Only a few have an infallible three-dimensional memory as regards the different approaches necessary for treating fractures by internal fixation. Thus there is a real need for a reference book on the approaches to the extremities. This is true both for emergency situations and for the "evening before" preoperative planning. Thomas Ruedi was one of the early AO teachers, founder members and a gifted trauma surgeon. He is also a wonderful artist and an unusual illustrator. This modification of Judet's approach was described by Ruedi in 1968. He has authored numerous AO books and manuals, many of them illustrated by himself and these books form essential reading for all trauma surgeons across the world.

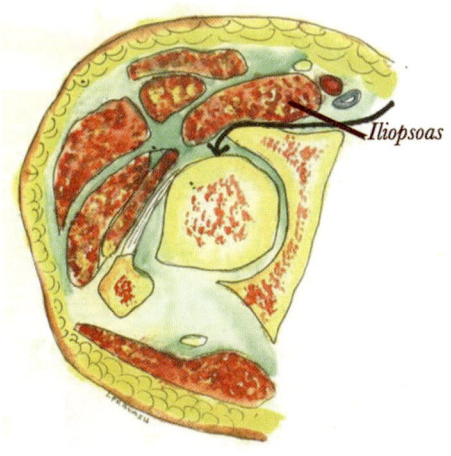

Iliopsoas

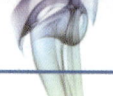

Plane

Between iliopsoas and the pelvic wall, after osteotomy of anterosuperior iliac spine.

Access provided

One of the most extensive acetabular exposures giving access to:

- Interior of hemipelvis
- Iliac crest
- Exterior of pelvic crest
- Sciatic notch inferomedially
- Symphysis pubis anteriorly
- Ala of sacrum posteriorly

Dislocation

Hip can be dislocated superiorly, anteriorly or posteriorly, depending on the requirements of the area of acetabulum to be exposed.

Position and draping

Supine with sandbag under buttock.

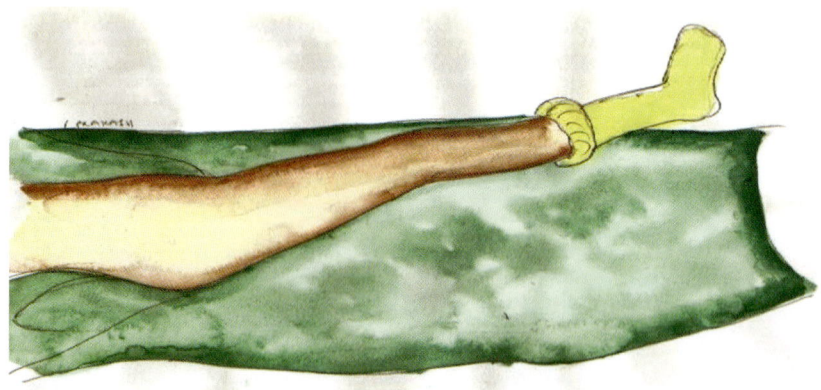

Incision

Long incision from posterior iliac crest to symphysis pubis, which is curved distally.

Osteotomy of ASIS along with anterior half of iliac crest.

Fascia along the inferior border of inguinal ligament is incised.

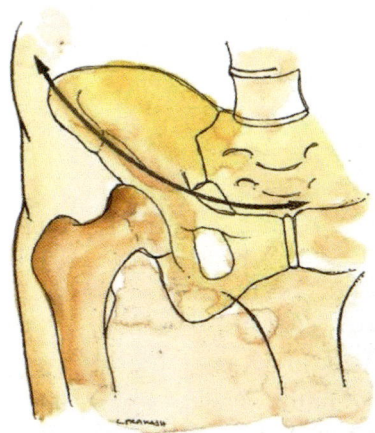

Ruedi approach is a litter inferior

The iliac sliver, ASIS, inguinal ligament, and external abdominal musculature are retracted superiorly and medially.

The lateral cutaneous nerve of the thigh is identified and protected.

Iliopsoas muscle mass and the femoral neurovascular bundles are identified and separated as with Judet approach.

In males, the spermatic cord is protected, and the supero-medial aspect of pubic ramus is stripped, leaving a decent strip for reattachment.

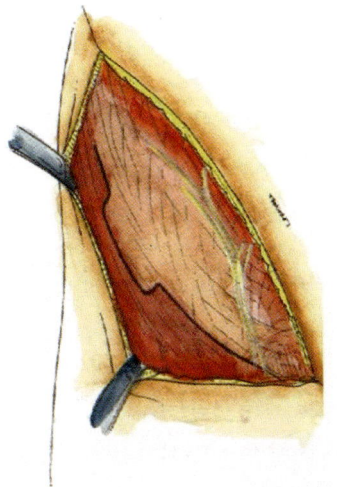

Deep incision before ASIS osteotomy

The approach can be extended to the other side of midline, to expose the whole anterior brim of pelvis in complex pelvis injuries.

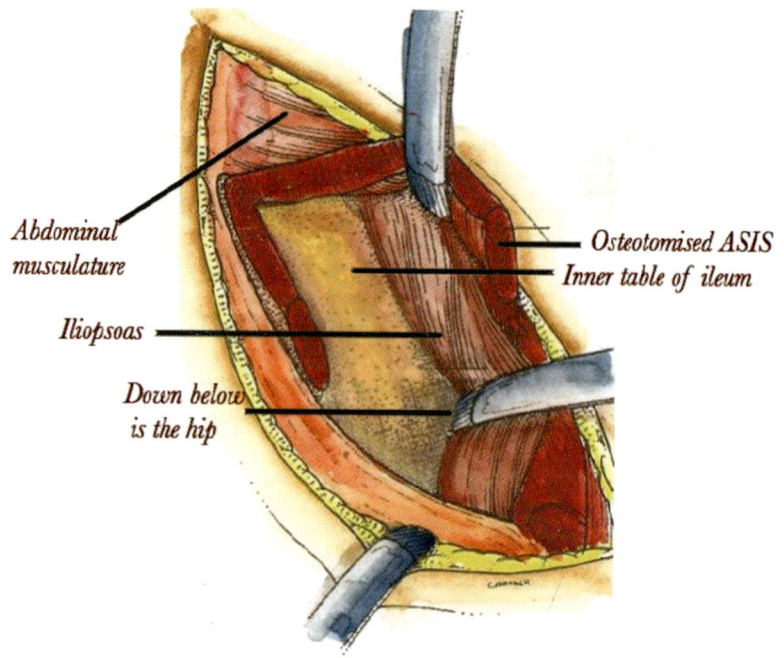

Abdominal musculature

Osteotomised ASIS

Inner table of ileum

Iliopsoas

Down below is the hip

Indications
- Pelvic fractures, except those involving sacrum.
- Fractures of the anterior column.
- Superior pubic ramus fractures.
- Floating symphysis pubis or disruption of symphysis pubis.

Advantages
- Excellent field of exposure from one side to the other, especially in anterior column fractures.
- Good clean cosmetic scar.

Disadvantages
- Difficult and technically demanding operation.
- Lateral cutaneous nerve is in danger; irritating complications occur, if it is cut.
- External iliac and femoral vessels have to be carefully protected.

Extended Iliofemoral Approach by Judet and Letournel

History

Émile Letournel, born in 1927, was an outstanding French surgeon of his times. He joined Judet in 1954, and was a pioneer in the study of acetabular fractures.

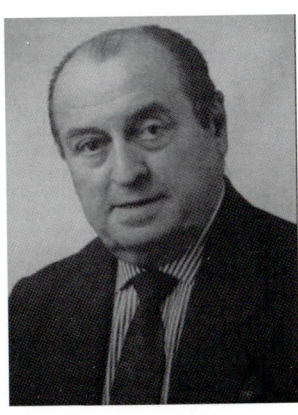

Professor Letournel was recognized as the conclusive source of extensive experience and innovative techniques in the management of severe pelvic and acetabular trauma. His lifelong contributions to the understanding of the complex acetabular fractures and techniques required to treat these difficult injuries have defined the fundamental principles of these injury patterns. This incision was described in 1964.

Plane

- Between sartorius and tensor fascial lata inferiorly
- Subperiosteal elevation of Gluteus medius and minimus muscles.

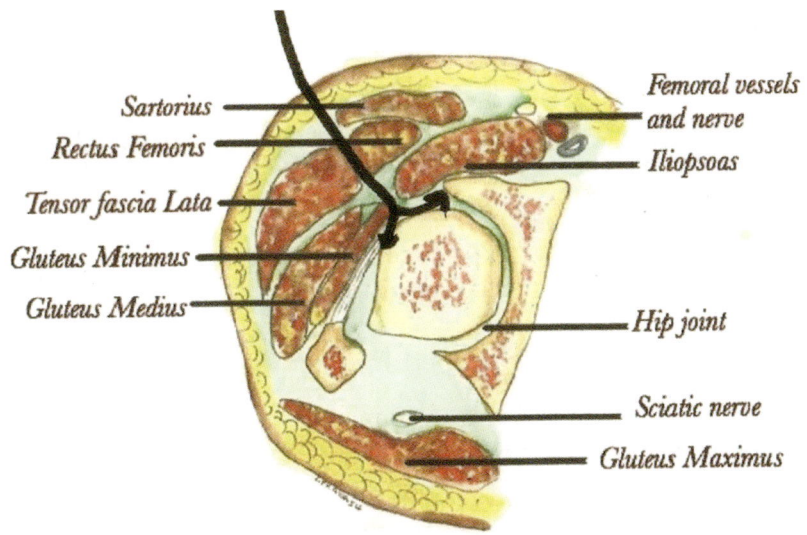

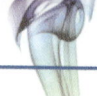

Access
- Posterior acetabular column
- Superior dome of acetabulum
- Anterior column as far back as iliopubic eminence

Dislocation
In any direction needed, except inferior

Position and draping
- Lateral position

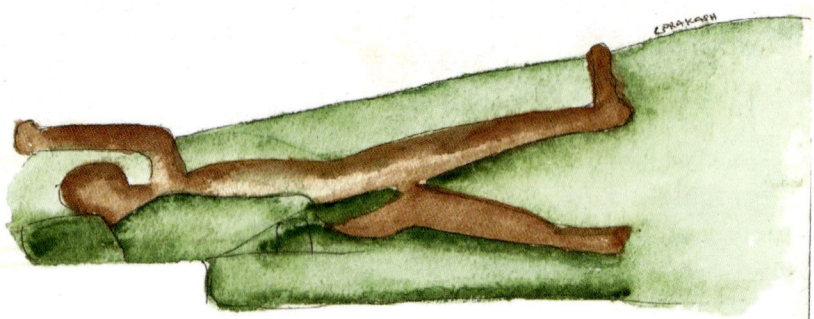

- Appropriate attachments on the operating table ensure a fixed lateral position.
- K wire with tensioned Ilizarov half ring in the distal transcondylar area to give good traction. (The original Letournel method advocates a Stienman pin and stirrups.)

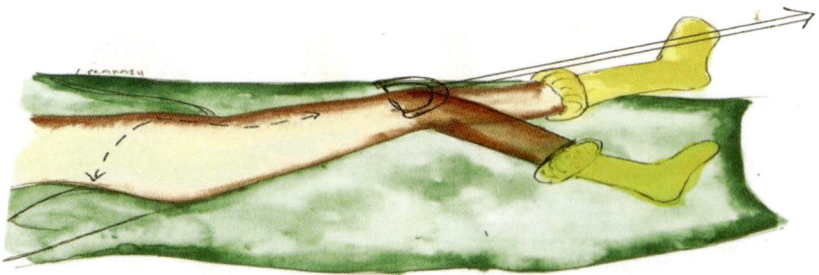

- The knee should be draped free and kept flexed to avoid stretching of the sciatic nerve.

Incision
- Along the anterior 80% of the iliac crest up to the ASIS.
- Curves to 90° at ASIS to go towards patella.

- Exposure up to a little below mid-thigh allows relaxation of structures and a better acetabular exposure.

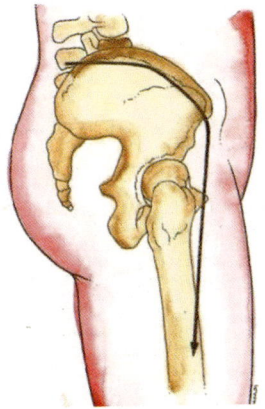

Skin incision for extended iliofemoral approach of Fudet and Letournel

Dissections

- Subperiosteal detachment of the gluteus medius and minimus from the outer wing of the ileum, right up to the sciatic notch, allowing them to be retracted posteriorly.
- The superior gluteal neurovascular bundle is identified and protected.
- The short lateral rotators are now detached with sufficient flaps for reattachment.

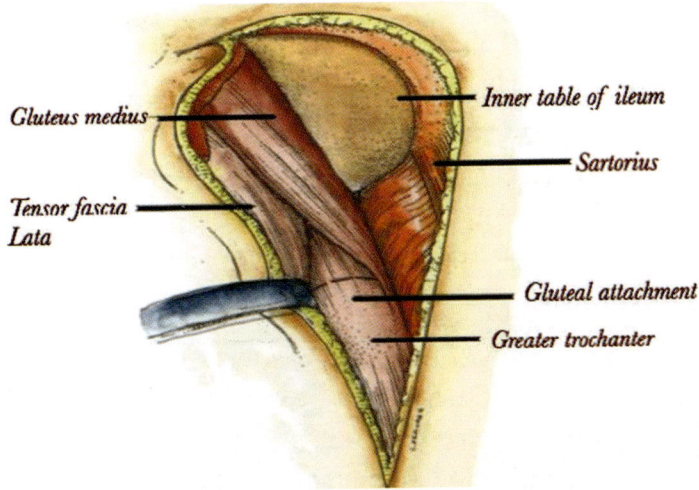

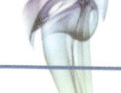

- Order of detachment of rotators is piriformis, superior gemellus, obturator internus, inferior gemellus and the quadratus femoris.

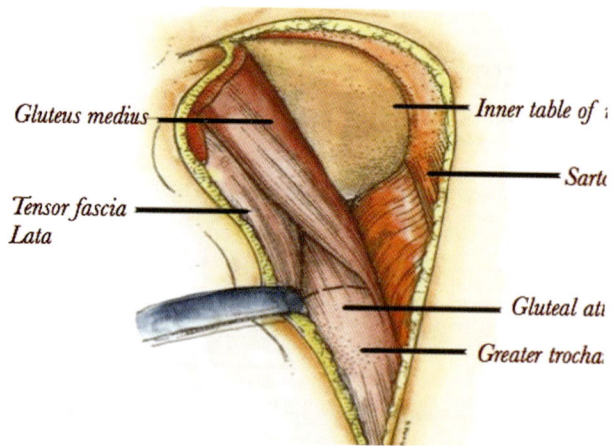

- Division and medial retraction of both heads of rectus femoris.
- Abdominal muscles are either detached from iliac crest, or the crest is osteotomized to deflect the bone with muscles.
- Flexion of the hip at this stage relaxes all the muscles and an extensive approach is achieved.

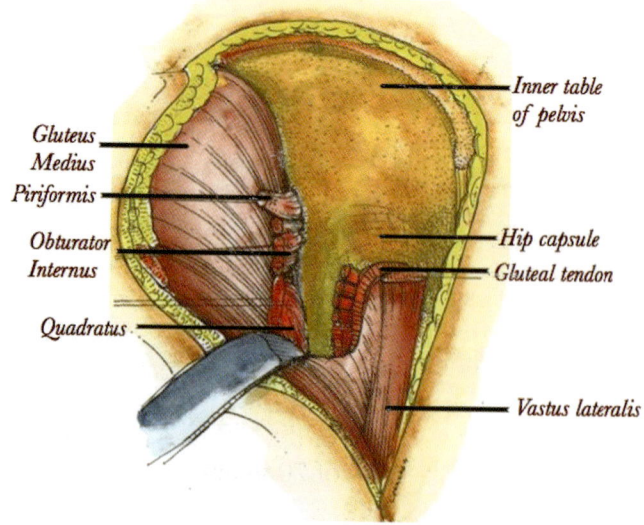

Extended iliofemoral approach

Indications
- Pelvic fractures, involving both columns.
- Fractures of the anterior column, superior dome.

Advantages
An extensive large exposure that can be extended in either direction.

Disadvantages
Anterior column exposure is limited to its superior parts.

Detachment of glutei needs proper reattachment and post-operative protection.

Anterior Approaches

History

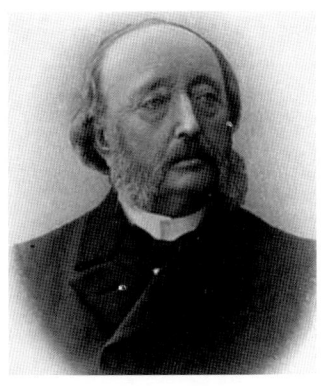

Watson-Jones in 1936 described an easy anterior approach with a more acceptable scar than the original Ollier's approach on which it was based.

Louis Xavier Édouard Léopold Ollier was born in Vans, Ardèche, France, where both his father and grandfather had been doctors. He initially studied Natural Science at Montpellier; in 1849, he was assistant in Botany in the faculty of medicine. He then became an intern of Lyon Hospital in 1851, graduated in medicine with distinction in 1856, and in 1857 obtained his doctorate at Paris based on histological studies of 400 malignant tumours.

In 1860, aged only 30, Ollier became the Chief Surgeon at the Hôtel-Dieu in Lyon, one of the oldest hospitals in Europe. When France was invaded by the Germans in 1870, he became head of the Lyons Ambulance. A meticulous and thorough surgeon, he soon attracted patients from all over the world.

In 1877, he was appointed professor of clinical surgery; in 1894, he was made commander of the Légion d'Honneur. Ollier died in Lyon in 1900 at the age of 70 years.

Ollier was revered for his role in the development of orthopaedic surgery in France. A monument was erected in his

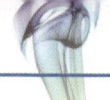

memory in the square outside his home. The Museum of Pathological Anatomy at the University of Lyon now bears his name.

Ollier was one of the first surgeons to employ an audit on his operative procedures, stating "It is in the certification and criticism of old results that is to be found the true consecration of operative methods which are intended to be used for purposes of conservative surgery."

The U shaped incision for anterolateral hip approach was described by him in 1881.

Ollier's original approach involved osteotomy of the greater trochanter after the U shaped incision. This approach has been abandoned for the more cosmetic linear skin incisions and easier transtrochanteric approaches. Here a few drawings show the approach, but the current anterolateral Watson Jones approach is described more fully subsequently.

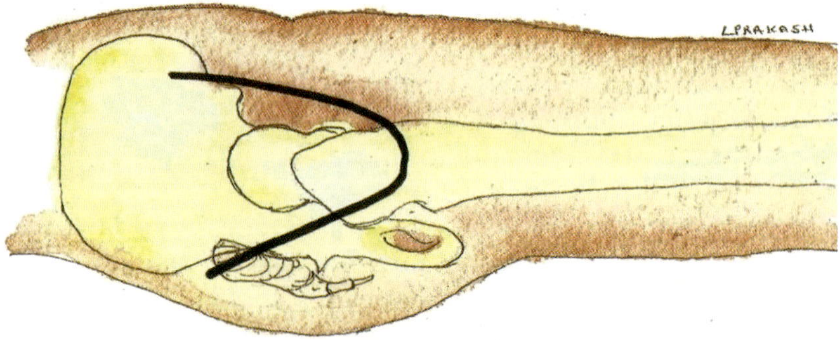

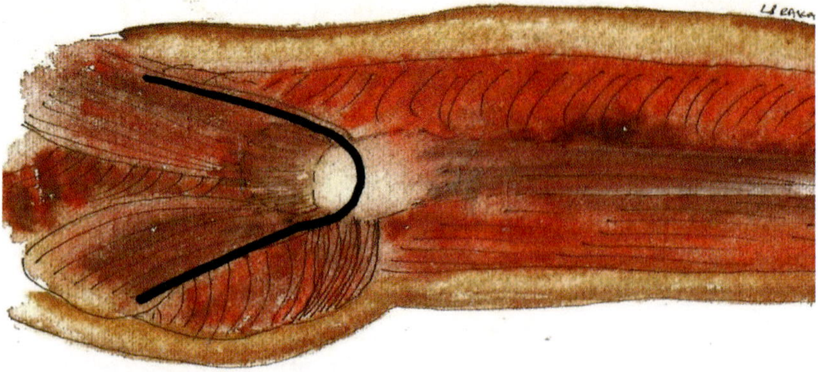

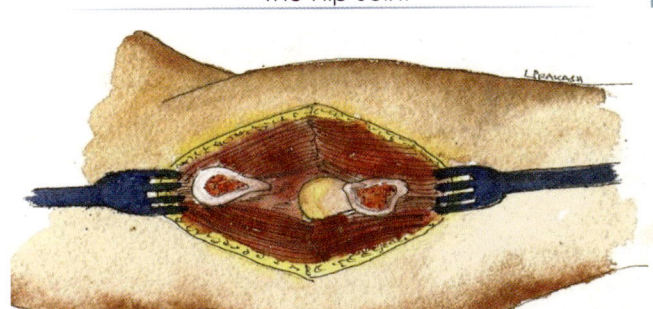

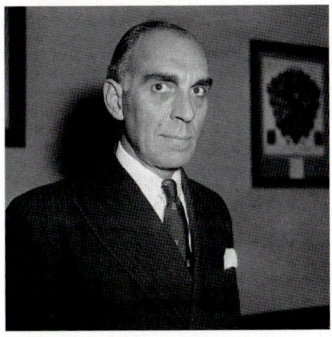

Sir Reginald Watson-Jones has been described as the pioneer scientist of the new era of orthopaedics in Britain.

Watson-Jones was born on March 4, 1902, to a school teacher and his wife. He graduated from the University of Liverpool in 1922 with a Bachelor's degree in science and went on to receive his medical education at the university's medical school. In 1926, he became one of the first surgeons to receive the MCh (Orth.) degree.

Following his education in Liverpool, he continued his training in London, where he met and impressed Sir Robert Jones, eventually becoming his protégé.

Shortly after the start of his orthopaedic career, Reginald Jones adopted his mother's maiden name and became Reginald Watson-Jones to distinguish himself from the many other Joneses practicing medicine in England at that time, including his mentor. Also, that period saw the beginning of a seemingly inexhaustible writing talent when the Journal of Bone and Joint Surgery (JBJS) accepted his first paper for publication in 1930. He would eventually publish two to three papers every year in numerous journals for decades.

Watson-Jones' excellent surgical abilities, combined with the exposure he received from his hospital appointments, allowed his practice to thrive. He eventually had a Packard limousine with chauffeur, a butler, a personal secretary and an office staff of five, according to his JBJS obituary.

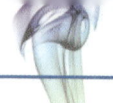

Plane
Between tensor fascia lata and gluteus medius and minimus.

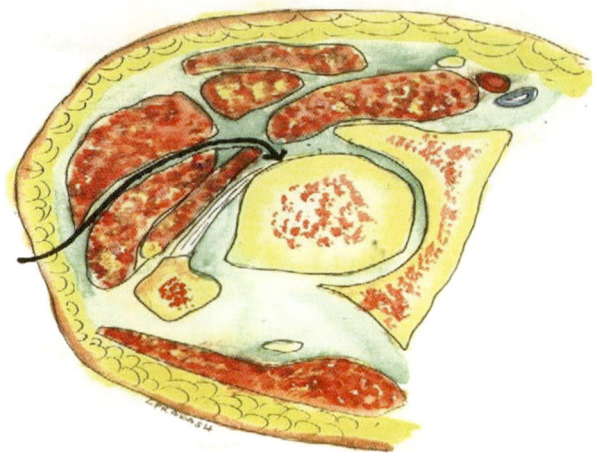

Access provided
- Lateral pelvic wall
- Anterior capsule of hip joint
- Acetabulum
- Proximal femur

Dislocation
Anterior

Position and draping
Supine with two small sandbags or rolled towels under both buttocks. The leg below the knee is draped free as the flexed knee acts as the fulcrum for dislocating and reducing the hip joint.

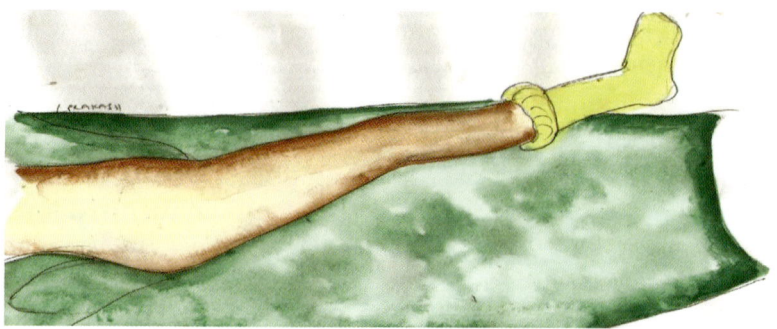

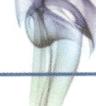

Incision

From a little above ASIS curving over trochanteric flare, descending down to thigh straight.

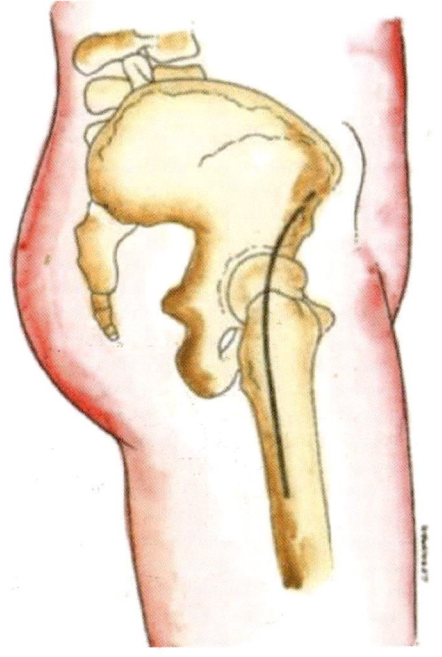

Modified Watson Jones approach

Dissections

Fascia lata is cut along the posterior border of trochanteric flare. This is split longitudinally parallel to the femur downwards and in the direction of ASIS upwards.

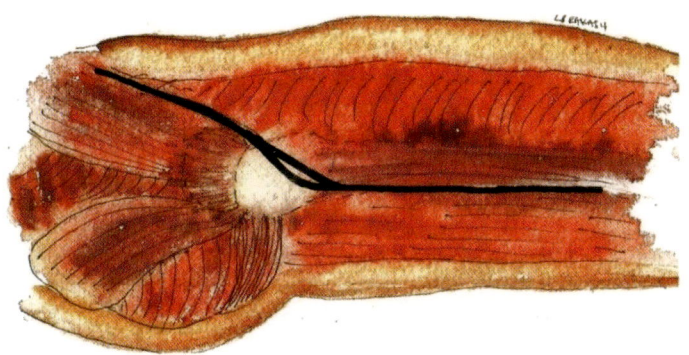

After clearing off the adipose tissue from vastus lateralis, the gap between gluteus medius and tensor fascia lata is identified.

Bleeders are cauterized on the way; gluteus medius and minimus attachments from greater trochanter are cut, leaving decent stubs for reattachment.

The rectus femoris is now elevated to visualize the anterior capsule of the hip. By externally rotating the hip, the capsule is stretched for incision to expose the hip joint.

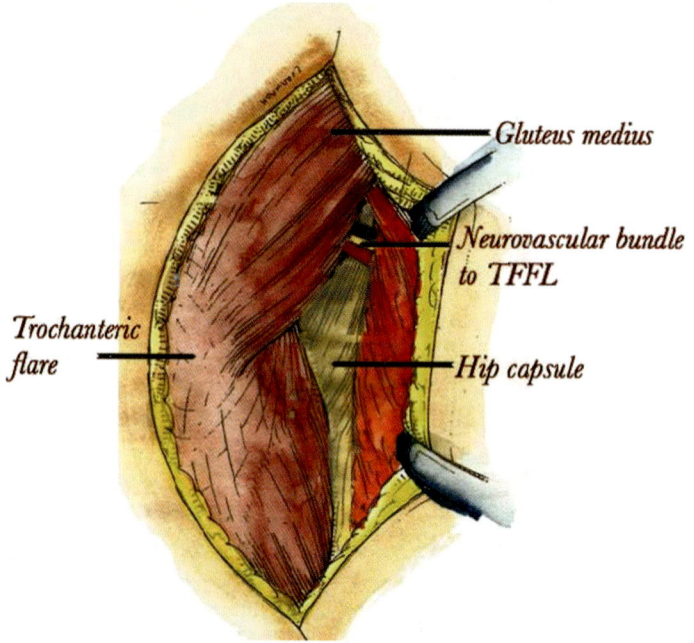

The vessels and nerve to tensor fascia lata are preserved to the maximum extent.

A T shaped incision in the capsule exposes the hip joint. By using the flexed knee and leg as the long arm of the lever, abduction and external rotation of the flexed knee dislocates the hip.

In osteoarthritic hips or deeply seated heads, it may not be possible to dislocate the hip easily. One must desist from forcible attempts to dislocate the head at this stage, because it may lead to a spiral fracture of femur.

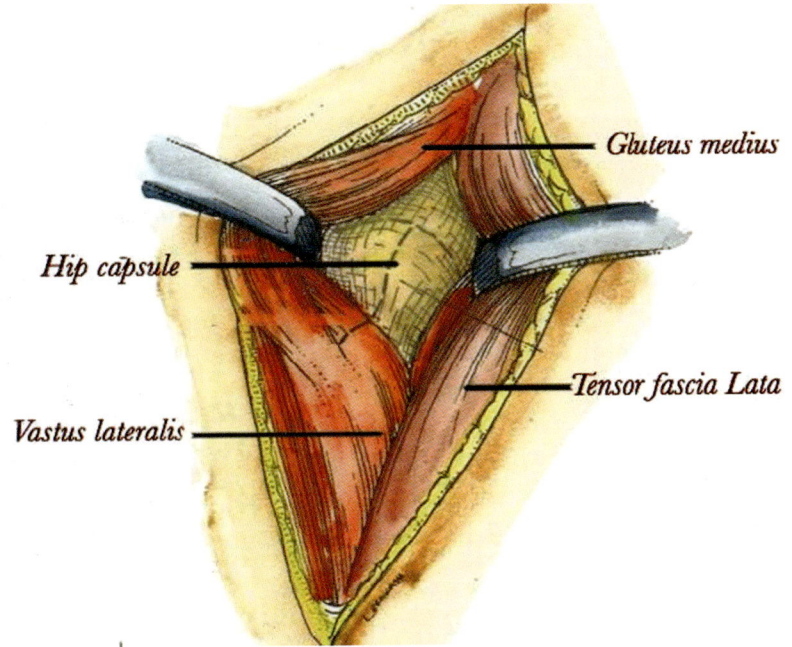

Gluteus medius

Hip capsule

Tensor fascia Lata

Vastus lateralis

If the exposure is made for total hip replacement, it may be a good idea to cut the neck, and remove the head, after retracting the trochanter.

Indications
- Open reduction and internal fixation of fractures of neck of femur.
- Hemiarthroplasty and bipolar.
- Total hip replacement.
- For capsular release with psoas tenotomy.
- The approach is not recommended for revision arthroplasties.

Advantages
- Preservation of abductor mechanism allows rapid rehabilitation and weight bearing.
- Orientation of femoral stem is easier as the anterior border of lesser trochanter can be used to decide the version of the stem.
- No vital structures in the way, except way superiorly.

Disadvantages
- Damage to neurovascular bundle to tensor fascia lata.

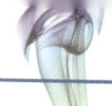

- Rather limited exposure to acetabulum for reaming and screw placement in cementless hips.
- Poor exposure of femoral neck.
- This approach was popularized by Maurice Muller for his total hip replacement.

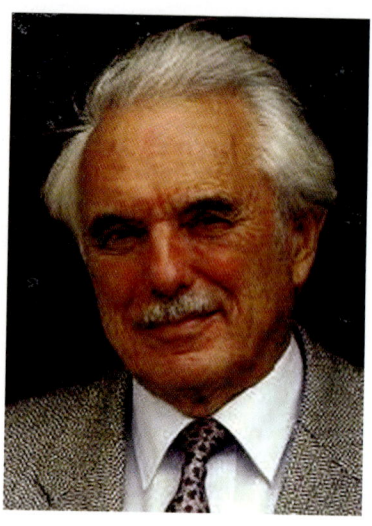

Maurice Muller, a pioneering hip surgeon, was named surgeon of the century by SICOT in 2002.

Born on 28 March 1918, Muller was a surgeon, inventor, scientist, designer, biomechanical engineer, and a very skilled magician. I have had the pleasure of watching him perform startling magic tricks.

He was born and had his early schooling in Biel, Switzerland. He had his medical studies in various Swiss universities, and finally received his MD from University of Zurich in 1946.

After spending his initial years serving the poor in Ethopia, he returned to Switzerland, to work in its various hospitals. He was professor at University of Berne, and chief orthopaedic surgeon at Inselspital in Berne.

His interest in internal fixation of fractures stemmed from observing results of Gerhad Kuntchner and Robert Danis, the pioneers of intramedullary and plate fixation. After developing his own instrumentation and implant designs, he founded the AO Foundation with three other Swiss colleagues in 1958.

In the early 1960s, he developed a strong interest in hip replacements and visited Sir John Charnley in Wrightington, UK. After spending some time there, he returned with a set of instruments and began performing hip replacements in Berne. Though extremely pleased by the results of hip replacements per se, he was a tad dissatisfied with a high postoperative dislocation rate, which he attributed to a small head size used in Charnley hips and the lateral transtrochanteric approach, which, in his opinion, considerably weakened the abductor mechanism.

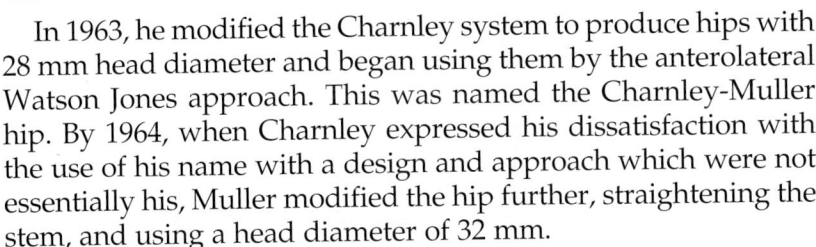

In 1963, he modified the Charnley system to produce hips with 28 mm head diameter and began using them by the anterolateral Watson Jones approach. This was named the Charnley-Muller hip. By 1964, when Charnley expressed his dissatisfaction with the use of his name with a design and approach which were not essentially his, Muller modified the hip further, straightening the stem, and using a head diameter of 32 mm.

In 1967, he founded another company Protek AG to market his Muller hips. He was a rich man by his retirement and became a great patron of arts, donating close to eighty million Swiss francs for the cause of building an art museum dedicated to a Swiss painter.

One of the lesser known facts about Muller is that apart from his medical writings, he has also published a few articles in magic magazines, explaining secrets of certain card tricks that he had conceived.

Transgluteal Lateral Approach

History

First described in 1954 by Osborne and McFarland, the cleavage was through the gluteus medius proximally and vastus lateralis distally. This was later modified by Hardinge for total hip replacement.

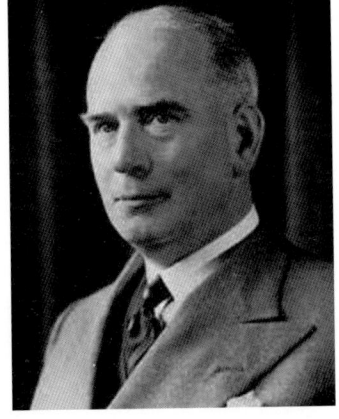

Bryan Leslie McFarland 1900–1963

Professor Bryan McFarland was the director of orthopaedic studies and professor of orthopaedic surgery in the University of Liverpool, past president of the British Orthopaedic Association, vice-president of the Royal College of Surgeons of Edinburgh, and president of the International Orthopaedic Society.

Born and brought up in Liverpool, Bryan's life was spent in Merseyside, first at the Wallasey Grammar School and then the medical school of the University of Liverpool. He was one of the first candidates to become master of orthopaedic surgery in 1926, gained the fellowship of the Royal College of Surgeons of Edinburgh in 1928. 20 years later, in recognition of clinical and

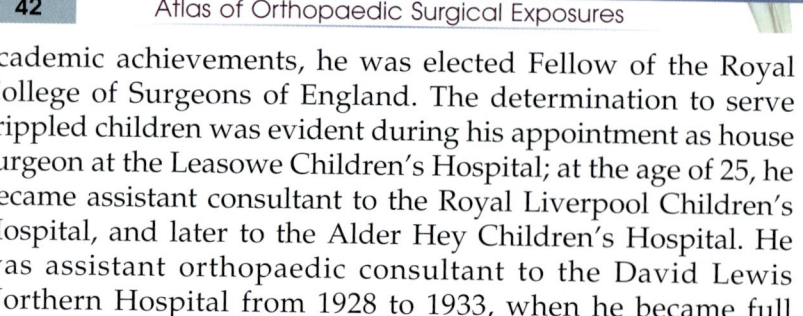

academic achievements, he was elected Fellow of the Royal College of Surgeons of England. The determination to serve crippled children was evident during his appointment as house surgeon at the Leasowe Children's Hospital; at the age of 25, he became assistant consultant to the Royal Liverpool Children's Hospital, and later to the Alder Hey Children's Hospital. He was assistant orthopaedic consultant to the David Lewis Northern Hospital from 1928 to 1933, when he became full consultant orthopaedic surgeon to Robert Jones's own hospital, the Royal Southern.

In earlier years, Bryan's teaching of undergraduate and postgraduate students was overshadowed by the powerful personality of the late Professor McMurray, whom he served loyally and faithfully as clinical lecturer; but on succession in 1948 as director of orthopaedic studies, and later in the professorial chair of the University, his magnitude of vision blossomed and his great qualities of surgical, academic and scientific brilliance emerged.

The distinction he added to this historic school of orthopaedics will be treasured with pride and affection by MCh(Orth) graduates, not only in Great Britain, but in other countries throughout the world.

An excellent marksman, he was passionate about wild fowl hunts. He would leave home at 3.00 am to arrive in Anglesey before dawn for wild fowl shooting. It was not until after the age of 40 that he became an enthusiastic fisherman, but so thorough was his preparation and practice that he could equal the skill of any professional angler.

Mr Kevin Hardinge, a practicing consultant orthopaedic surgeon in Manchester, has worked in Wrightingtom with Sir John Charnley and in Exeter with Mr Robin Ling. He is still active in orthopaedics in Manchester. An MCh (Orth) from Liverpool, he described his classical transgluteal approach based on Osborne and MacFarland's incision in 1982.

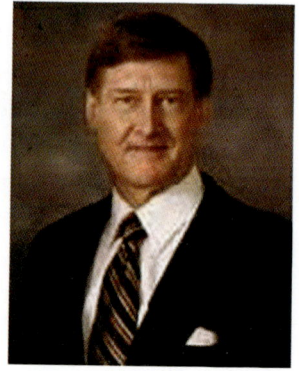

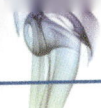

Plane
Single flap of gluteus medius, its periosteal attachment, and vastus lateralis are lifted as a single layer from the anterior part of the trochanter.

Access provided
- Excellent 360° approach to the acetabulum.
- Decent approach to proximal femur.

Dislocation
The hip is dislocated anteriorly by externally rotating the limb using the flexed knee as a fulcrum.

Position and draping
The positioning depends on the surgeon's familiarity and comforts, and the patient can either be in supine or lateral position. If supine, the operative hip is raised with a small pillow. In lateral position, the patient is strapped to back rests and sandbags to keep the pelvis steady during the entire surgery.

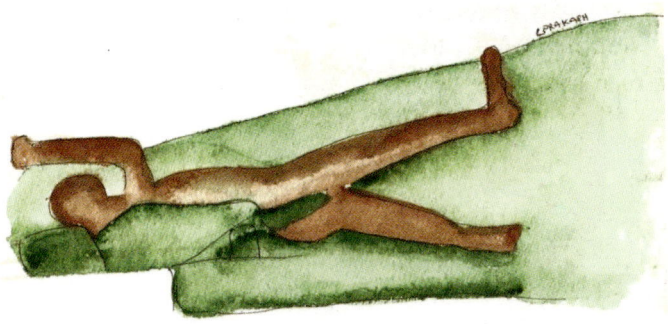

The limb is draped free and the knee should flex comfortably to provide a good lever arm for generous internal and external rotations of the hip joint during the surgery.

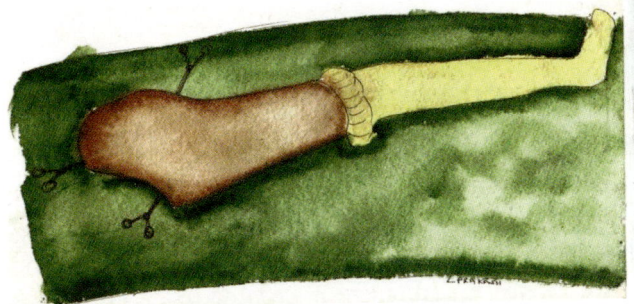

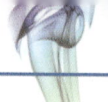

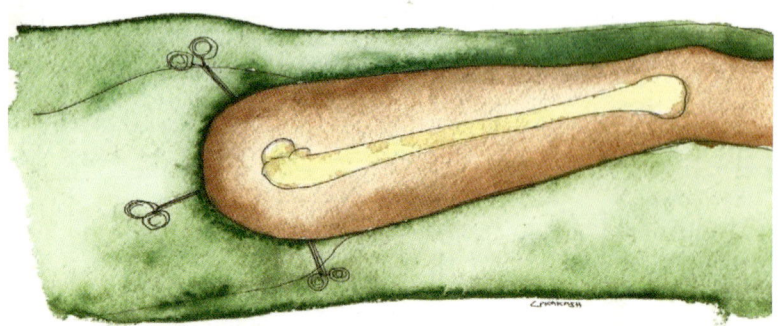

Incision
Straight mid-lateral incision, extending 5 cm up and down from the midpoint of the greater trochanter.

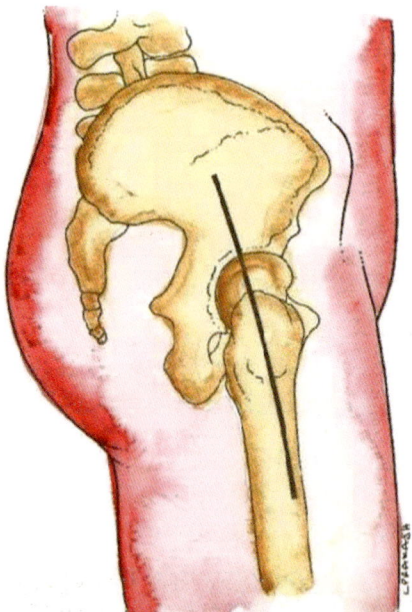

Straight incision for a Hardinage approach

Dissections
Subcutaneous tissue is incised in the same line as skin.

Glistening white tensor fascia lata is identified over greater trochanter. Using a cutting diathermy, a bone deep incision is made on the posterior margin of greater trochanter.

The attachment of gluteus medius to the greater trochanter is visualized by full internal rotation of the hip.

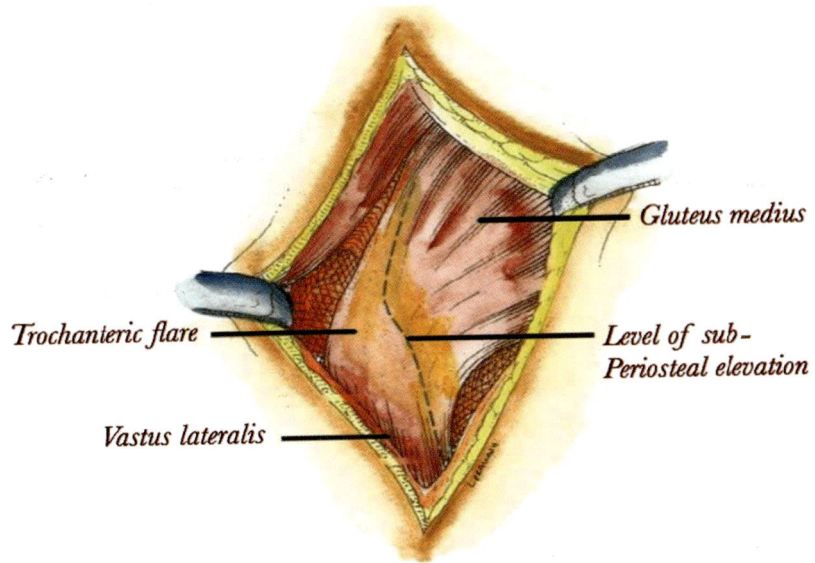

- Gluteus medius

Trochanteric flare —

Level of sub-
Periosteal elevation

Vastus lateralis —

The whole width of gluteus medius is identified, and the muscle is split in line of its fibres at the junction of its anterior and middle thirds.

Now using a very sharp chisel, the entire subperiosteal flap on the anterior aspect of the trochanter is lifted as a single flap and deflected anteriorly, starting with gluteus medius proximally, and the fascia of the vastus lateralis distally.

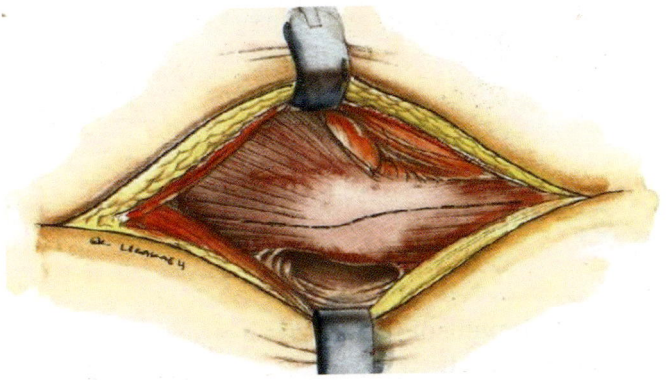

The entire gluteal structures are lifted as one flap

The tendon of gluteus medius is now detached, and the hip capsule below is cut with a T shaped incision.

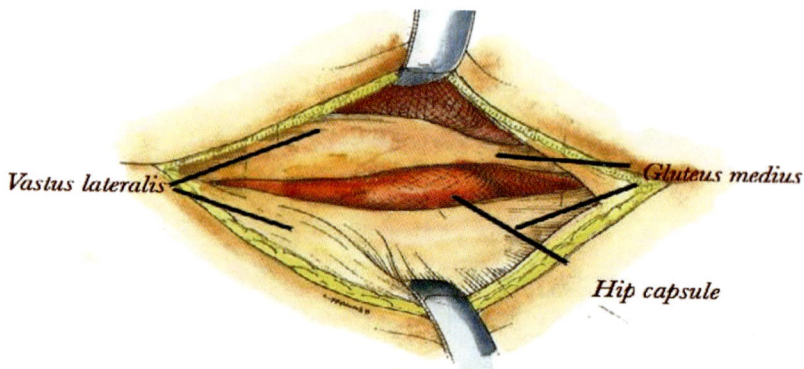

Vastus lateralis — — *Gluteus medius*

Hip capsule

Level of cleavage in Hardinge

The transverse branch lateral circumflex femoral artery has to be located deep to the vastus lateralis and cauterized to avoid persistant bleeding.

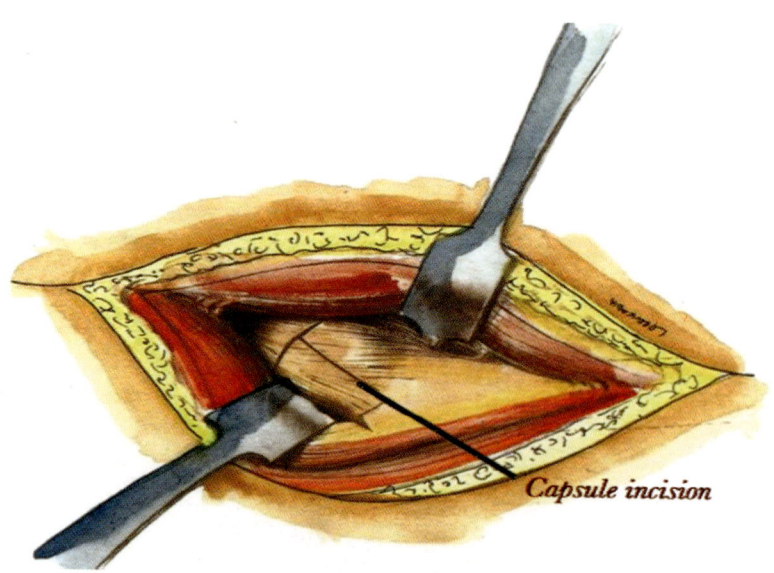

Capsule incision

Judicious placement of Hohmann retractors allows a full vision of the capsule, and a fairly extensive capsular dissection can be done.

Now the hip can be dislocated by external rotation. An easy method is to keep the flexed knee on the opposite thigh. If the head does not come out, additional capsular releases may be performed.

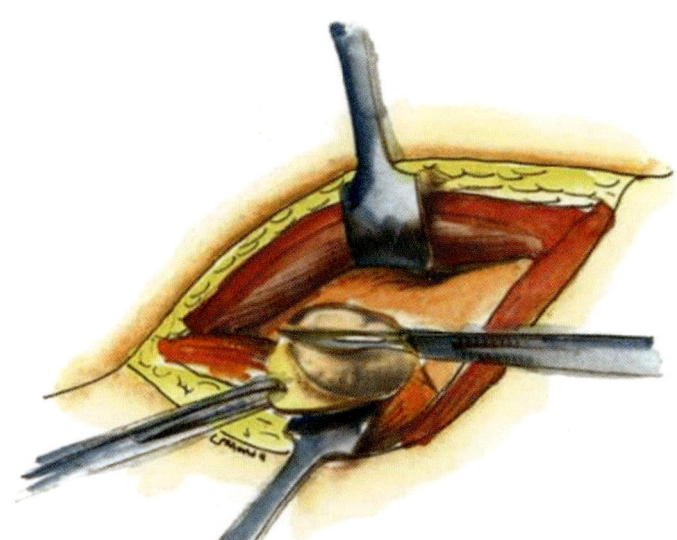

Capsular excision to expose head

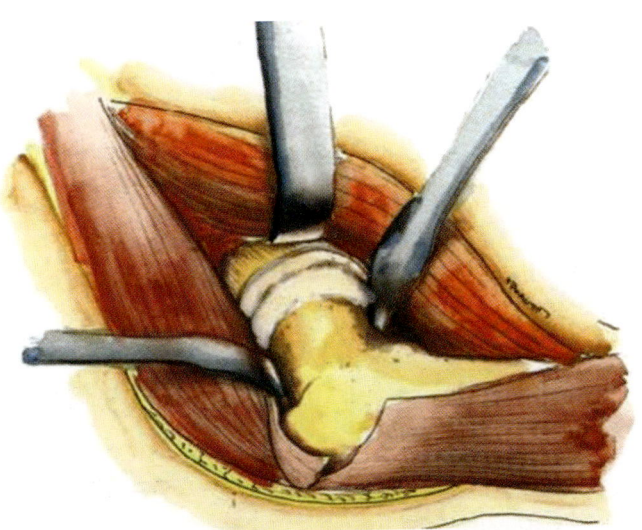

External rotation to dislocate the head

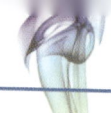

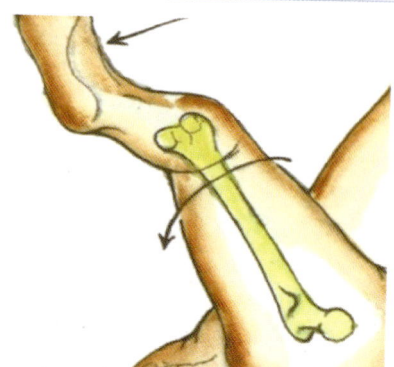

External rotation will dislocate the head

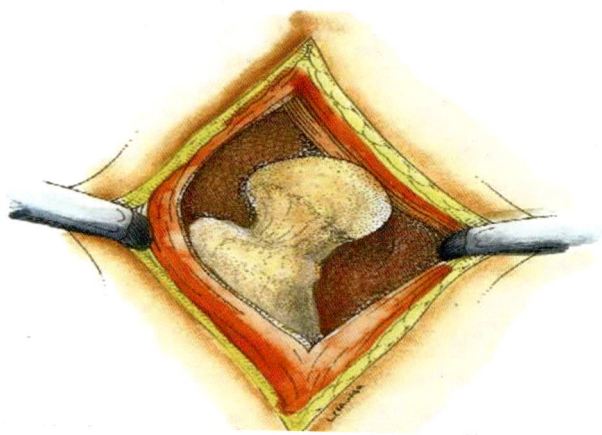

Head dislocated in the Hardinge approach

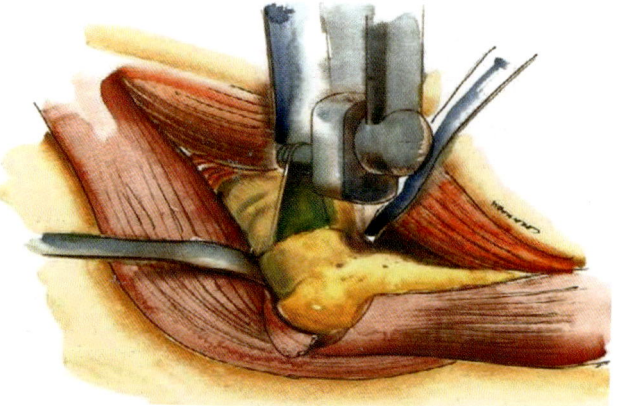

In case the hip end is fused, neck is osteotomized first

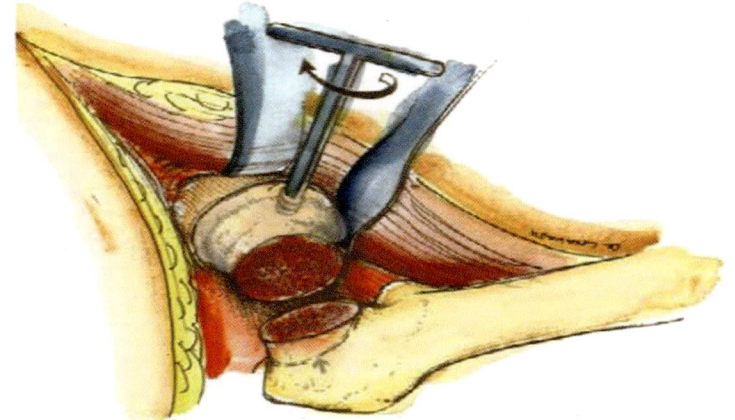

The cut head is removed with a cork screw

Indications
- Hemiarthroplasty
- Total hip replacement
- Revision hip replacement, especially if the patient is fixed in a lateral position.

Advantages
- Excellent exposure.
- Supine position allows perfect cup placement.
- Preservation of greater trochanter allows rapid return to work.

Disadvantages
- Slightly increased blood loss.
- Gluteal weakness postoperatively.

Charnley's Transtrochanteric Approach

History
Sir John Charnley (1911 to 1982)
He is probably the greatest hip surgeon of all times and it was his ceaseless toil that produced the Total Hip Replacement. I quote from Mr Wroblowsli's article about him:

"Charnley's contributions to orthopaedic sciences and surgery are so vast that it

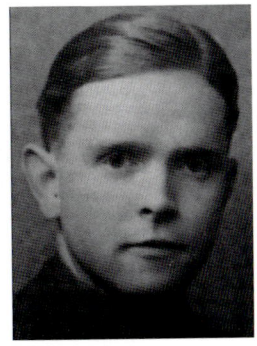

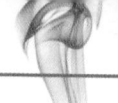

would be difficult to do justice when attempting to present more than a mere outline. Three aspects form a main theme: trauma, fusion of joints by compression methods and total hip arthroplasty."

The Closed Treatment of Common Fractures, first published in 1950, went to three editions and three reprints, the third one 40 years after the volume was first published! Justice will not be done by attempting even to summarize the volume, which has become, as intended by Charnley, the vade mecum of a practising trauma surgeon. Charnley's objective is clearly stated in the preface 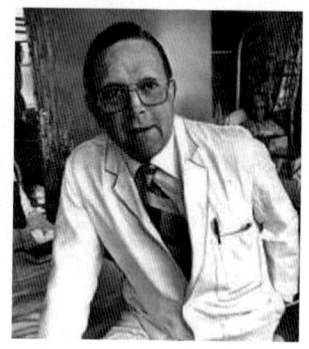 to the first edition:...*An attempt is here made to re-emphasize the non-operative method, and to show that far from being a crude and uncertain art, the manipulative treatment of fractures can be resolved into something of a science.*

Yet Charnley was not slow to admit that certain fractures, as of the tibia, proved difficult and had to be treated by internal fixation.

In 1961, Charnley wrote: *"There is a tendency to imagine that serious research nowadays can only come out of a laboratory, and the contributions from the pure act of thinking on clinical facts ended with the great clinicians of the past. In the training of young surgeons?...?the attempt to foster the habit of making clinical observations and questioning accepted beliefs ought to start from the earliest moment.?*

Published in 1953, *Compression Arthrodesis* is a monumental work on the physiology, principles and practice of cancellous bone union under compression. *"A few observations on the human body are often of more value than a large series of experiments on animals. It has rightly been said that every surgical operation is a biological experiment."*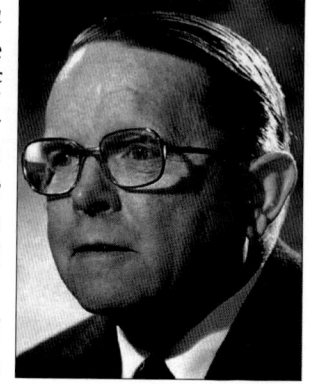

Although not as popular a method of treatment as it used to be before the

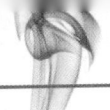

advent of total joint arthroplasty, the principles remain valid and are almost certainly the basis of formation of the Association for the Study of Osteo-synthesis, the *Arbeitsgemeinschaft fur osteosynthesefragen* Group with their very detailed description of operative treatment and compression fixation of fractures.

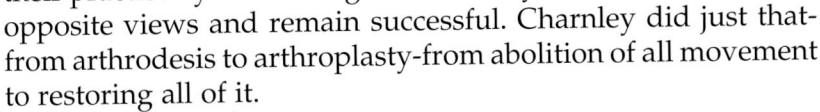

Few individuals are capable of changing their practice by advocating diametrically opposite views and remain successful. Charnley did just that-from arthrodesis to arthroplasty-from abolition of all movement to restoring all of it.

From 1962 onwards, Charnley committed his energies to hip replacement surgery with a full-time practice at Wrightington Hospital. And here began his breathtaking and monumental work in arthroplasty.

Charnley himself did suffer trials and tribulations when developing his hip replacement, but he never gave up and finally, in November 1962, the Charnley hip replacement became practical reality and has become the gold standard for this form of treatment. Clinical and radiographic success of this procedure is now approaching 50 years of follow-up.

Total dedication to all aspects demanded by this type of surgery consumed Charnley's time. Development of the clean air enclosure, total body exhaust suits and the instrument tray system are the essential aspects to reduce deep infection in this type of surgery. Prospective documentation, the establishment of a Centre for Hip Surgery and the collection of numerous post-mortem specimens bequeathed by his patients in order to study the histology of the bone-cement interface, show clearly how farseeing Charnley's ideas were.

Charnley's contribution to orthopaedic surgery was recognized both nationally and internationally with numerous awards, including a Knighthood in 1977.

Plane

Transtrochanteric

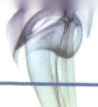

Access provided

A very wide access for both acetabulum and upper femur in all directions.

Dislocation

Anterior or posterior depending on the surgeon's choice.

Position and draping

Once again, depending on the surgeon's choice, the patient can be placed supine or in lateral position. A slightly increased hip manoeuvrability in lateral position makes it the position of choice in revision arthroplasty.

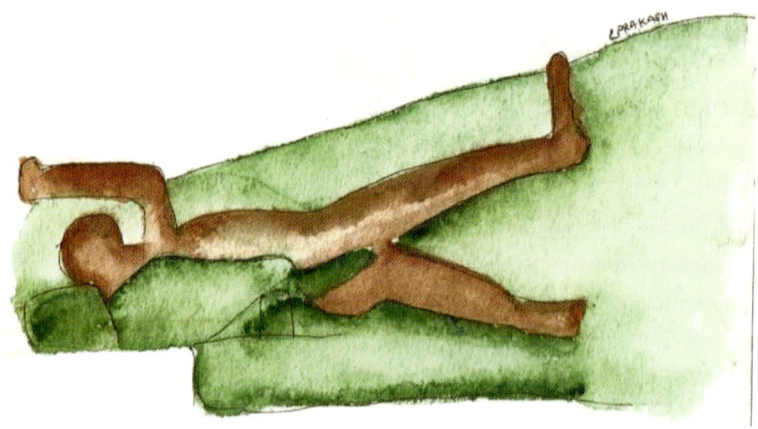

The leg is draped free for easy hip manoeuvrability.

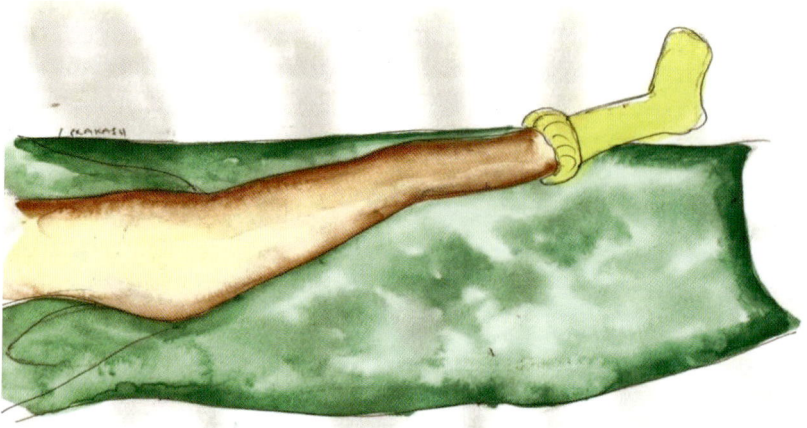

Incision

Straight incision centred over trochanter extending 5 cm proximally and distally.

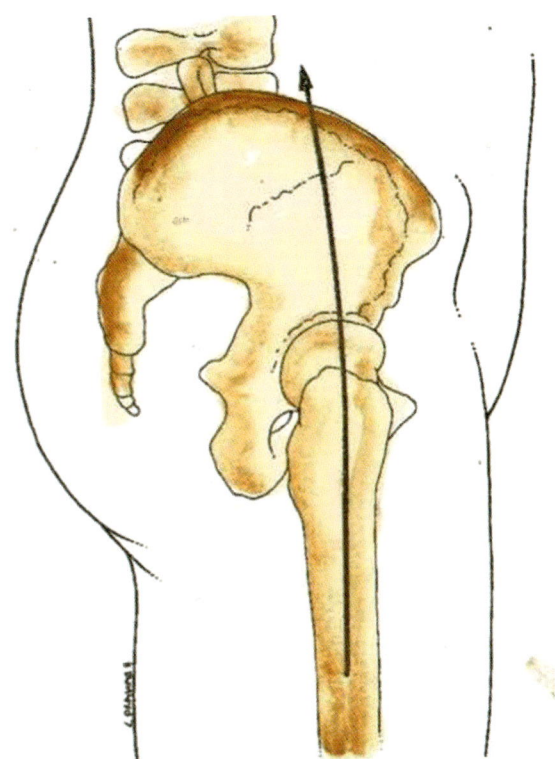

Charnley's transtrochanteric approach

Dissections

The fascia lata is divided in skin line. The gap between tensor fascia lata and gluteus medius is explored till the hip capsule.

The posterior margin of the gluteus medius is now identified and a curved forceps is introduced directly over the capsule coming from the anterior to posterior fibres of gluteus medius.

The limb is internally rotated and abducted to guide the tip of the curved forceps to emerge correctly.

The anterior half of origin of the vastus lateralis is now erased with a cutting diathermy, going bone deep and a part of vastus lateralis is now deflected out.

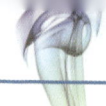

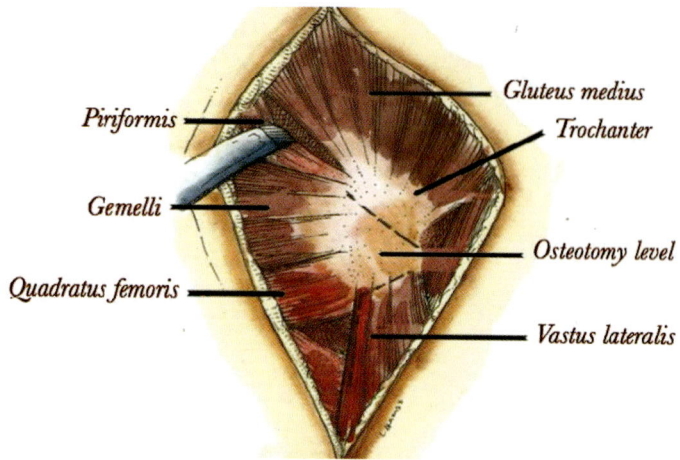

Gluteus medius

Trochanter

Piriformis

Gemelli

Quadratus femoris

Osteotomy level

Vastus lateralis

Osteotomy level in Charnley approach

The trochanteric osteotomy is now performed. The curved artery forceps may be used to pull out a Gigli saw which can then be seesawed. Else a Steinmann pin pushed into the trochanter gives a wedge-shaped Chevron osteotomy for better reattachment.

Some surgeons use small sharp chisels, while others use a power saw. The important point to remember is to include the posterior aspect of the greater trochanter as well. The piece should not be too small to make reattachment difficult.

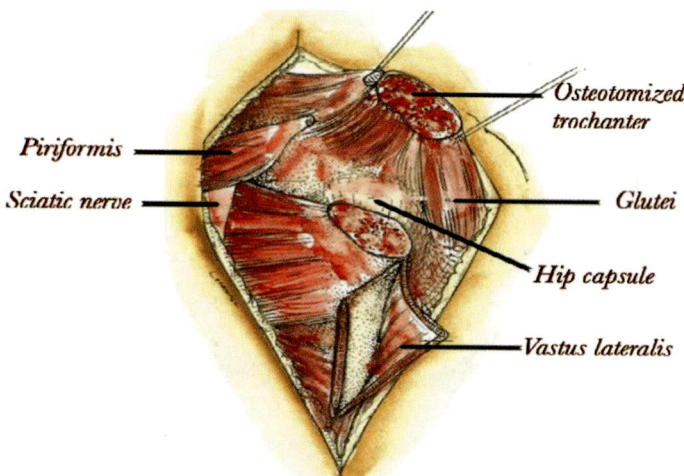

Osteotomized trochanter

Piriformis

Sciatic nerve

Glutei

Hip capsule

Vastus lateralis

Trochanteric osteotomy gives a really wide exposure

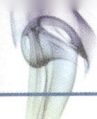

Deflection of the osteotomized trochanter exposes piriformis, which is divided to reach the hip capsule.

The capsule is cut or excised to expose the hip. Dislocation is easy by external rotation and abduction.

The trochanter is reattached either by tension band wires or by a couple of lag screws.

The following drawings redrawn from Charnley's book describe the master's steps.

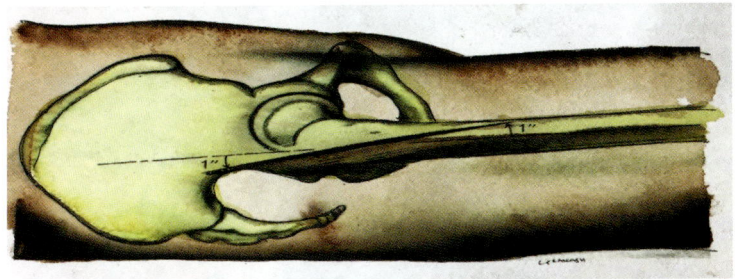

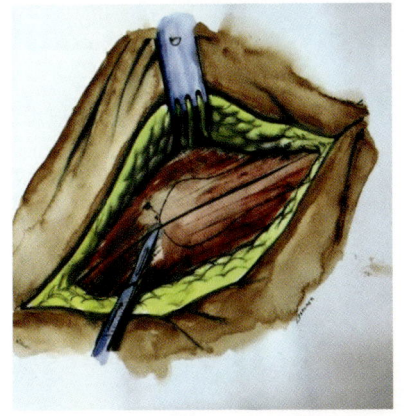

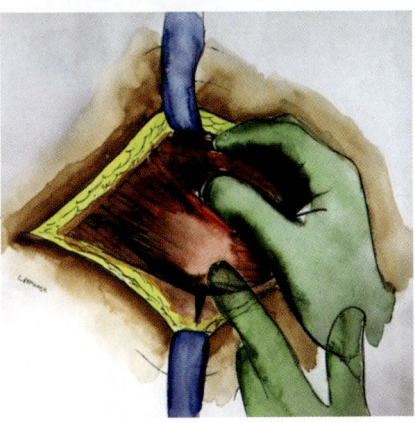

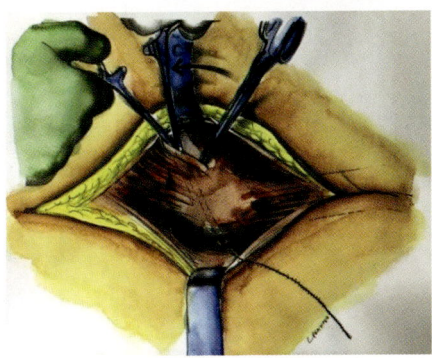

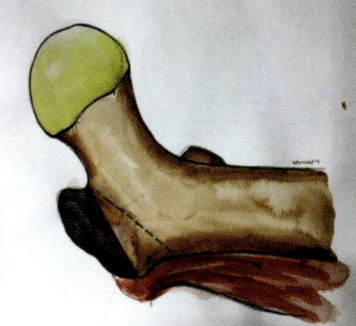

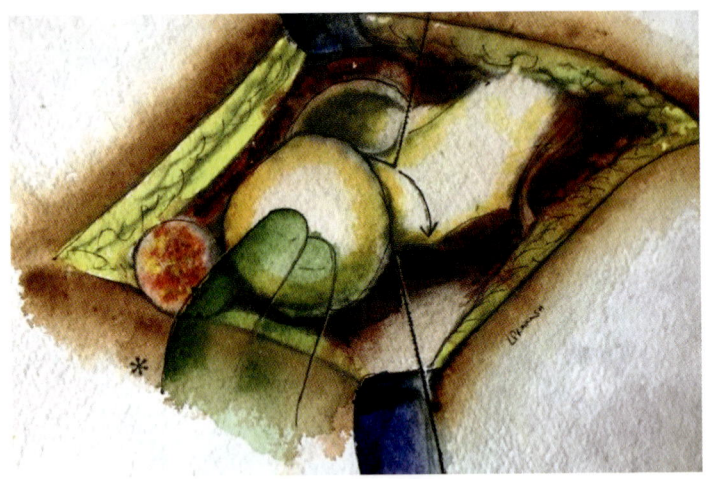

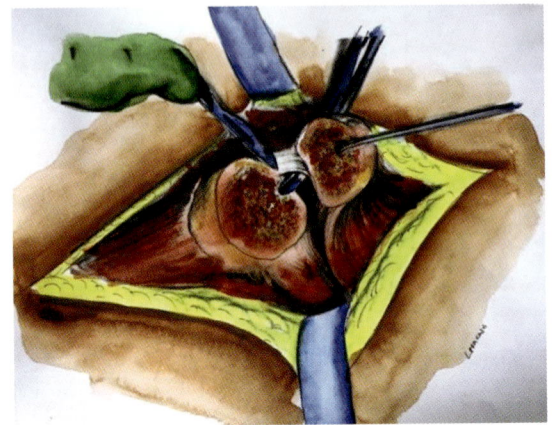

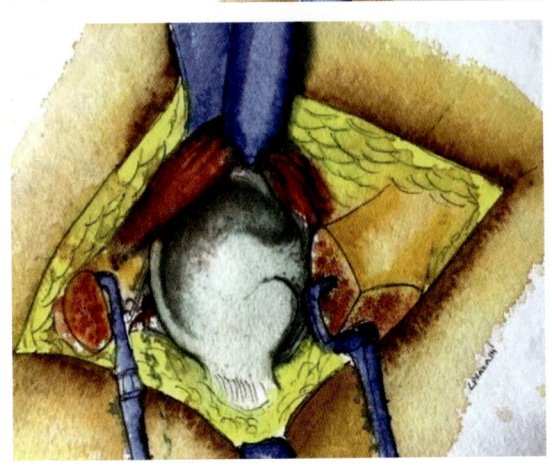

Indications

Primary and revision hip replacements, especially difficult and complex hips.

Advantages

- Widest exposure of hip.
- Gluteus medius and minimus remain undamaged.
- Distalisation of the trochanter can tighten the abductor lever arm and improve postoperative function.

Disadvantages

- Increased blood loss
- Slower recovery
- Trochanteric problems, non-unions and bursitis.

Extended Transtrochanteric Approach

History

The approach was described by Ruedi in 1984 along with his other AO colleagues, and was principally meant for complex pelvic acetabular injuries.

Plane

Transtrochanteric approach, where stripping muscles from pelvis exposes the pelvis from anterior column right up to iliopubic eminence.

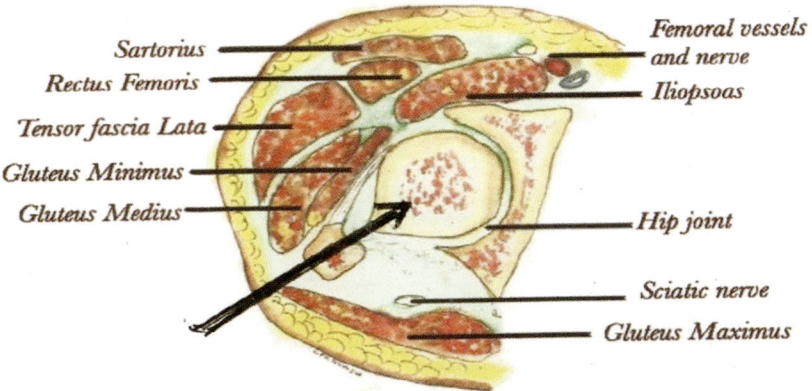

Anatomical planes for hip approach

Access provided
- Posterior column
- Superior acetabular dome
- Anterior column
- Iliopubic area

Dislocation

Anterior, posterior or inferior, depending on the fracture type and fixation needs.

Position and draping

In lateral position, the patient is strapped to back rests and sand-bags to keep the pelvis steady during the entire surgery. The limb is draped free and the knee should flex comfortably to provide a good lever arm for generous internal and external rotations of the hip joint during surgery.

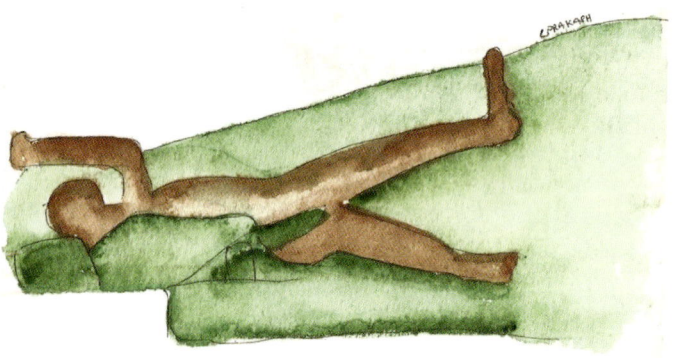

A distal femoral pin traction on an Ilizarov half ring or a Bohler's stirrup will allow traction to be applied when needed.

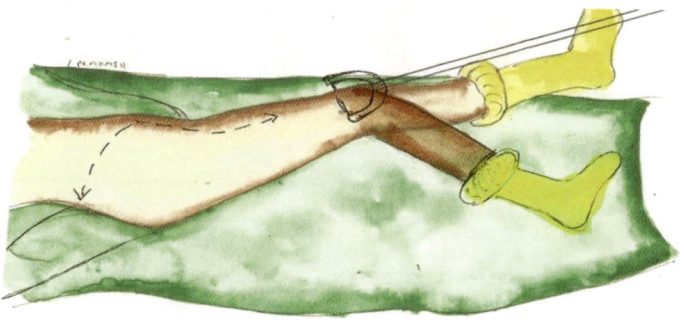

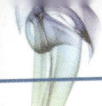
Incision

The three landmarks to be kept in mind are iliac crest, posterior border of trochanteric flare and the lateral border of patella.

The skin incision is a straight line centred over greater trochanter extending almost equally upwards and down-wards.

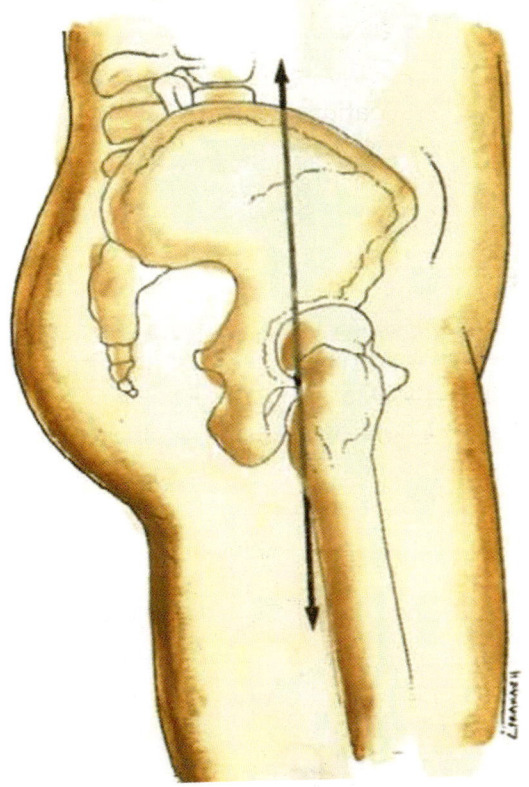

Extensive transtrochanteric approach

Dissections

Subcutaneous fat and fascia are dissected a little more extensively in the proximal part of the incision than the distal part. The gluteus medius is exposed as far as iliac crest.

A high skin incision allows it to be retracted in a thick flap to allow a T incision in the gluteus medius dividing the iliotibial tract towards front and back a little below the iliac crest.

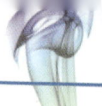

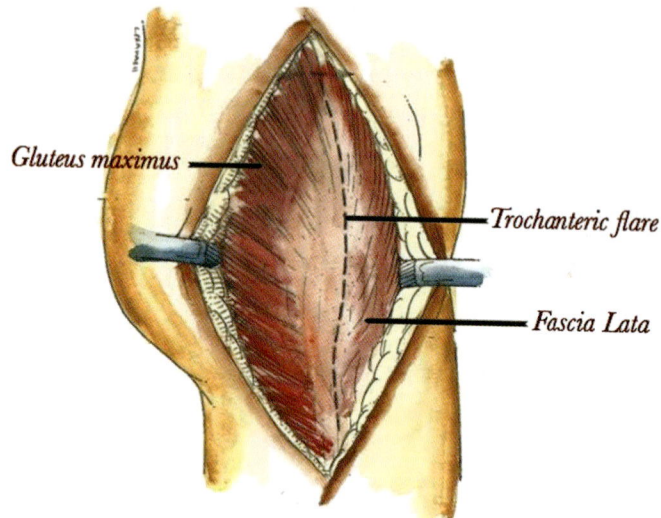

Deep fascia is raised as flaps from the underlying muscles. The posterior flap contains the gluteus maximus. Iliotibial tract is detached from upper gluteus medius.

Gluteus medius, short lateral rotators, and vastus lateralis are identified.

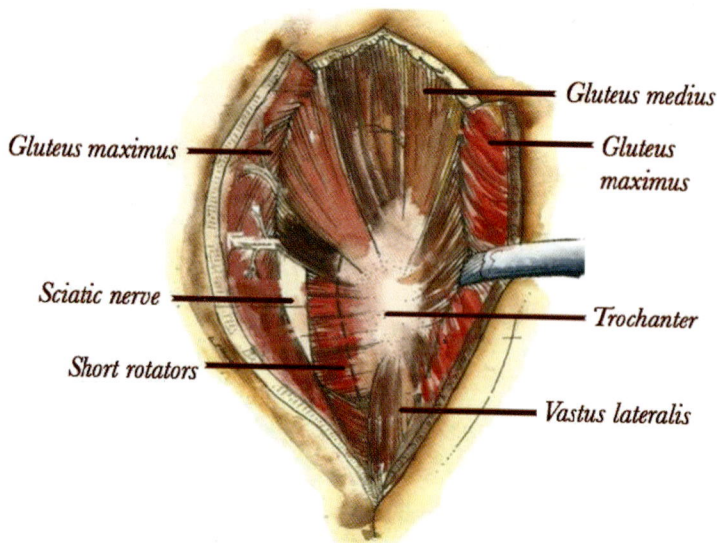

Gluteus maximus is split

Greater trochanter is now osteotomized, to allow gluteus medius and minimus to be subperiosteally elevated from ASIS to sciatic notch.

The superior neurovascular bundle is identified and protected. This is the only remaining supply for the remaining muscle belly and the muscle mass has to be frequently replaced back till it perfuses red again.

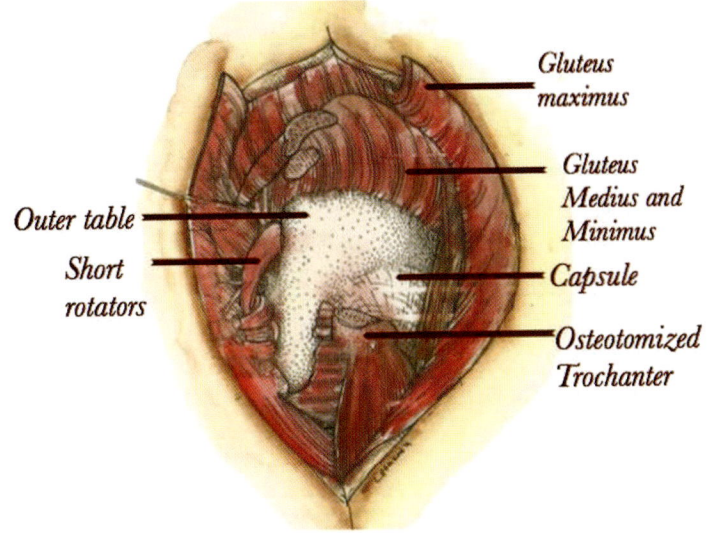

Outer table
Short rotators

Gluteus maximus

Gluteus Medius and Minimus

Capsule

Osteotomized Trochanter

Ruedi's approach

Small lateral rotators are now detached from posterior border of greater trochanter leaving sufficient mass for reattachment. Their posterior retraction protects sciatic nerve.

Anterior column is accessed by dividing the straight and reflected head of rectus femoris.

Osteotomy of iliac crest will give additional access, if needed.

Flexion of the hip and subperiosteal erasure of iliacus muscle from inner table allows palpation of inner surface of acetabulum to check reduction.

The iliac crest is reattached with lag screws, and trochanter with screws, clamps or wires. The lateral rotators are reattached before closure.

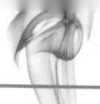

Indications

- Pelvic fractures, including those involving sacrum.
- Fractures of the anterior column.
- Superior pubic ramus fractures.
- Floating symphysis pubis or disruption of symphysis pubis.

Advantages

- Excellent field of exposure from one side to the other, especially in anterior column fractures.
- Good clean cosmetic scar.

Disadvantages

- Difficult and technically demanding operation.
- Superior gluteal vessels have to be carefully protected, and the muscle mass repeatedly perfused intraoperatively.
- Increased blood loss.
- Osteotomies have to be fixed back.

Posterior Approaches

History

Von Langenbeck in 1874, and Kocher in 1887 described posterior approaches with minor differences. Frequency of foot drop and sciatic injuries made these approaches unpopular until 1950, when Gibson decribed his variation. In 1957, Moore described his modification for insertion of his prosthesis. From the 1960s, the direct posterolateral approach has become the most popular approach for most hemiarthroplasties, and total replacements of hip.

Bernhard Rudolf Konrad von Langenbeck, the nephew of the anatomist and surgeon Konrad Johann Martin Langenbeck, studied in Göttingen where he received his doctorate in 1835. He began his career as a lecturer in physiology and pathological anatomy in Göttingen in 1838.

Langenbeck became extraordinary professor in Göttingen, and in 1842 was called to the chair of surgery in Kiel, where he was also director of the Friedrich Hospital.

Later he became the physician to the general staff – General Stabsarzt – then Physician General (Generalarzt) and consulting surgeon—and that same year was raised to the nobility.

His experiences from field hospitals were laid down in numerous papers. His fields of interest were resection of joints as well as gunshot wounds and their treatment. He was a great innovator and developed several surgical instruments.

In surgery, apart from his hip approach, Langenbeck made important contributions in the development of plastic surgery, and manipulations of the contracted knee joint in contractures with percutaneous tenotomies. He is also remembered for his operation of cleft palate published in 1861.

For years, Langenbeck was the undisputed leader of German surgery and is best known today as the "father of the surgical residency". He developed a system whereby new medical graduates would live at the hospital as they gradually assumed a greater role in the day-to-day care and supervision of surgical patients. Among his most well-known "house staff" were such illustrious surgeons as Christian Albert Theodor Billroth and Emil Theodor Kocher.

The brilliance of his house staff model was acknowledged by Sir William Osler and William Stewart Halsted, who quickly co-opted his concept into the teaching system of the departments of medicine and surgery respectively, at the Johns Hopkins University Hospital in the late 19th century.

From orthopaedics to ENT, from maxillofacial to arthrolysis, from medical training to apprenticeship, from design to instruments making, his contributions to the field of medicine were phenomenal. In 1864, he was knighted for his services during the Danish war. He was a highly recognized and very popular teacher, drawing large flocks of students to the University of Berlin during his tenure.

Emil Theodor Kocher: Emil Theodor Kocher (1841–1917, Bern) was the Swiss surgeon who won the 1909 Nobel prize for Physiology or Medicine for his work on the thyroid gland.

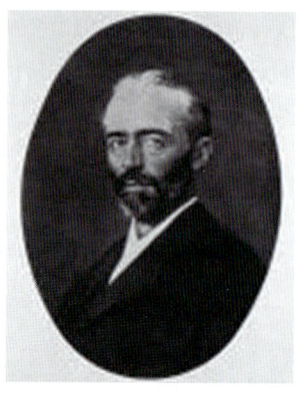

After qualifying in medicine at the University of Bern in 1865, Kocher studied in Berlin, London, Paris, and Vienna, where he was a pupil of Theodor Billroth. In 1872, he became professor of clinical surgery at Bern, remaining head of the surgical clinic for 45 years.

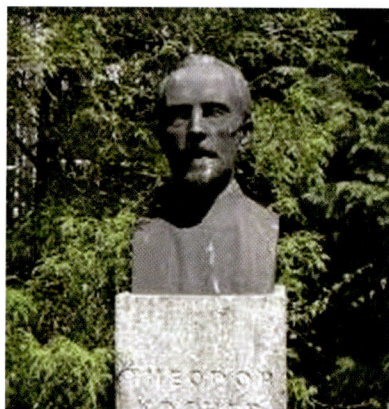
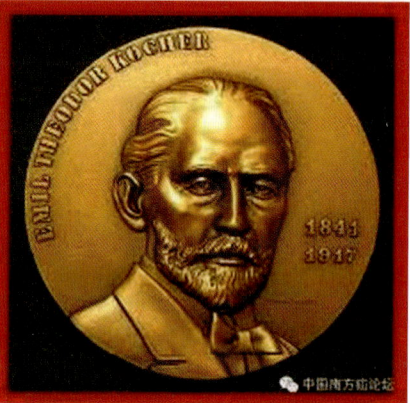

There Kocher became the first surgeon to excise the thyroid gland in the treatment of goitre (1876). In 1883, he announced his discovery of a characteristic cretinoid pattern in patients after total excision of the thyroid gland; when a portion of the gland was left intact, however, there were only transitory signs of the pathological pattern.

His other surgical contributions include a method for reducing dislocations of the shoulder and techniques for surgery on hip, stomach, the lungs, the tongue, and the cranial nerves and for hernia. In surgical practice, he adopted the principles of complete asepsis introduced by Joseph Lister. He also devised many new surgical techniques, instruments, and appliances. The forceps and incision (in gallbladder surgery) that bear his name remain in general use.

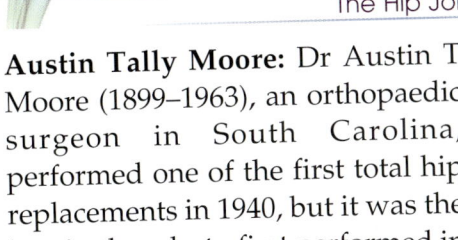

Austin Tally Moore: Dr Austin T Moore (1899–1963), an orthopaedic surgeon in South Carolina, performed one of the first total hip replacements in 1940, but it was the hemiarthroplasty first performed in 1942, to which he lent his name.

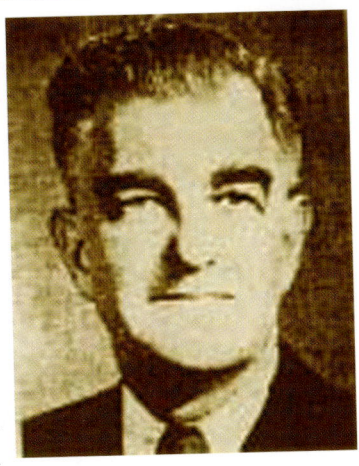

After completing medical school in 1924 from South Carolina, Moore worked in various hospitals till 1939, when he founded Moore Clinic in Columbia. He was also the surgeon of the psychiatric hospital in the city of Columbia, which had 7,000 beds. Fractures of the neck of the femur are frequent among older patients who are often in bad general state.

Moore thought of a revolutionary process of fixing the femoral head in such fractures, whereby the metal head would be carried by a stem driven into the medullary canal of the femur. In 1952, he designed an improvement that featured a fenestrated stem to allow bone ingrowth. Both designs were produced in collaboration with Howmedica Inc. (at the time, Austenal Laboratories, now merged with Stryker® Corporation).

These were the first hip arthroplasty products that were widely distributed. They eventually became legendary and are still widely used for replacement of the femoral head and neck, especially following femoral neck fractures in the elderly. Moore described his method of implanting the prosthesis in JBJS in 1957, the year I was born.

Moore's Southern Approach

Plane
The fibres of gluteus maximus are split and small lateral rotators are detached from trochanteric attachment, leaving enough bits for reattachment.

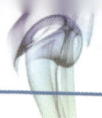

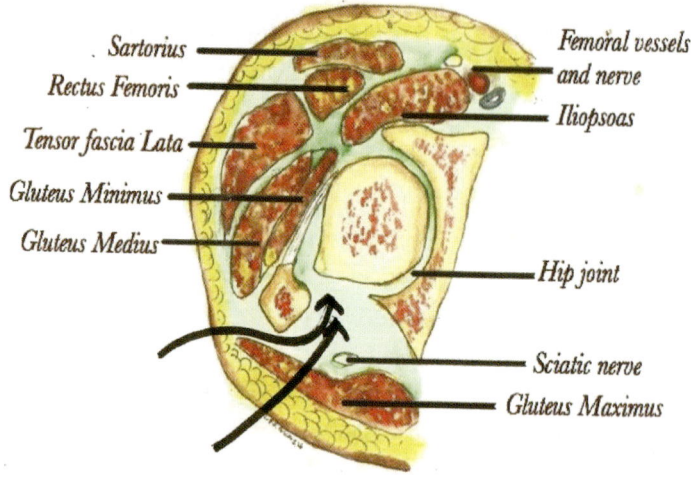

Sartorius

Rectus Femoris

Tensor fascia Lata

Gluteus Minimus

Gluteus Medius

Femoral vessels and nerve

Iliopsoas

Hip joint

Sciatic nerve

Gluteus Maximus

Access provided
- Hip joint, especially posterior superior aspect
- The sciatic nerve
- Neck of femur
- Lesser trochanter

Dislocation
Posterior

Position and draping:
Original Moore's position was semiprone with sandbags under the affected ASIS. Later modifications placed the patient in the lateral position, stabilized in place by supports, clamps and sandbags.

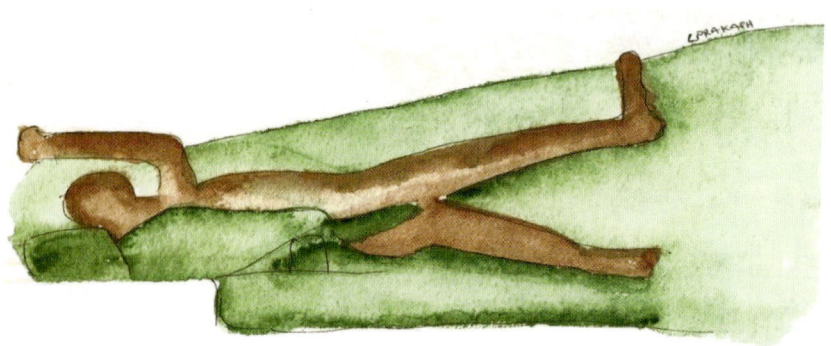

Incision
Begins 7.5 cm below the posterosuperior iliac spine, extends to trochanteric flare and then curves along the lateral border of thigh.

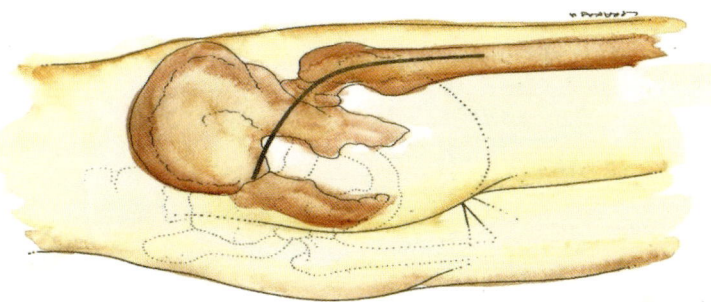

Dissections
The fascia lata is divided over the greater trochanter and carried in both directions in the line of skin incision.

The fibres of gluteus maximus are separated by blunt dissection to expose the small lateral rotators. The sciatic nerve comes on the lateral side, while the inferior gluteal vessels are near the proximal most portion of the incision.

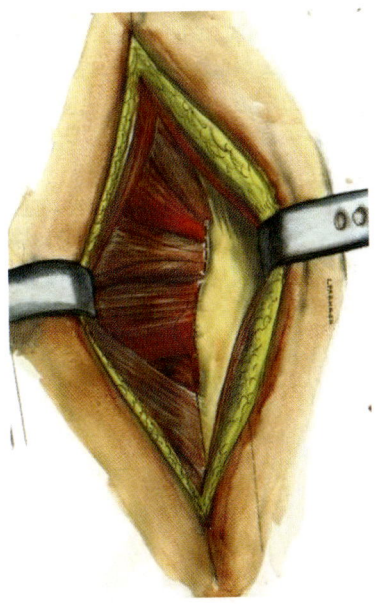
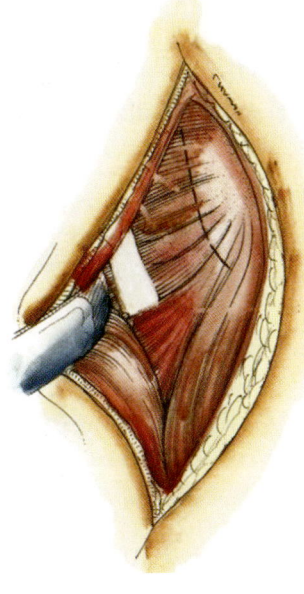

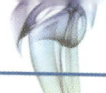

The small lateral rotators are now divided close to their insertion into the trochanter, leaving enough attachments for repair.

This exposes the hip joint capsule, which can be incised in a T fashion. The femoral head and neck will be visible at this stage.

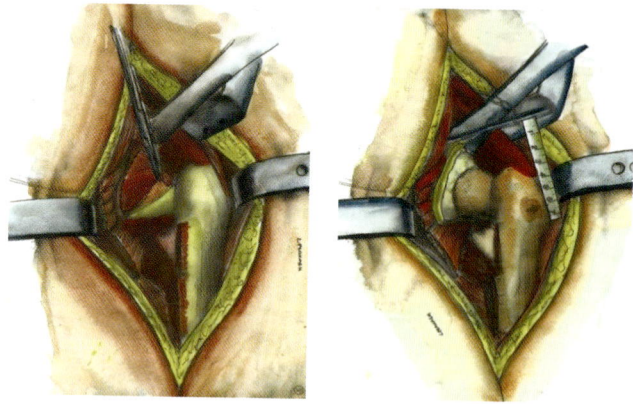

Internal rotation of the leg, using the bent knee as a lever arm, dislocates the hip easily and provides a complete exposure of the acetabulum, which can be visualized using properly placed Hohmann retractors.

Closure

It is important to ensure that the lateral rotators are re-attached precisely using the stay sutures applied earlier. It is a good idea to place the suction drain over the joint and then suture the small lateral rotators above it.

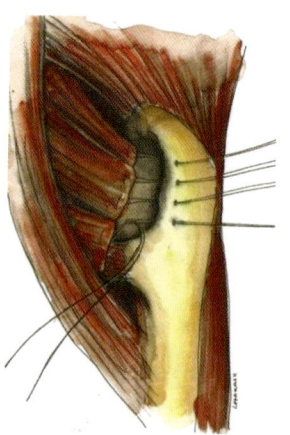
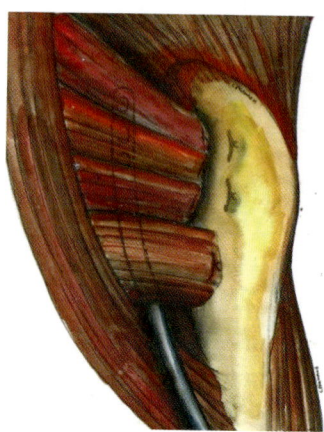

Indications

Originally described for unipolar arthroplasty, this remains the most satisfactory approach for that problem even today.

It can also be used for posterior column pelvis and posterior acetabular fractures.

Advantages

Easy and quick exposure through almost bloodless fields and planes.

Easy dislocation of the hip.

This is probably the best approach for unipolar and bipolar hips.

Provides an excellent access to the posterior lip and the posterior column of the acetabulum.

Disadvantages

Sciatic nerve injury and foot drop due to neuropraxia in case of excessive lateral exposure.

Injury to inferior gluteal vessels.

Dependant incision with associated problems.

Slightly higher risk of postoperative infection and dislocation.

Acetabular exposure is a little less adequate than with lateral approaches.

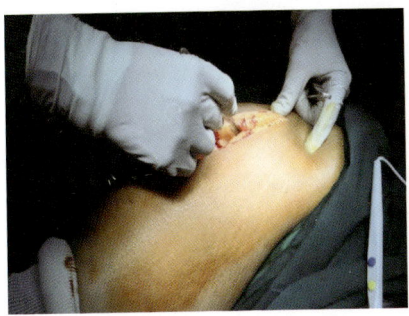
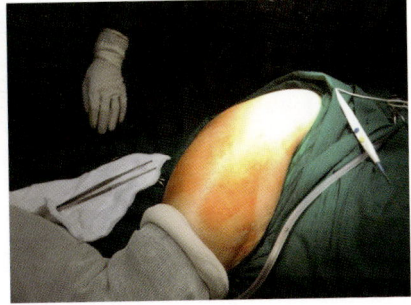

Position, draping and skin incision

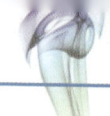

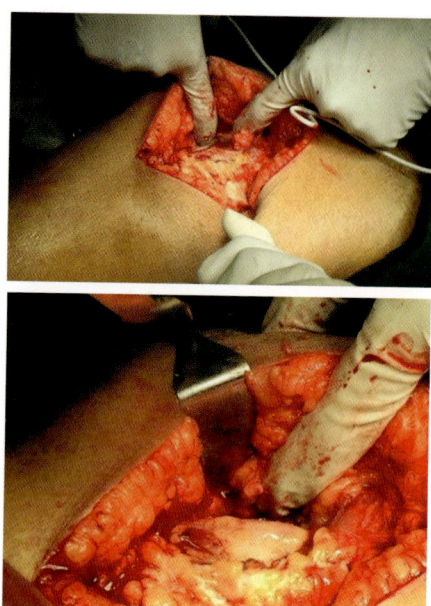

The small lateral rotators are cut and hip capsule is exposed.

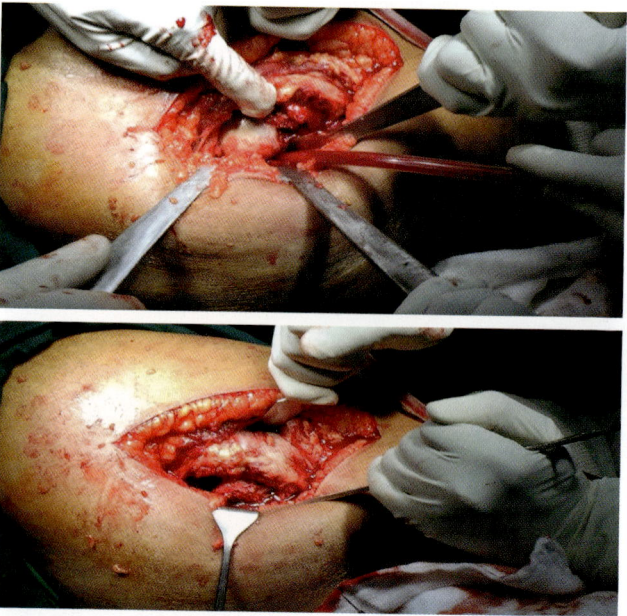

The hip joint is exposed by internally rotating the limb, and the broken head is removed.

The Standard Lateral Approach

This is the preferred and most commonly used approach for total hip replacements, and is a modification of Moore's approach with a slightly more lateral straight incision. It has the advantage of making the approach less dependant and avoids postoperative oedema. It provides the same excellent approach as the Classic Moore's Southern approach, but at the same time has a lesser rate of postoperative complications.

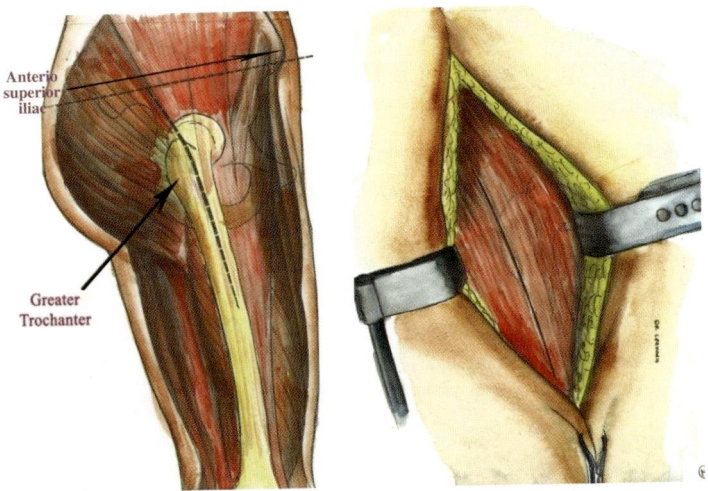

Anterior superior iliac

Greater Trochanter

Plane

The fibres of gluteus maximus are split and small lateral rotators are detached from trochanteric attachment, leaving enough bits for reattachment.

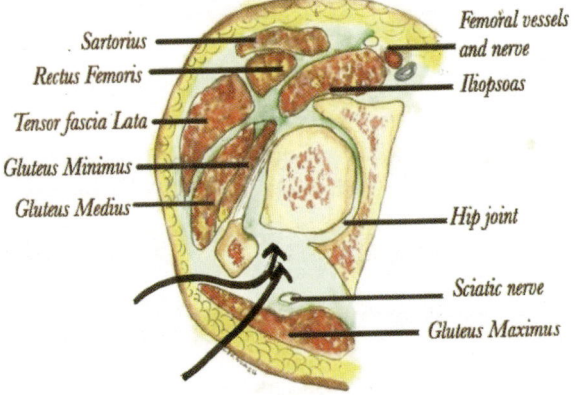

Sartorius

Rectus Femoris

Tensor fascia Lata

Gluteus Minimus

Gluteus Medius

Femoral vessels and nerve

Iliopsoas

Hip joint

Sciatic nerve

Gluteus Maximus

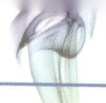

Access provided
- Hip joint, especially posterior aspect
- Neck of femur
- Lesser trochanter
- Acetabulum

Dislocation
Posterior

Position and draping
A lateral position with sandbags and table attachments to keep the patient stable. The leg is draped free for manipulations and dislocations.

The knee is flexed and kept flexed throughout the procedure to ensure that sciatic nerve is kept in relaxation during the entire period.

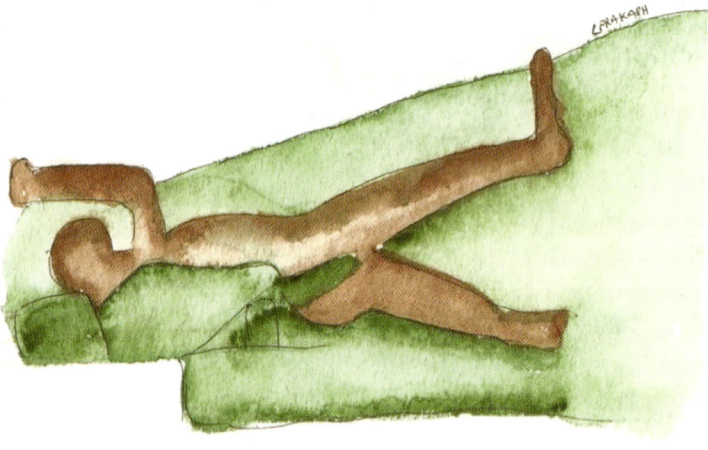

Incision
Straight midlateral or slightly posterolateral incision centred on posterior aspect of greater trochanter extending superiorly to iliac crest about 7.5 cm below trochanteric flare. In revisions, the incision can be extended both superiorly and inferiorly.

Dissections
The fascia lata is divided over the greater trochanter and a finger inserted to separate it from the gluteal fibres. The deep incision is carried in both directions in the line of skin incision.

The fibres of gluteus maximus are separated by blunt dissection to expose the small lateral rotators. The sciatic nerve comes on the lateral side, while the inferior gluteal vessels are near the proximal most portion of the incision.

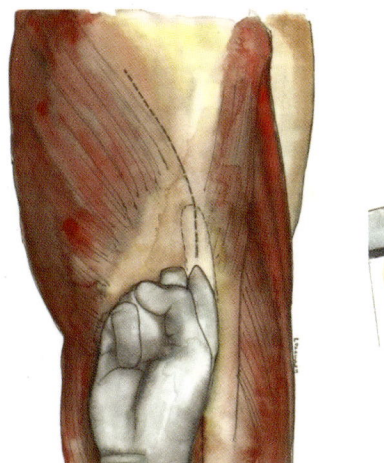 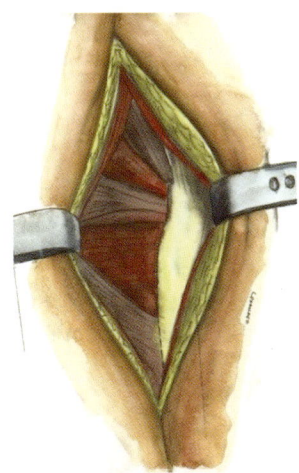

Sciatic nerve may not always be visualized, but its position should be always kept in mind. The fatty areolar tissue over the small lateral rotators is cleared by pushing it with a pad.

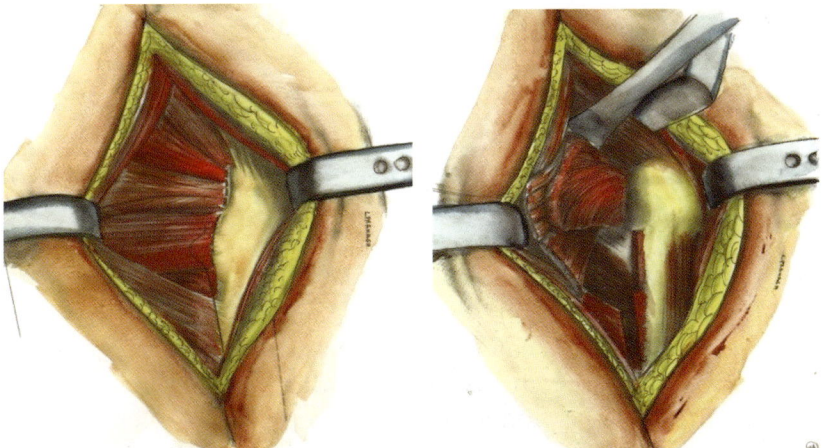

The hip is now internally rotated; this stretches the attachment of the lateral rotators and they can be now detached, leaving adequate bits for reattachment. Stay sutures in the lateral rotators allow the whole belly to be retracted.

This unit of small lateral rotators retracted posteriorly acts as a soft tissue sleeve to protect the sciatic nerve. The medial circumflex femoral artery (at the uppermost part of the exposure) needs to be identified and either ligated or coagulated.

If additional exposure is desired, gluteus maximus is detached from its femoral attachment.

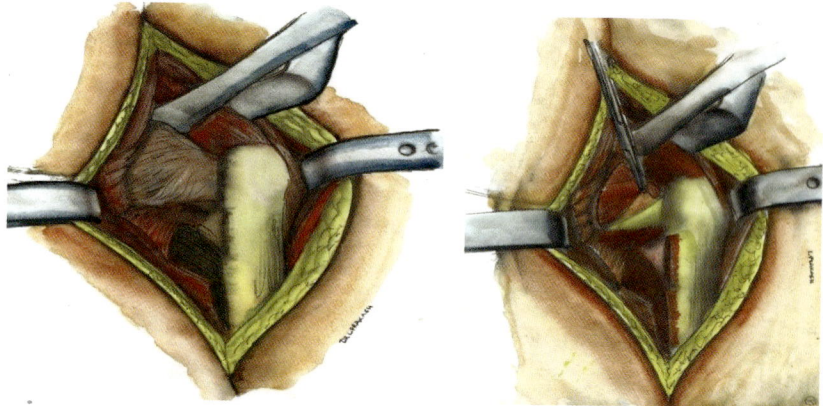

At this stage, the capsule is incised along the femoral neck and the hip is exposed.

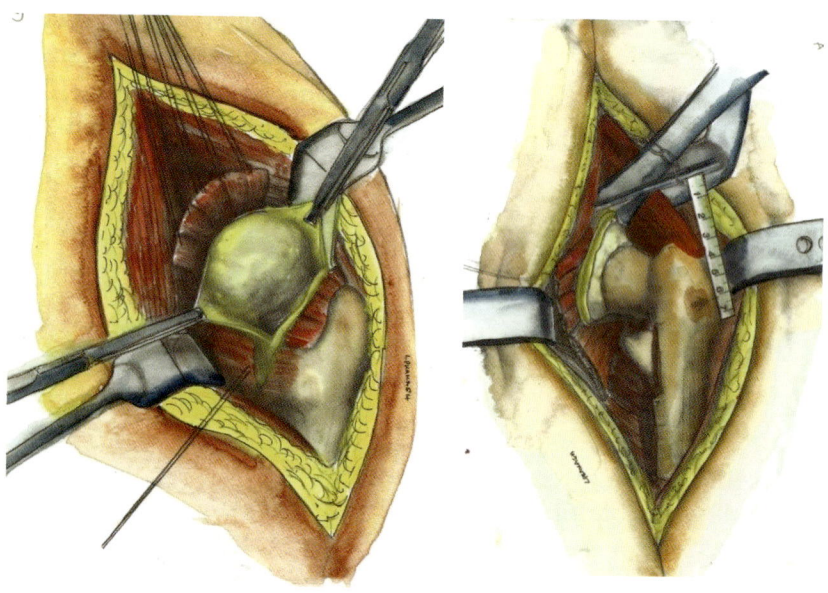

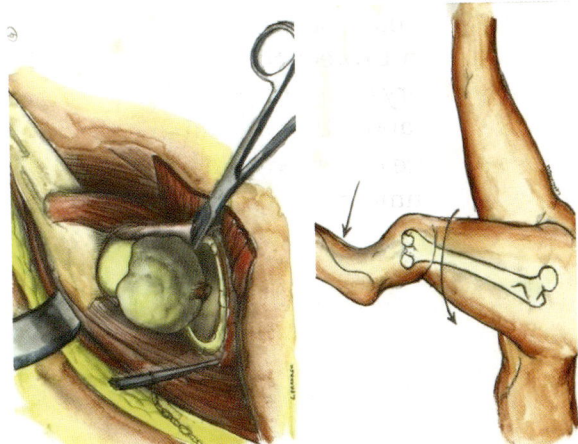

The hip is dislocated by flexion, adduction and internal rotation of the hip.

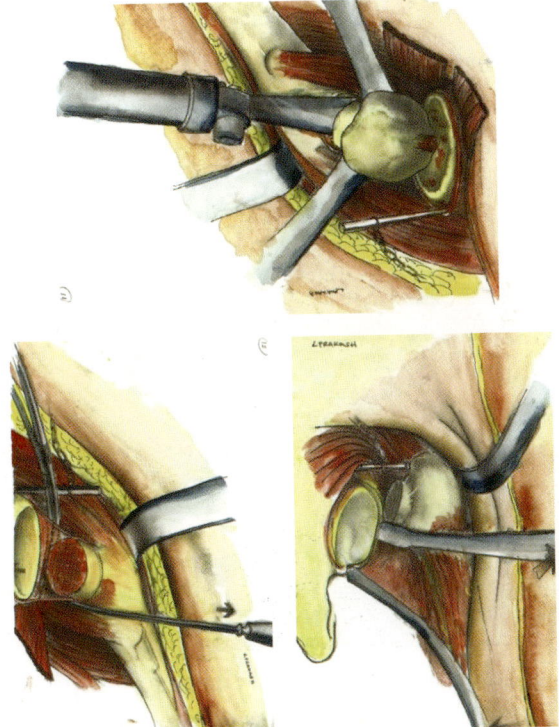

Appropriate and judicious placement of Hohmann retractors expose the whole of acetabulum.

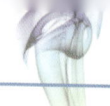

Indications

Monopolar, bipolar, and total hip replacements.

Revision hip replacements.

Fracture with posterior dislocation of the hip, especially with transacetabular posterior column fractures.

Exploration of sciatic nerve.

Drainage of septic arthritis of the hip joint.

Advantages

Easy quick approach through relatively bloodless fields and planes.

Easy dislocation of hip with extreme manoeuvrability.

Decent exposure for acetabular reaming.

Disadvantages

Increased risk of dislocation and infection.

Positionally dependant area subject to tissue oedema and associated complications.

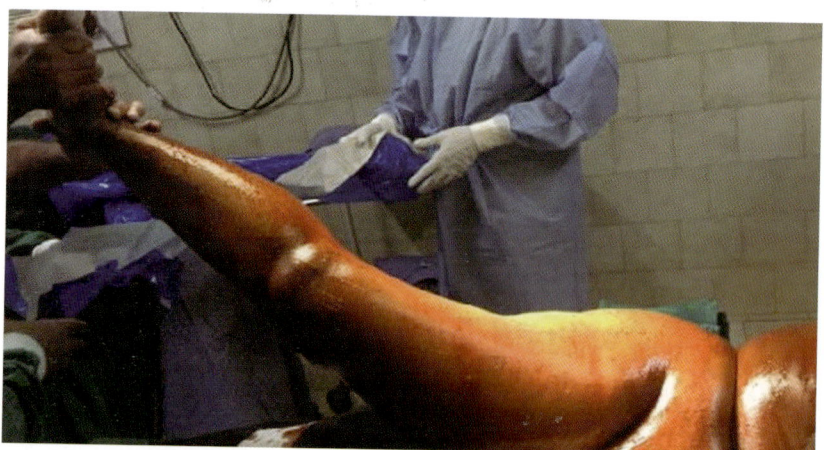

The patient is strapped in a dead lateral position.

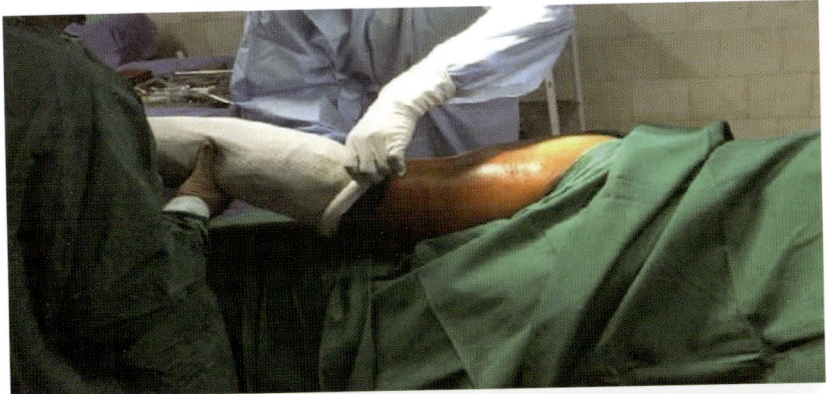

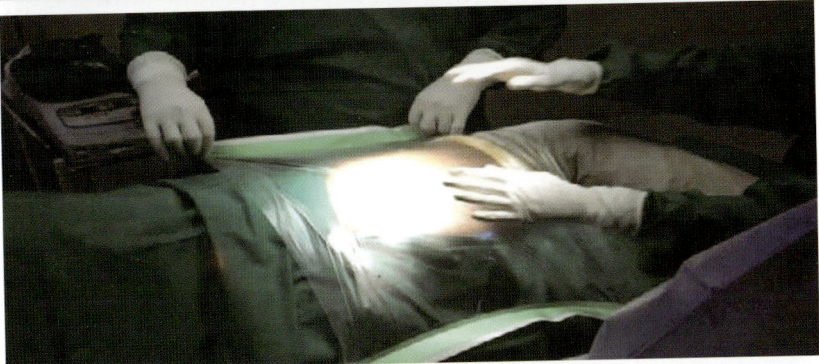

Draping and preparation.

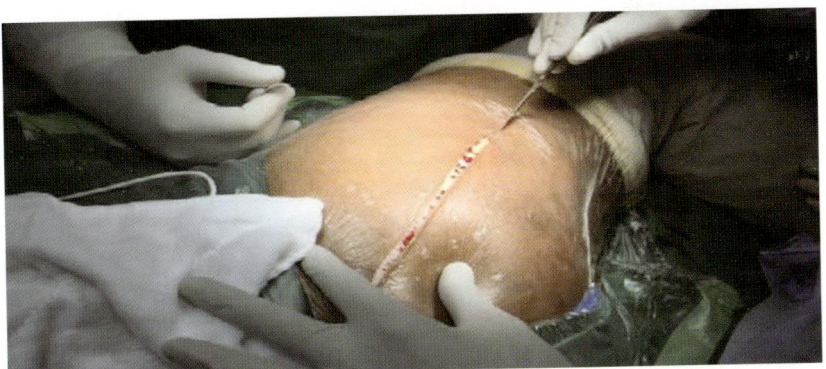

Skin incision

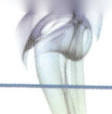

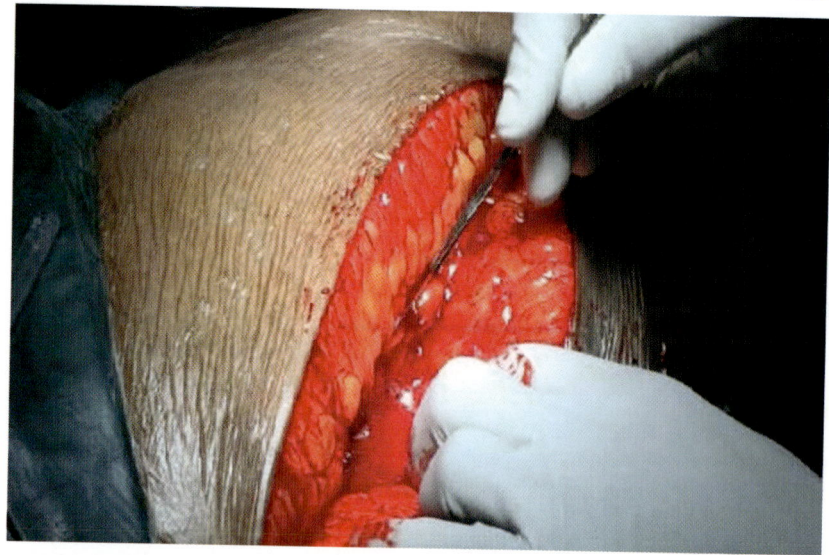

Subcutaneous fat and deep fascia cut in the same line.

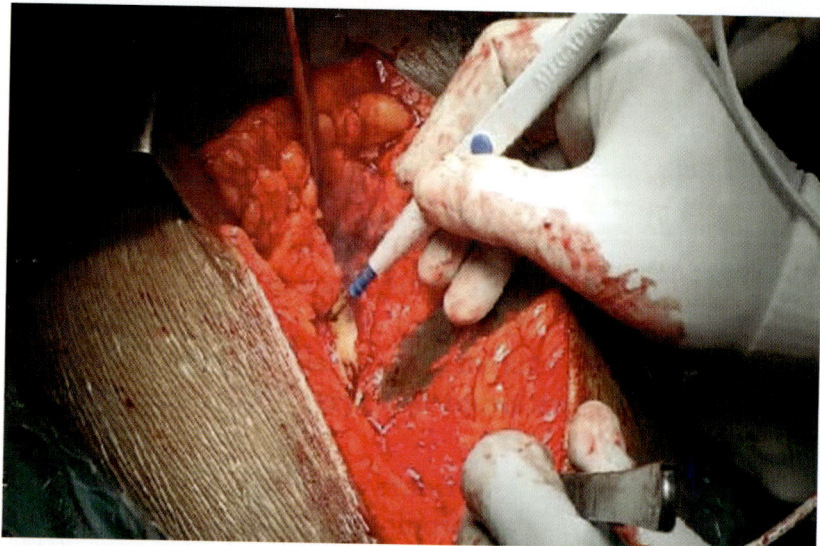

The fat is incised in the line of skin incision, and the fibres of glutei are split to expose the small lateral rotators of the hip.

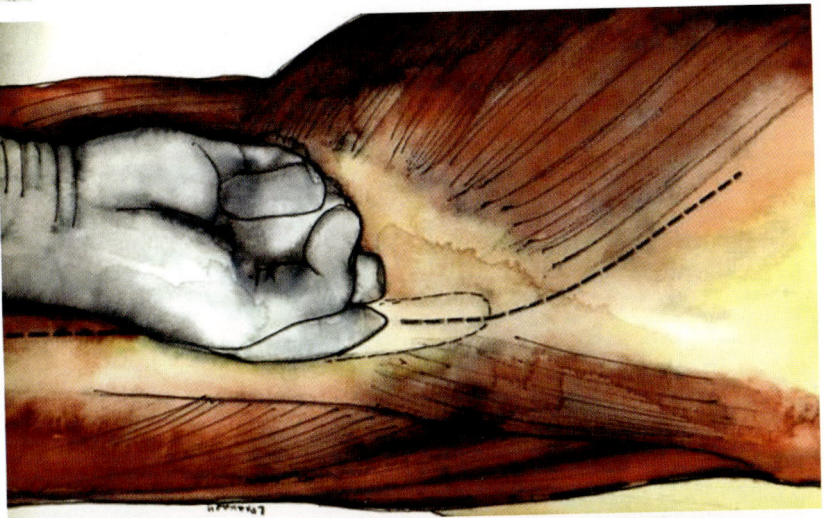

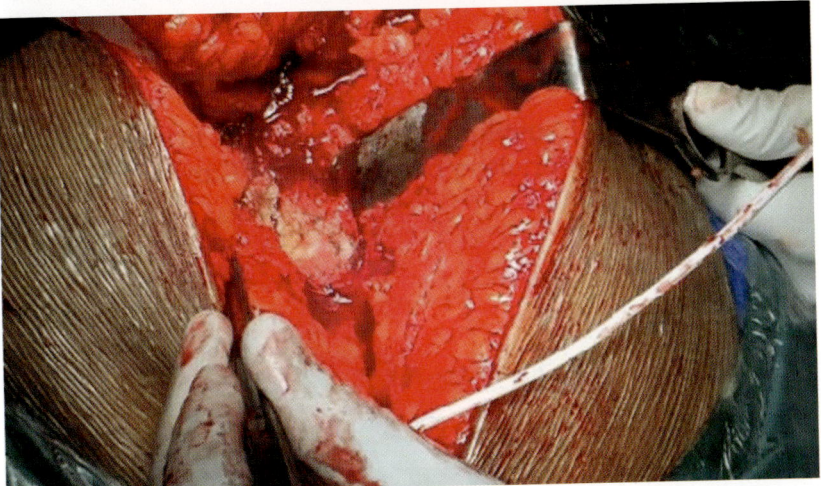

The assistant now internally rotates the hip and this tightens the short rotators.

The muscle bellies of quadratus femoris, superior and inferior gemelli, and piriformis are identified.

The lowermost part of the incision has the superior branch of lateral femoral circumflex artery, which has to be located and coagulated.

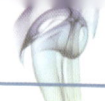

This vessel lies a little deep and will keep on oozing and irritating the surgeon is not dealt with early.

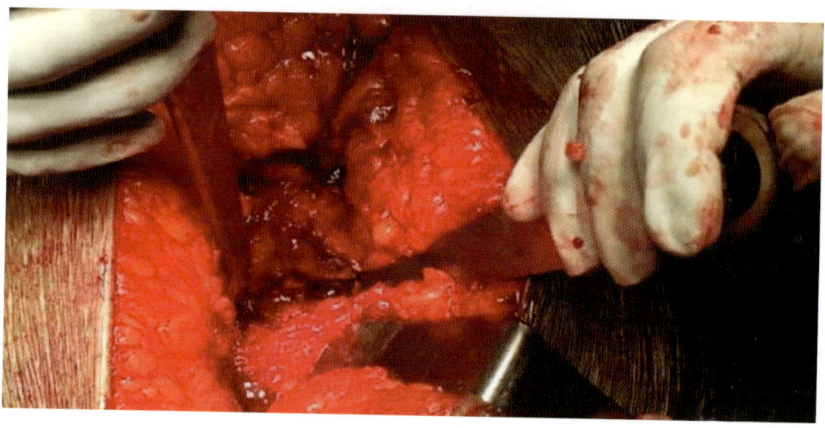

The short lateral rotators are now cut, leaving an attachment to the trochanteric flare for subsequent reattachment.

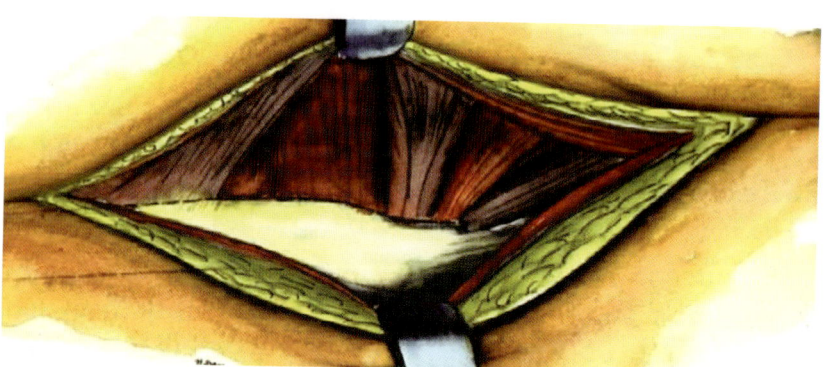

The inferior part, if piriformis, is detached as well.

If the hip appears tight, additional soft tissue releases are performed.

The assistant internally rotates the hip, using the flexed knee as a lever, and this manoeuvre tightens the short rotators, making them prominent.

Some surgeons use stay sutures in the rotators to facilitate reattachment.

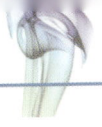

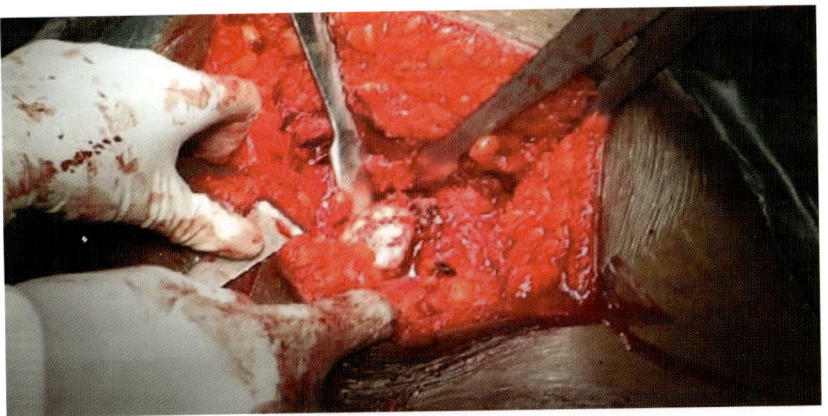

A gentle rocking movement of the flexed knee towards internal rotation exposes larger areas of the head.

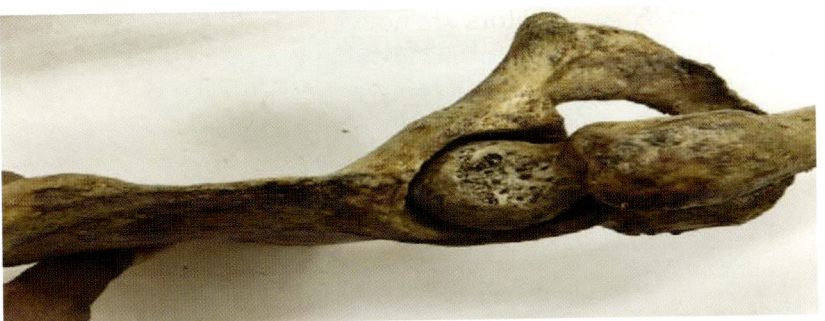

The surgeon levers out the head, as the assistant continues to slowly externally rotate the hip.

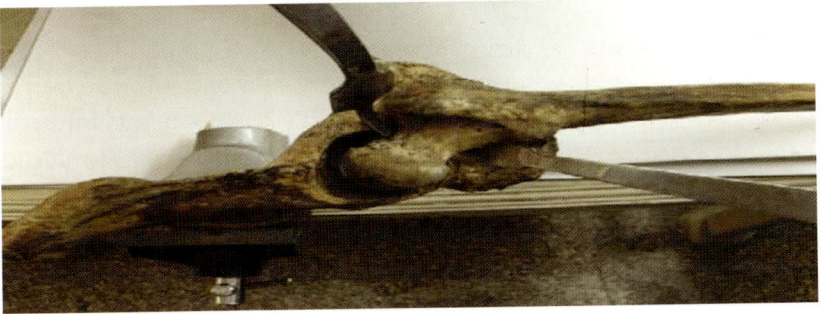

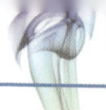

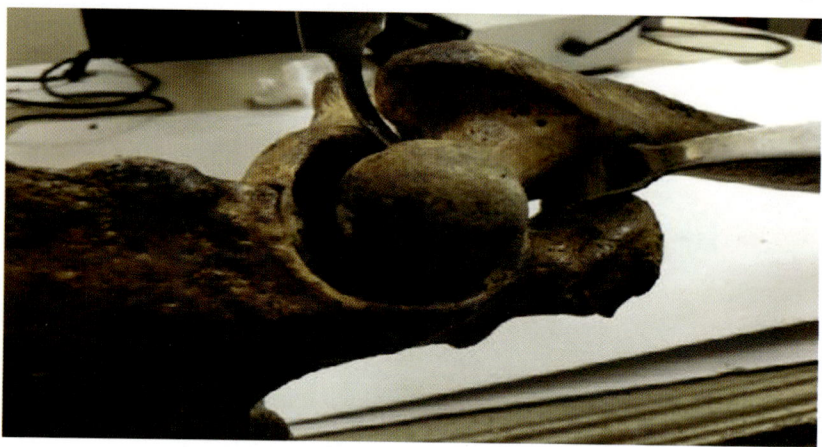

Additional soft tissue releases are done to facilitate an easy dislocation of the head. Hohmann retractors placed above and below the neck help this manoeuvre.

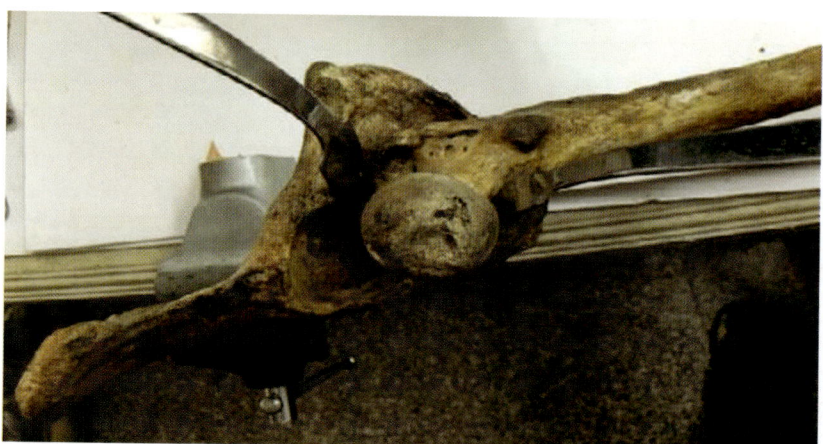

The assistant should not use excessive force during internal rotation, especially in patients with osteoporosis and rheumatoid arthritis, because there is a risk of spiral fracture of the shaft of femur.

As the limb is internally rotated, greater areas of the head become exposed.

Adduction and further internal rotation dislocates the hip joint.

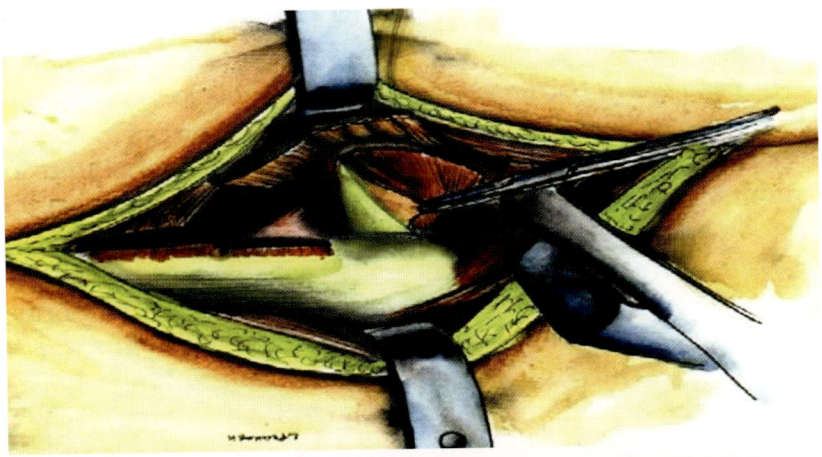

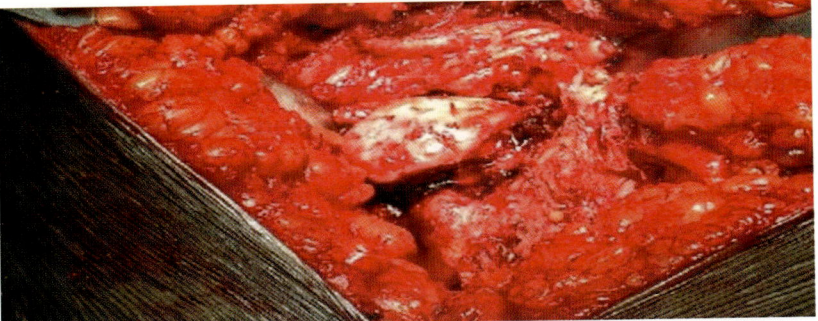

The dislocated head is now visualized completely.

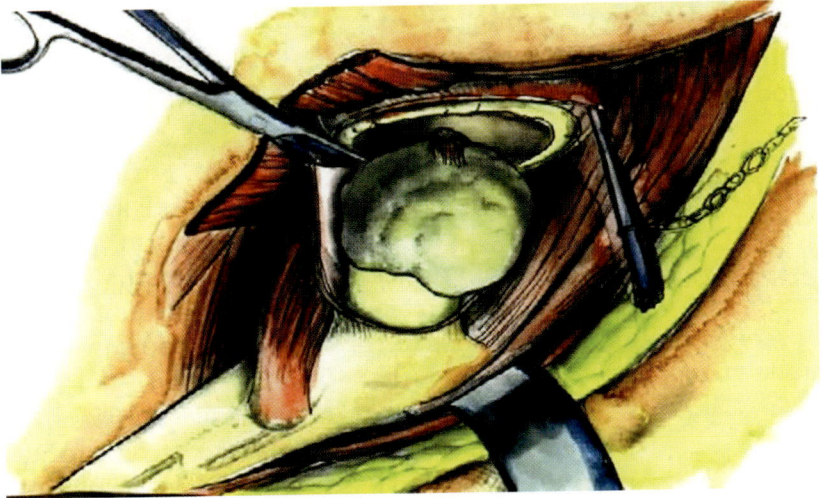

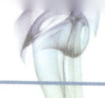

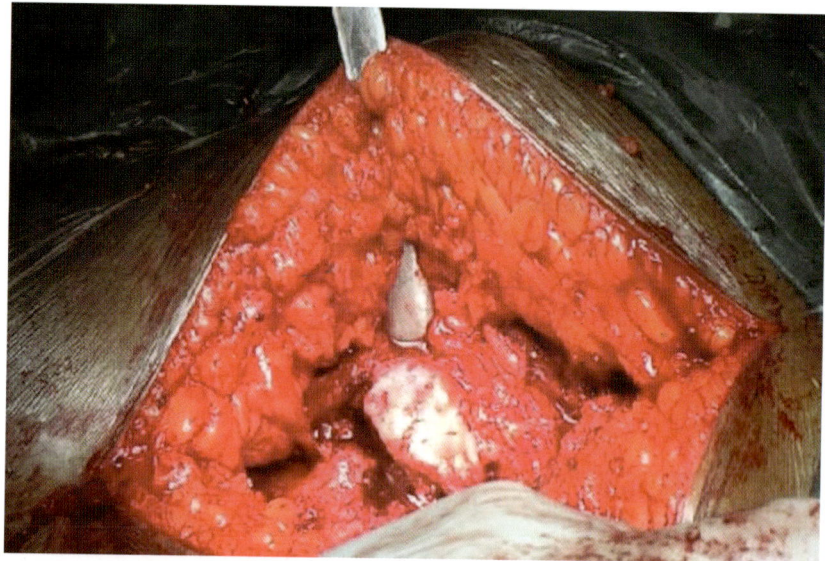

In this case, the head is completely deformed, and over-hanging osteophytes are hiding the neck.

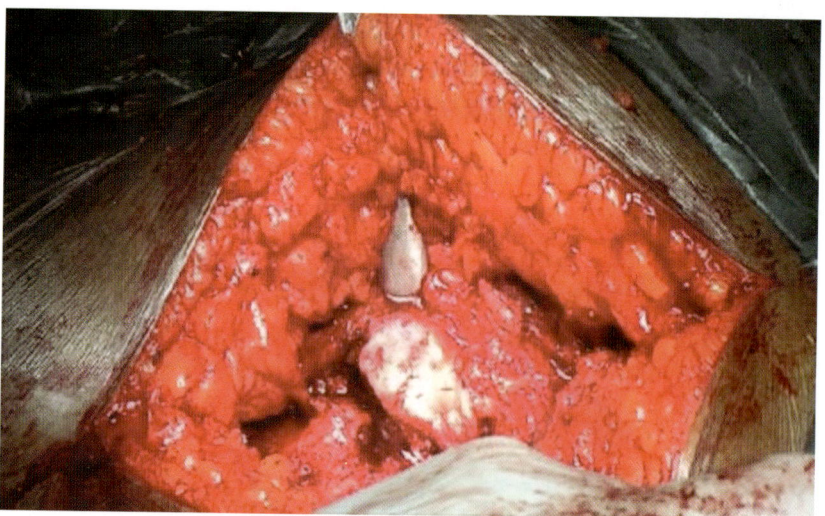

Appropriately placed Hohmann retractors will allow the head to be visualized in its entire extent.

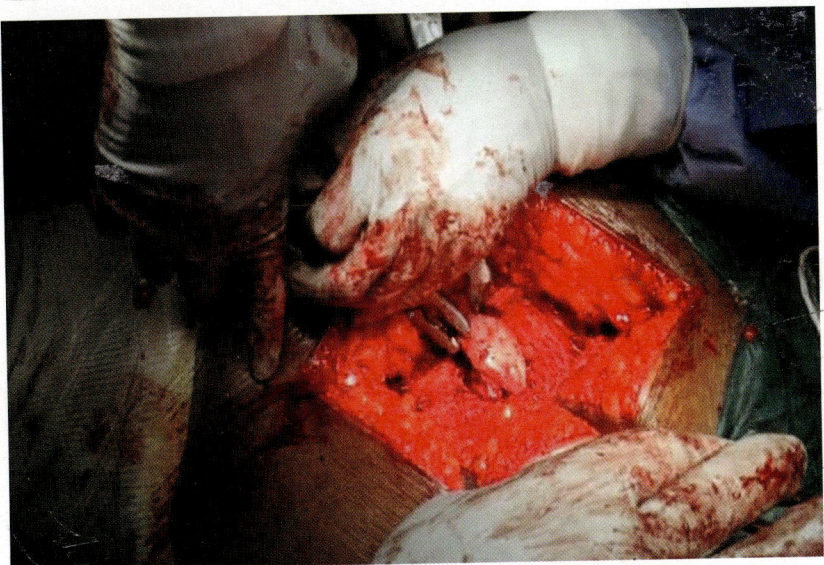

The overhanging osteophytes are nibbled to allow a proper visualization of the neck.

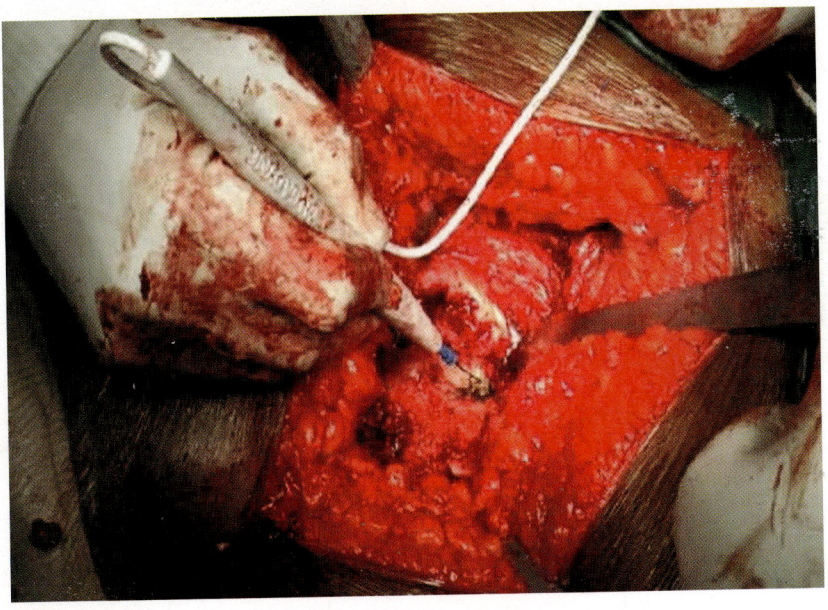

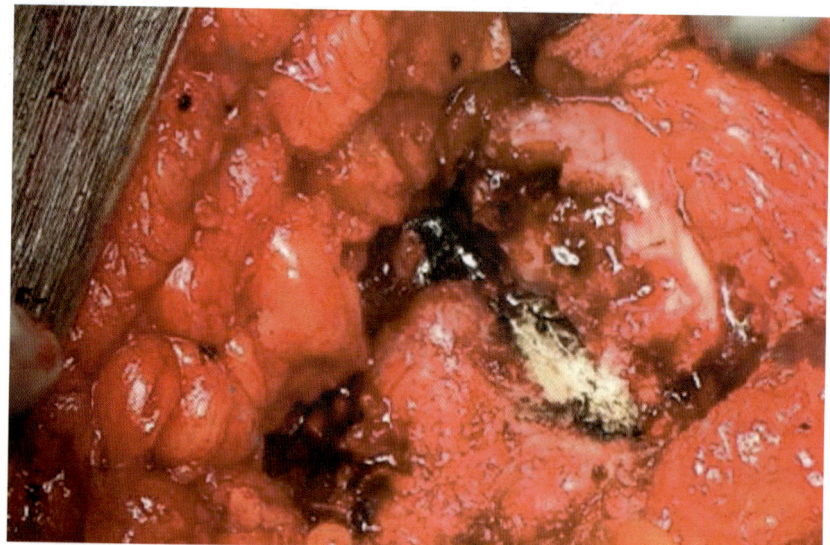

Using a cutting diathermy, the line of correct neck osteotomy is marked. Many companies provide templates for marking the correct cut angle.

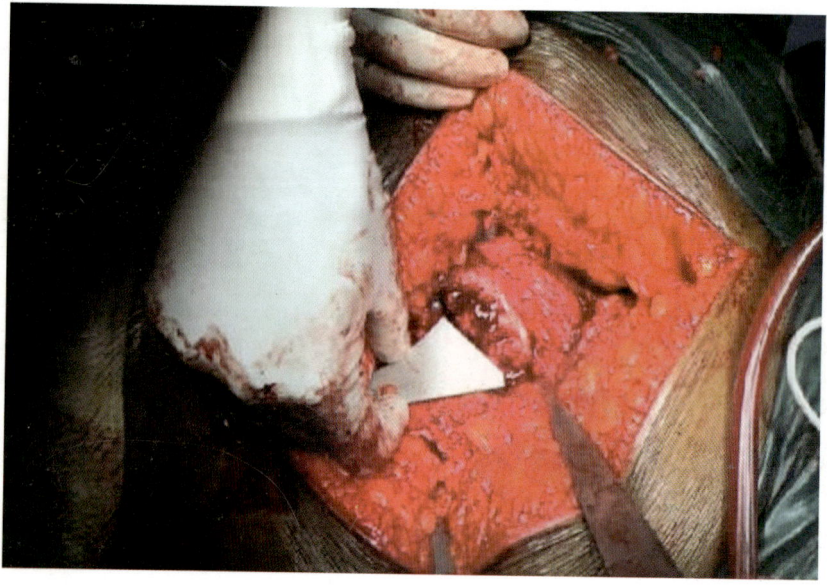

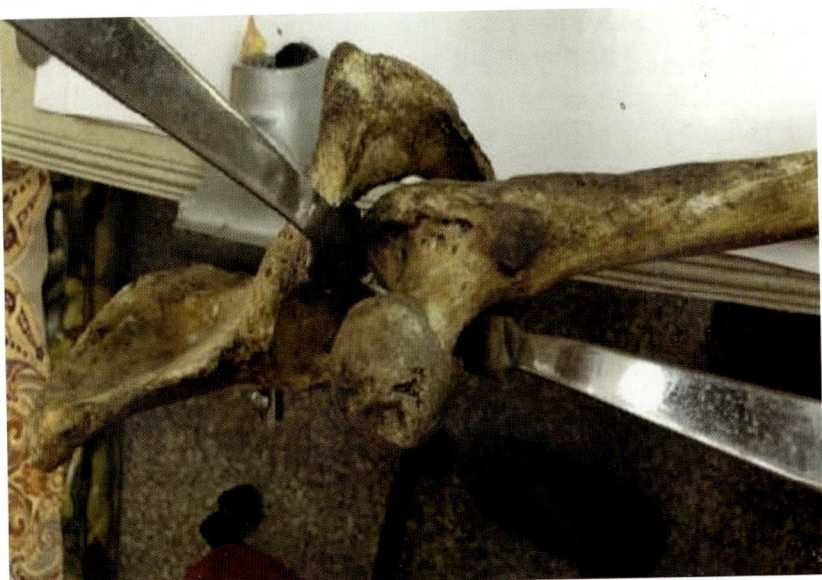

Some surgeons use a trial prosthesis aligned with the femoral shaft for marking the cut, instead of using a template.

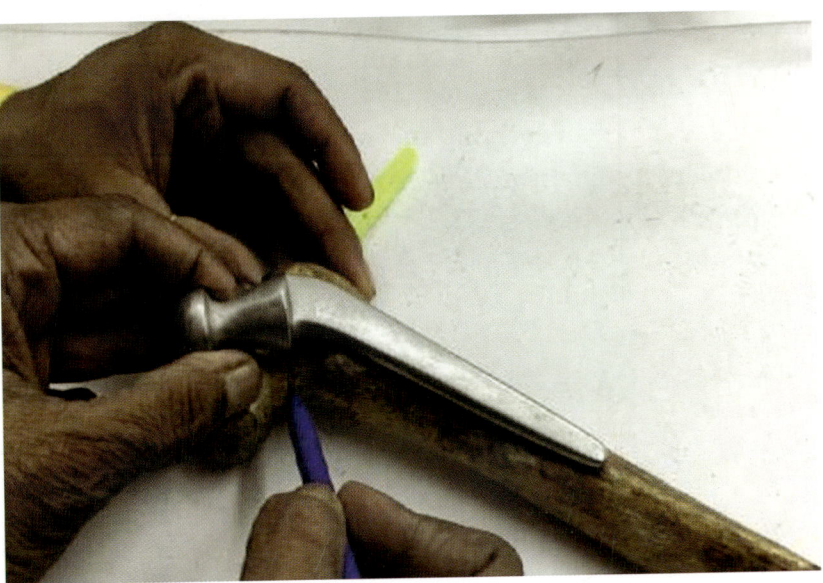

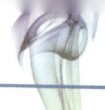

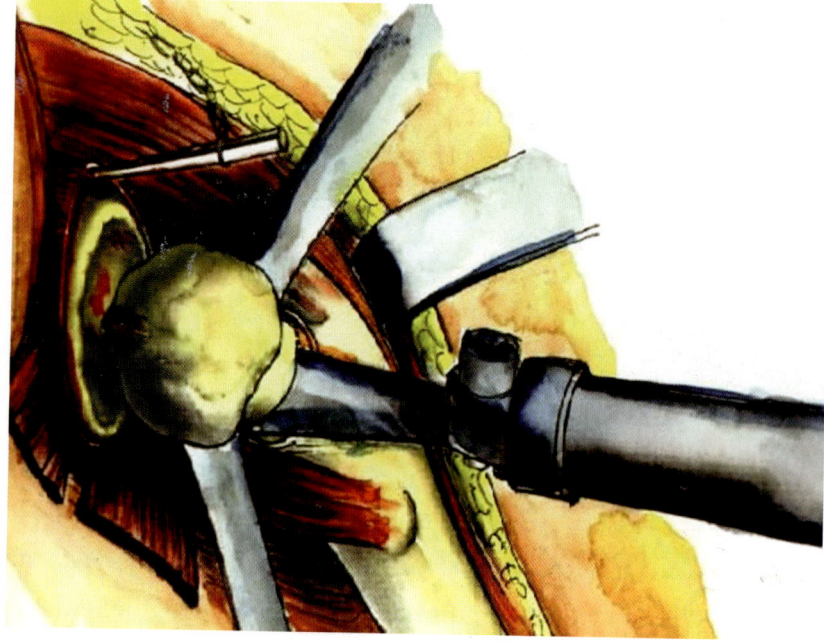

The inferior point of the cut should be 1 cm above the lesser trochanter, and go upwards at an angle of about 40° towards the greater trochanter.

As the version angle differs in different hips, it is best to follow the version angle of each hip during the procedure.

Hohmann retractors on either side of the neck will allow for support as the oscillating saw is used to cut the neck.

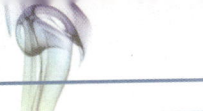
With a power saw, the neck is osteotomized at the correct angle.

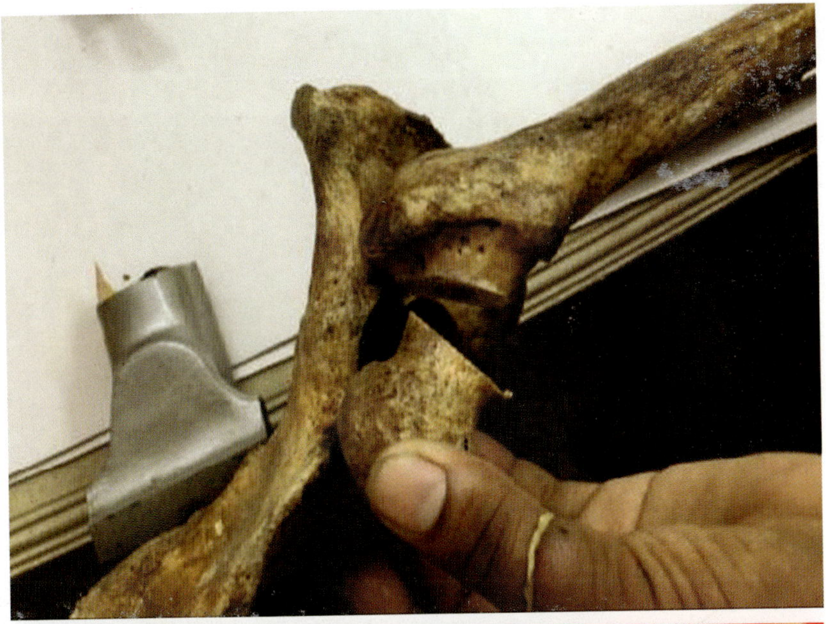

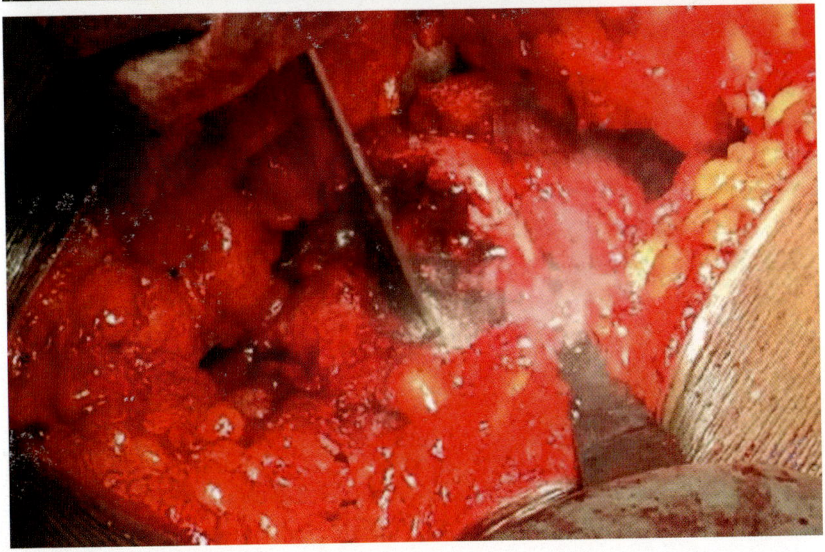

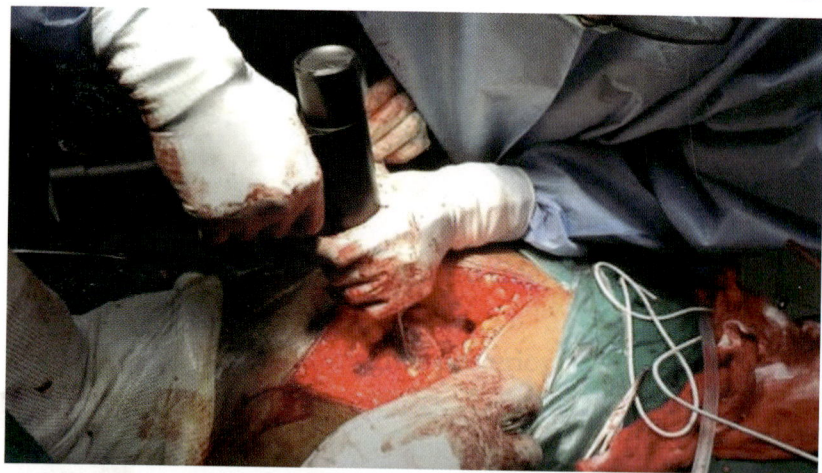

The head is now removed and measured. However, in such deformed heads, it is better to measure the acetabulum.

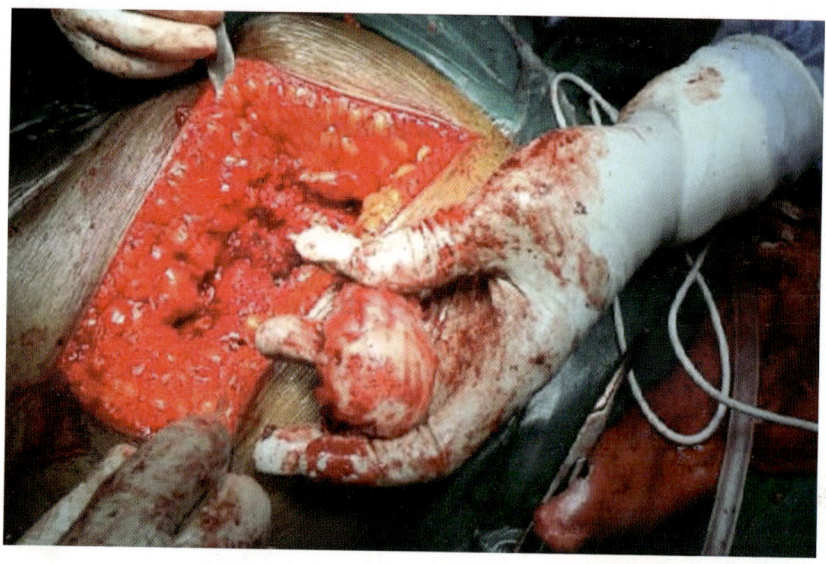

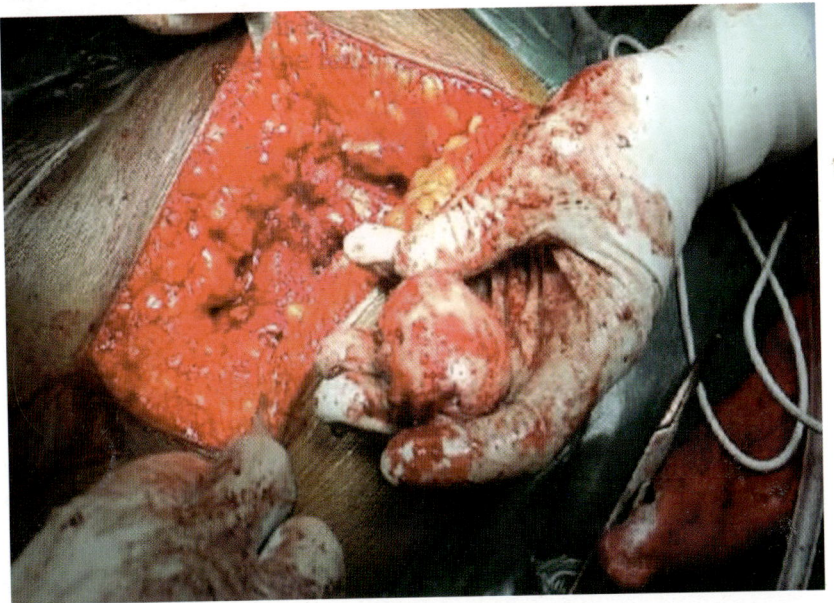

Examination of the deformities of the head tell us about the shape of the acetabulum and would guide the surgeon towards the correct areas to be reamed.

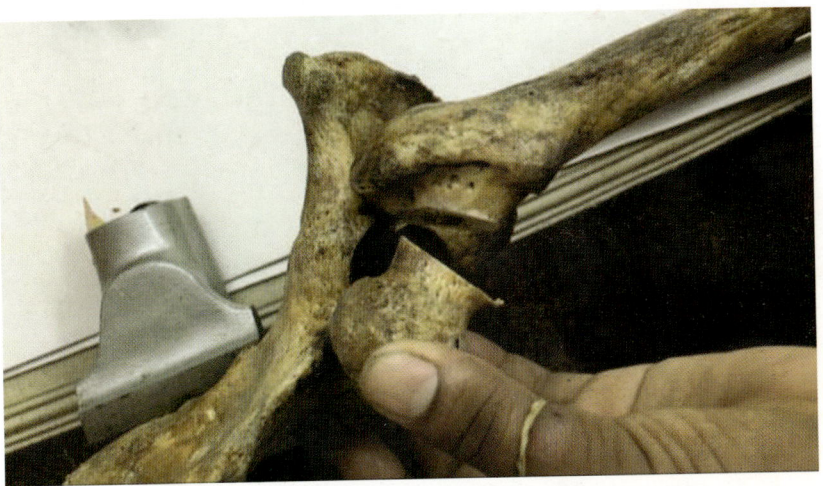

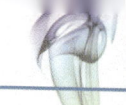

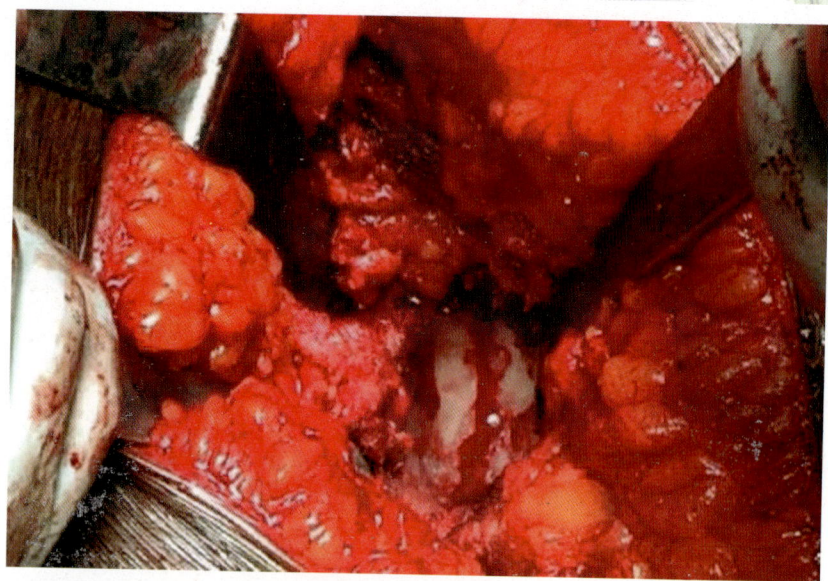

Judicious placement of Hohmann retractors will ensure that the femur is pushed out of the way and the acetabulum is visualized 360°.

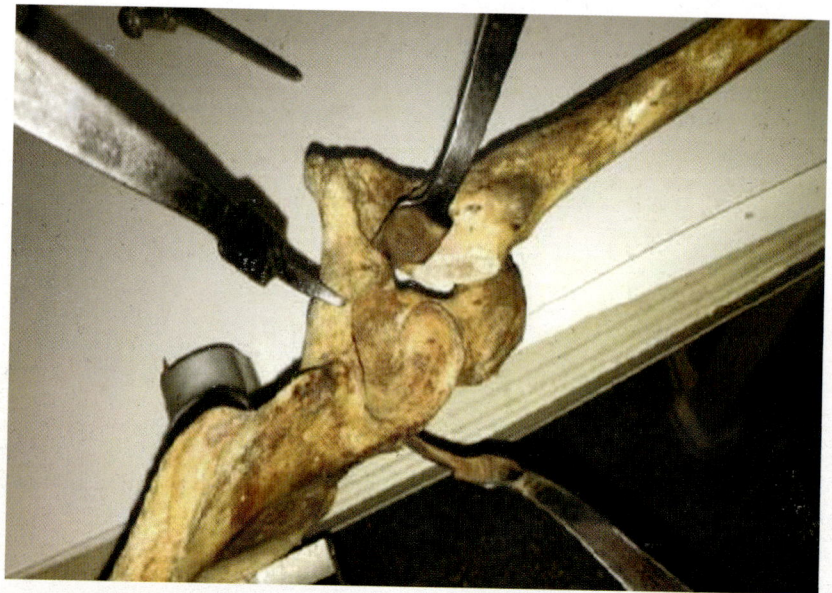

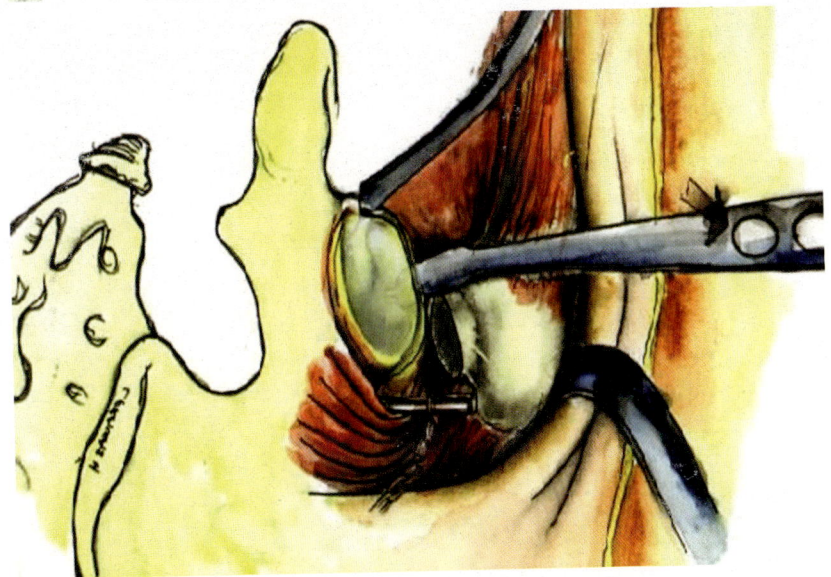

The acetabulum is inspected to evaluate its true extent and to distinguish between the true acetabulum and the false (with which subluxed heads usually articulate).

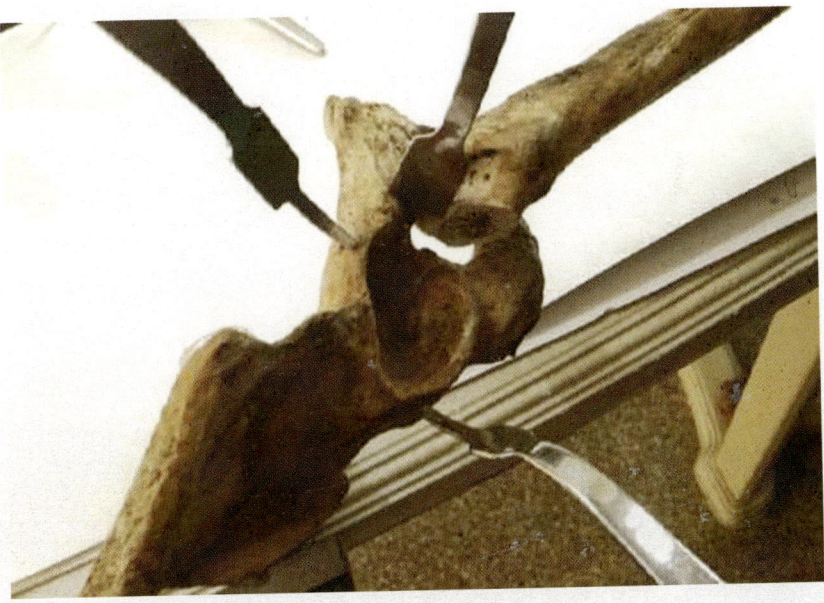

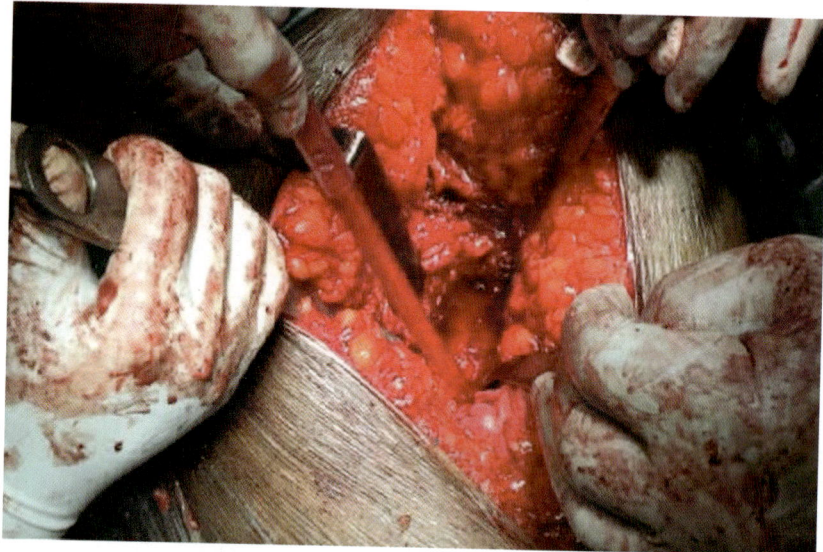

The hip capsule and surrounding soft tissue are now excised to allow the use of acetabular scraper spoons to scoop and clean the interior of the socket.

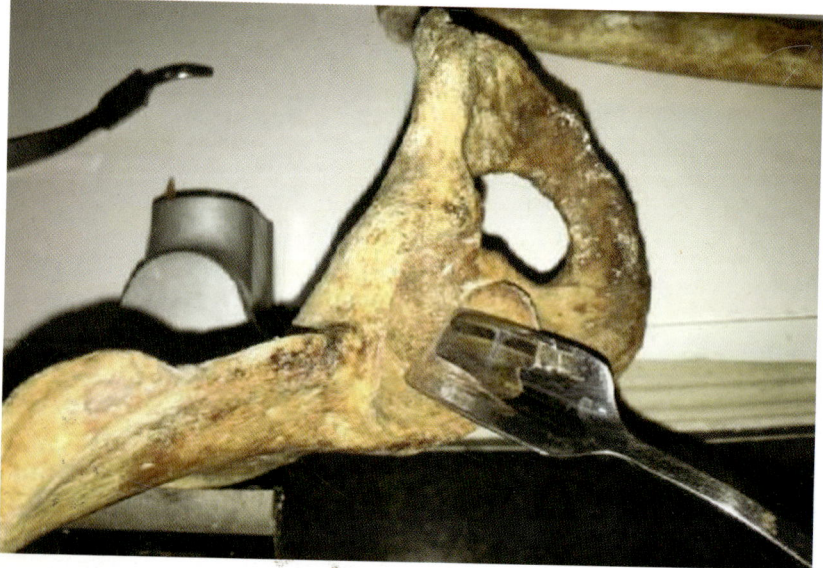

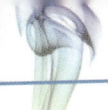

Medial Ludloff Approach

History

Karl Ludloff (1864–1945): *Karl Ludloff* studied in Jena, Würzburg, Munich, and Strassburg. He received his doctorate in Jena in 1894 and worked as assistant at the Physiological Institute in Königsberg, and the surgical clinics in Königsberg and Breslau. He began his surgical career in 1900, became the chief surgeon in 1906, and director of the University Clinic for Orthopaedic Surgery in Frankfurt, where he was appointed professor in 1919.

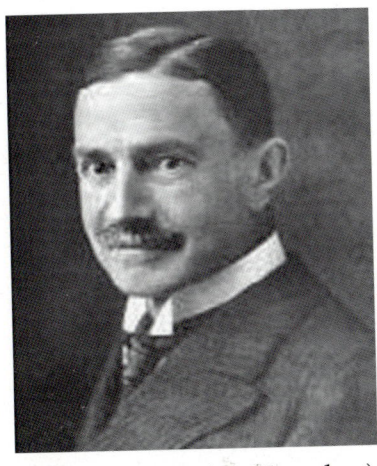

On February 10, 1916, The New York Times (via London) reported from the convention of the German Orthopaedic Society, then in session in Berlin. (At that time, the United States was still not at war with Germany.) The headline was "CUT NERVES UNITED IN LIFELESS LIMBS. False Hand Controlled by Upper Arm Muscles. Another German War Invention."

Obviously impressed by the achievements of the surgeons gathered in Berlin, The New York Times reported:

Dr Ferdinand Sauerbruch, Professor of Surgery at Zürich University, showed the delegates an artificial hand which was able to grasp objects of all forms and to lift weights up to 22 lb (10 kg). The hand and all the fingers are controlled by muscular action in the upper arm, which is prepared for such work by two operations. The muscular power afterward is transmitted to the hands through a system of wires and pulleys.

Dr Karl Ludloff, Professor of Surgery at Breslau University, described a method for uniting severed nerves and receiving the muscular action of nerveless limbs. He pointed out that the natural tendency of severed ends of nerves to reunite was hindered by the fact that the cicatrized new flesh between them was impervious to growing nerve fibres.

Professor Ludloff said he restored the connection by a piece of an artery of an ox filled with gelatine, through which nerves readily grew, even bridging gaps of several inches. After several

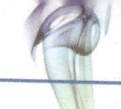

weeks, crippled limbs regained their motor activity. The Professor said that many cases had been successfully treated where permanent lameness would have followed.

Dr Karl Ludloff was a brilliant scientist, innovator, engineer, designer of instrumentation, and also an imaginative surgeon who invented many techniques. He first described the adductor approach in 1908. His classical publication in 1939 in The American Journal of Orthopaedic Surgery on his medial incision is a classic that needs to be read in its original form to be appreciated.

It is indeed unfortunate that I couldn't find a picture of this great man, so his description alone will have to do!!

Access
- Medial hip capsule
- Lesser trochanter
- Medial and inferior acetabular border.

Dislocation
Anterior

Position
- Supine
- Leg draped free
- Hip is abducted and externally rotated to make adductors taut.
- Perineum is well prepared. Scrotum is taped back in a male.

Plane
Between adductor longus and brevis straight to hip joint. Division of iliopsoas facilitates exposure.

Incision
From pubic tubercle downwards over adductor longus for about 10 to 12.5 cm.

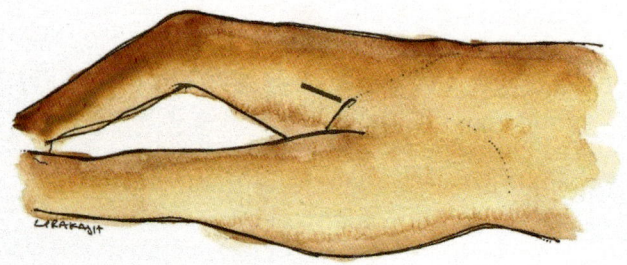

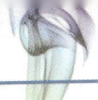

Dissections

- Deep fascia is incised over adductor longus.
- This muscle is detached from its insertion, if tight.
- The plane between adductor longus and brevis is developed.
- The obturator nerve is identified and protected. It lies in front of adductor brevis.
- Flexion, abduction, external rotation of the hip, by keeping the heel on the opposite knee will stretch the capsule for incision or excision.

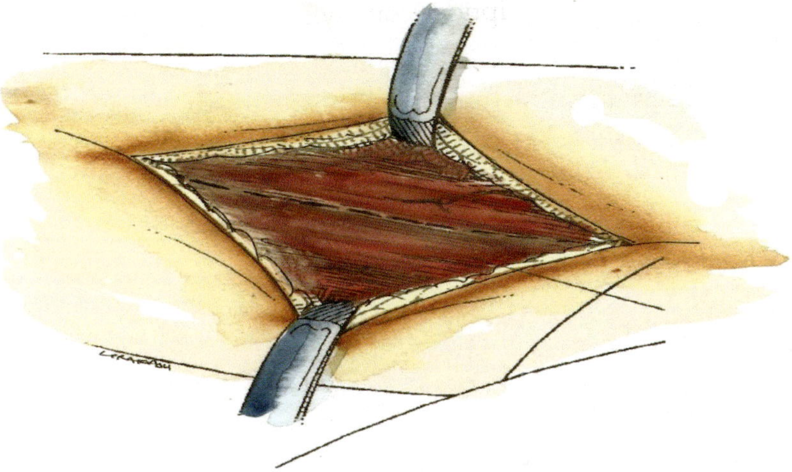

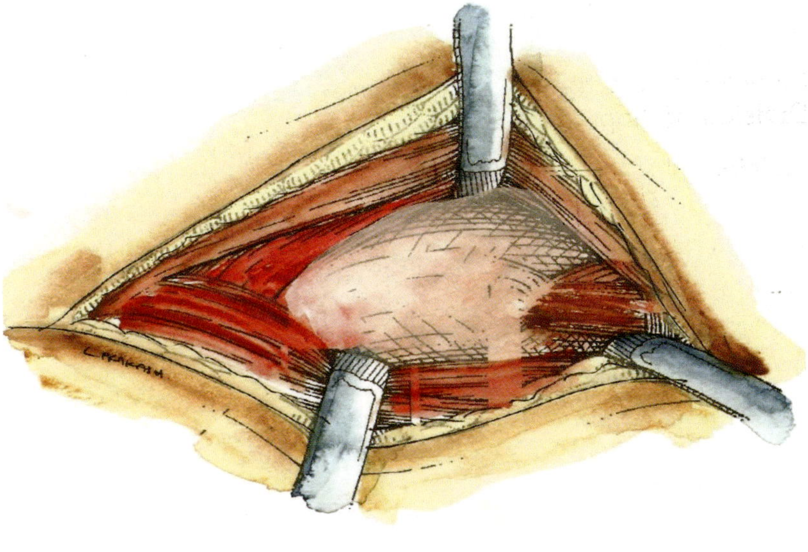

Indications
- Approach of lesser trochanter, e.g. osteoid osteoma.
- Hip exposures accompanied with psoas tenotomies and adductor releases.
- Pathology to inferior acetabulum.

Advantages
- Short bloodless exposure
- Direct access to lesser trochanter
- Early quick postoperative recovery

Disadvantages
- Extremely limited exposure to medial hip joint.
- Being close to perineum, the area is relatively unclean.
- Unsuitable for CDH due to limited blood supply. In addition, anteromedial dislocation places the head at risk of avascular necrosis.

3

The Femur

I call the femur a shy and covered bone, as opposed to the proud and subcutaneous tibia. The almost straight bone is covered by muscles all around, giving multiple planes of access and exposure. The following structures need familiarity in their topographical and locational identification, to protect them during surgery.

- The long saphenous vein
- The sciatic nerve
- Posterior cutaneous nerve of the thigh
- Femoral neurovascular bundle

The femur is encircled by flexors anteriorly, extensors posteriorly, adductors medially and abductors laterally. The femoral neurovascular bundle is anteromedial, while the sciatic nerve is posterolateral.

The femur can be approached from all four directions and also in between. The following pictures show the anatomy and the various important structures.

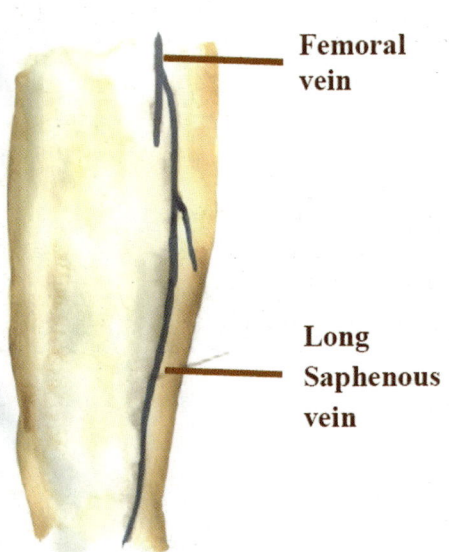

Femoral vein

Long Saphenous vein

Entering the thigh from the posterior aspect of medial condyle, the long saphenous vein travels medially upwards, becoming thicker as more tributaries join it.

At the saphenous hiatus in the upper third of the thigh, it empties into the femoral vein after perforating the femoral sheath.

The vein is susceptible for injury in medial approaches.

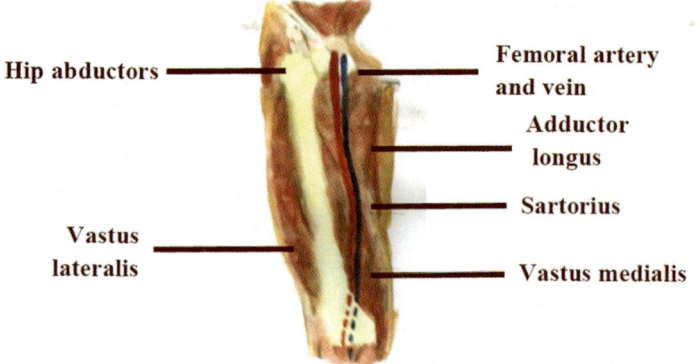

Hip abductors

Femoral artery and vein

Adductor longus

Sartorius

Vastus lateralis

Vastus medialis

The femoral artery emerges from the femoral triangle, travels in the subsartorial canal medial and posterior to femoral shaft; at the junction of proximal two-thirds and the distal third, it enters the adductor hiatus and becomes the popliteal artery.

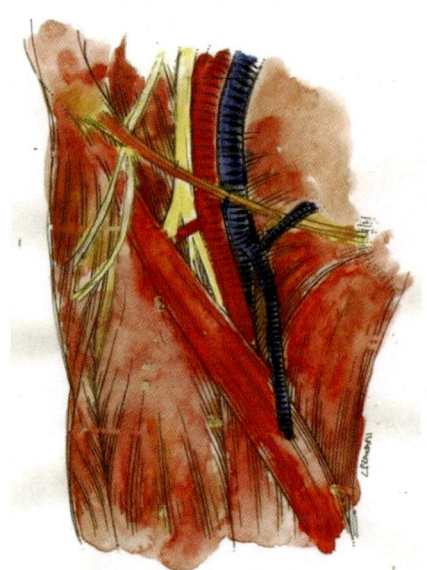

The femoral neurovascular structures are susceptible to injuries in proximal and medial exposures of femur.

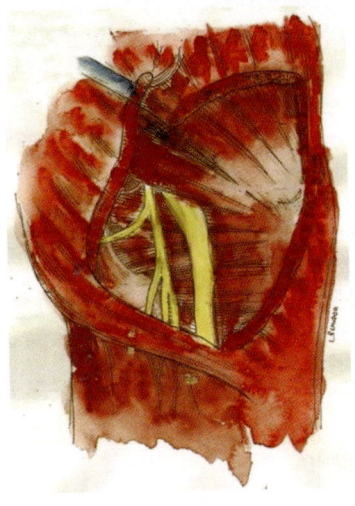

The sciatic nerve exits the pelvis through the greater sciatic notch, then travels over the short lateral rotators and leaves the gluteal area at the lower border of quadratus femoris. Above this, it is covered by gluteus maximus. This part is exposed during hip approaches.

Thereafter, it moves close to the posterior border of the femur.

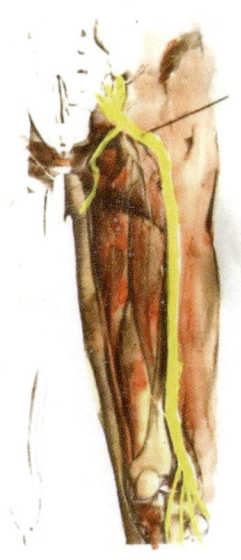

It passes under the cover of hamstrings, and then beneath the long head of biceps. Here the fibres clump into popliteal and tibial divisions. Biceps, semitendenosus, semimembranosus, and adductor magnus are supplied by tibial half, while those to short head of biceps from peroneal part. It divides into the tibial and peroneal branches on reaching the popliteal fossa.

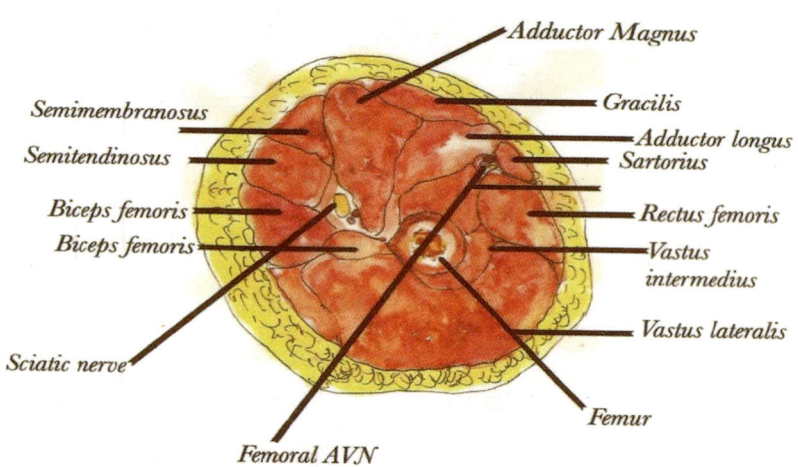

As seen in the cross-sectional drawing of the upper femur above, the sciatic nerve is posterior while femoral neurovascular bundle is anteromedial. The lateral corridor is reasonably safe, and allows a direct approach to the bone without many vital structures on the way.

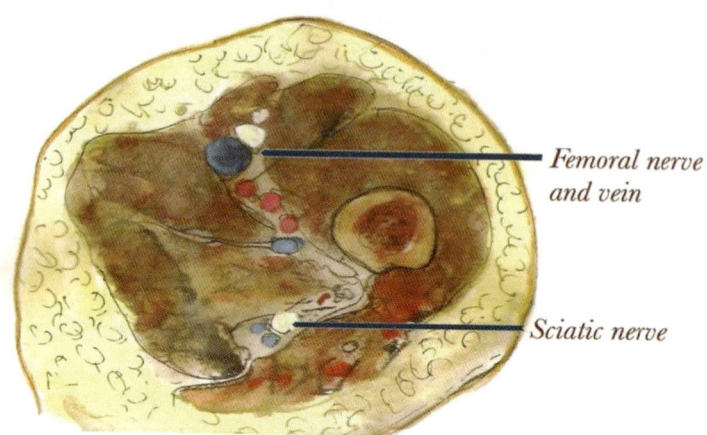

Section anatomy of upper femur

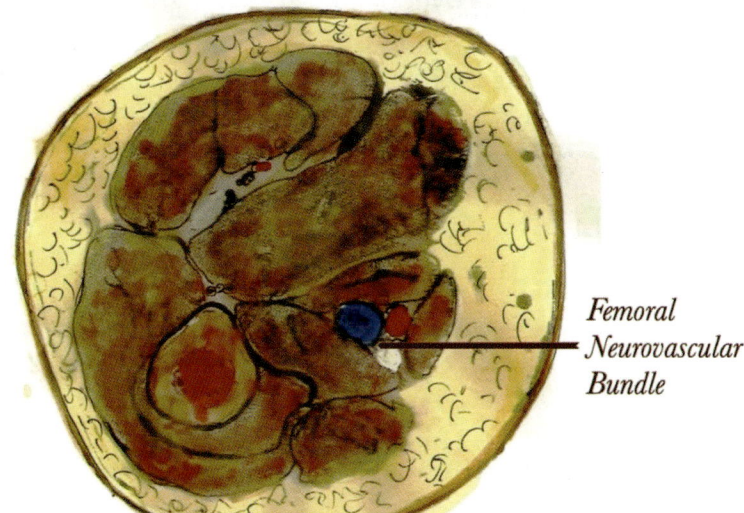

Femoral
Neurovascular
Bundle

Sectional anatomy of mid-femur

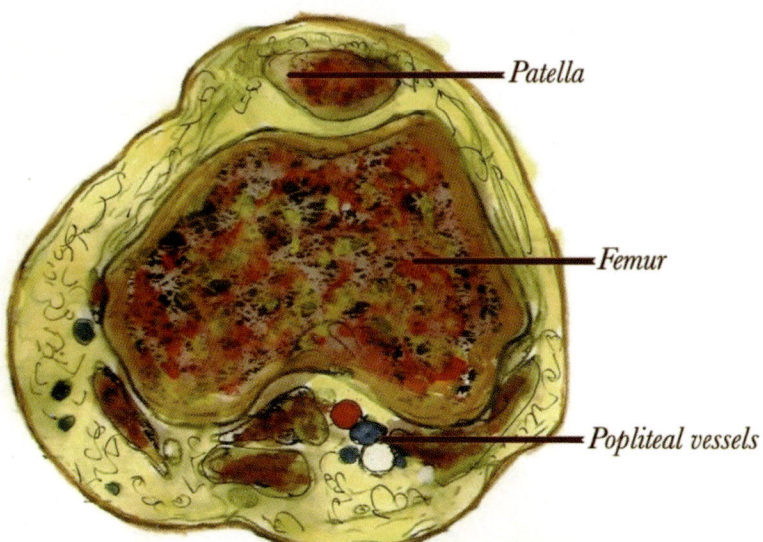

Patella

Femur

Popliteal vessels

Sectional anatomy of distal femur

From the tip of the greater trochanter, right down to the lateral border of lateral condyle, the femur is under non-vulnerable structures, without any major blood vessels or nerves. Lateral approach is the preferred one for most traumatic cases, especially in the middle third.

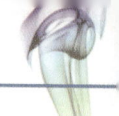

The femur can also be approached at various levels, anteriorly, medially or posterior, should the pathology dictate approach from that particular area.

History of Femoral Exposures

The history of femoral approaches and exposures is the history of surgery itself. The methods for approaching a fracture of femur from its lateral aspect and treatment of compound femoral fractures have been described in **Sushruta Samhita**, an ancient Sanskrit text. However, the history of modern surgical exposures to the femur can be firmly placed on the shoulders of four pillars: Professor **Arnold K. Henry** of Dublin, Ireland; **Gerhard Küntscher** of Germany; **Robert Danis** of Belgium; and the AO group of Switzerland founded by **Muller, Willeneggar,** and **Algower.**

Acharya Sushruta (around 600 BC) was a genius who has been glowingly recognized in the annals of medical science. Born to sage Vishwamitra and a disciple of sage **Atreya, Sushruta** practised around 600 BC, nearly 150 years before Hippocrates. East of the river Ganga was the city of Varanasi, where sage Sushruta headed the surgical department. Having learned anatomy from sage Atreya, Sushruta has documented in detail the first-ever surgical procedures ever written in his treatise *Sushruta Samhita*.

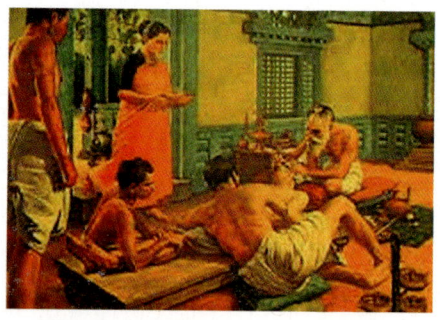

Sushruta Samhita, a unique encyclopaedia of surgery, indicates that he was probably the first surgeon to perform a rhinoplasty and earlobe reconstruction. In the same book, he prescribes treatment for 12 types of fractures and 6 types of dislocations.

His details on human embryology are simply amazing. Sushruta used 125 types of surgical instruments, including scalpels, lancets, needles, catheters and rectal speculums. He has also described a number of stitching methods, including the use of horse hair and fibres of bark as thread; he even details 300 types of operations. The beautiful oil painting by Raja Ravi Verma reproduced above is the most popular representation of this great surgeon performing an earlobe repair with horse hair. I have credited him with the first descriptions of femoral exposures; errors, if any, are entirely mine.

Professor AK Henry (1886–1962):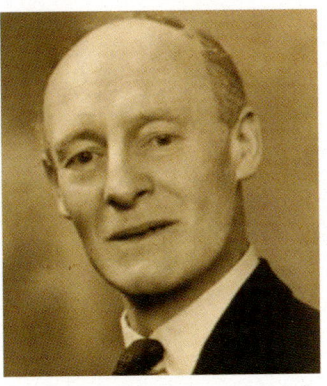
Professor Arnold K. Henry graduated from Trinity College in 1911 and obtained his fellowship of the Royal College of Surgeons in Ireland (RCSI) in 1914. In the First World War, he served as a surgeon in both the Serbian and French armies and was decorated by both. He was accompanied by his wife, Dr. Dorothy Milne Henry, a close collaborator and assistant.

Subsequent to this, he worked as a surgeon in Dublin, then as Professor of Surgery at the University of Cairo and at the Postgraduate Medical School at Hammersmith. In 1947, he returned to Dublin as Professor of Anatomy at the RCSI. Professor Henry was a trendsetter in many respects. At the time of his appointment to the college, he was a retired surgeon and not a "pure"anatomist. Consequently he was never at ease with the classroom, and swiftly abandoned this for teaching on the cadaver. His lectures were always very practical, demonstrating for example that the strap muscles of the neck were a barrier to surgical "damage". He also demonstrated in the cadaver that pulmonary emboli could be removed surgically, a technique that was long before its time.

His classic "Extensile Exposure Applied to Limb Surgery" is an absolutely amazing book and even today one cannot put it down, if he or she begins to read it.

I am copying below the first paragraph of his wonderful book and the wordplay speaks of his genius:

If, as one keeps on hearing, the sort of anatomy untastefully called 'gross' were really finished, this re-edition would count only as a further impertinence. But while its predecessor was received with unexpected kindliness, the not-intolerant climate held just the echo of a salutary

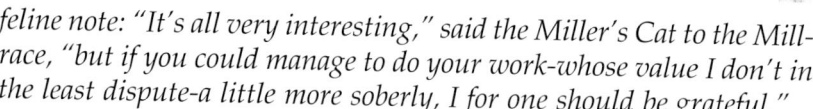

feline note: "It's all very interesting," said the Miller's Cat to the Mill-race, "but if you could manage to do your work-whose value I don't in the least dispute-a little more soberly, I for one should be grateful."

Meanwhile, however, Time, which finds ways of settling sobriety's *worse disorders, has not been idle. The present progress in surgery is so rapid that one year now is like a former hundred, and ten can leave us not outstripped but at the post. Even simple straight incisions have been altered, and I am most grateful for the chance of taking my impressions of their modern trends from a variety of patients, with scars long-healed and admirable, put at my disposal by the courtesy of Mr JC Sugars of the Adelaide Hospital, Dublin.*

He gets the undoubted credit for describing all exposures of femur together in one place and has detailed the anterior, anterio-lateral, and lateral approaches in detail.

Gerhard Küntscher (1900–1972): Gerhard Küntscher was born December 6, 1900 in Zwickau, Saxons, the son of a factory director. He studied medicine and the natural sciences at the universities of Würtzberg, Hamburg and Jena.

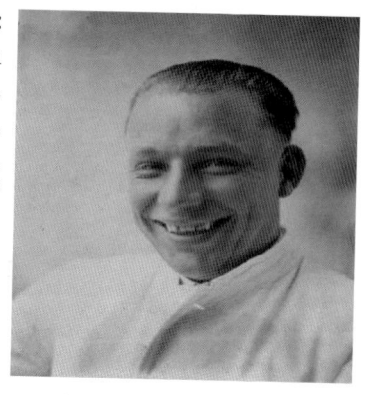

During World War II, Küntscher served as a surgeon on the Eastern Front; in 1946, he took charge of the surgical division of Kreis Hospital, Schleswig-Hesterberg. From 1957 until his statutory retirement in 1965, he was medical director of Hafen Hospital in Hamburg. After retirement, he established a centre for nailing in Spain in 1966, and became a visiting physician at St. Franziskus Hospital, Flensburg, where he continued to work until his death.

At the 64th meeting of the German Surgical Society in 1940, he attracted a great attention with his report "Medullary Nailing of Fractures", which was an important milestone in the operative treatment of fractures. From then on, the name Küntscher was associated with this specific surgical technique. The Küntscher nail must be included among the most ingenious inventions that German surgery brought forth in the last decades.

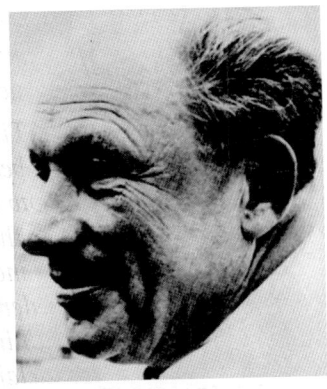

His revolutionary methods initially met with skepticism, but he was so convinced of his principles that he was soon able to persuade the German army to adopt his methods for treating war wounded soldiers. To the great amazement of the enemy armies, German soldiers nailed for fractures returned to the war front in 2 months as opposed to the British who needed 18 to 24 months!

His life was spent on intensive scientific investigations, animal experiments, and technical improvements of the instrumentation for closed medullary nailing. He was able to perform animal research outside the university only through considerable personal sacrifice. He managed to obtain the apparatus he needed through his friendly relationship with the Pohl Company.

An ingenious medical investigator, an exceptional surgeon, and an exemplary physician, he was also an outstanding draftsman, engineer, and physicist. On December 17, 1972, Professor Gerhard Küntscher died suddenly at his home in Glücksburg, West Germany. Death overtook him at his desk, as he worked on the completion of the manuscript of the new edition of his book "Practice of Medullary Nailing".

Another contemporary of Henry and Küntscher, Danis was the eldest son of a military veterinarian. He studied medicine at the Université libre de Bruxelles and started his surgical training after graduating in 1904 from Antoine Depage.

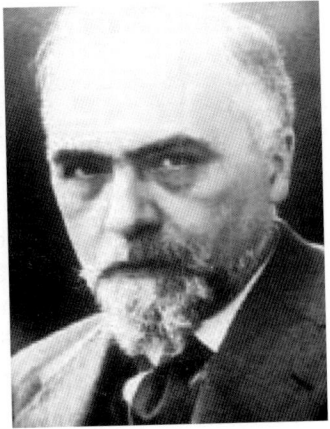

Initially interested in thoracic surgery, he designed a new significantly simpler and lighter apparatus for positive pressure ventilation at open lung surgery. He developed methods of regional anaesthesia, especially the lumbar and sacral nerve roots. He also developed regional anaesthesia in the face and numbing the ganglion through the mouth in order to perform surgery on the face and the eye. With his countryman Albin Lambotte, the Austrian Lorenz Böhler and the German Gerhard Küntscher, Danis was among the pioneers of Traumatology, by the AO Foundation are seen as role models.

One of the role models who was closely followed by Maurice Muller, Depage's approaches to limbs form the basis of the AO manual of limb exposures for trauma.

THE APPROACHES TO FEMUR

As described below, the anteromedial and posterior areas have vessels and nerves. Rest of the femur is easily approachable through safe corridors. The following are the commonly used approaches.

- Anterolateral
- Lateral
- Posterolateral
- Posterior
- Femur in medial popliteal area
- Femur in lateral popliteal area

Anterolateral Approach to Shaft of Femur

Access: This approach gives access to the anterior four-fifths of the femoral shaft.

Position: Supine with a sandbag under the buttock.

Incision: A straight line from the ASIS to the lateral patellar border.

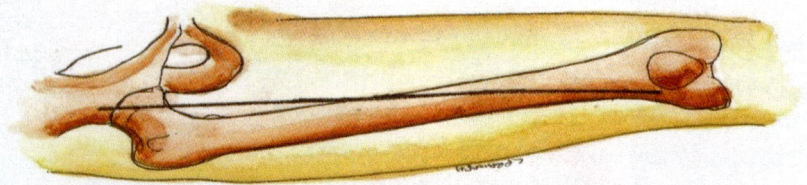

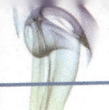

Plane: Between rectus femoris and vastus lateralis.

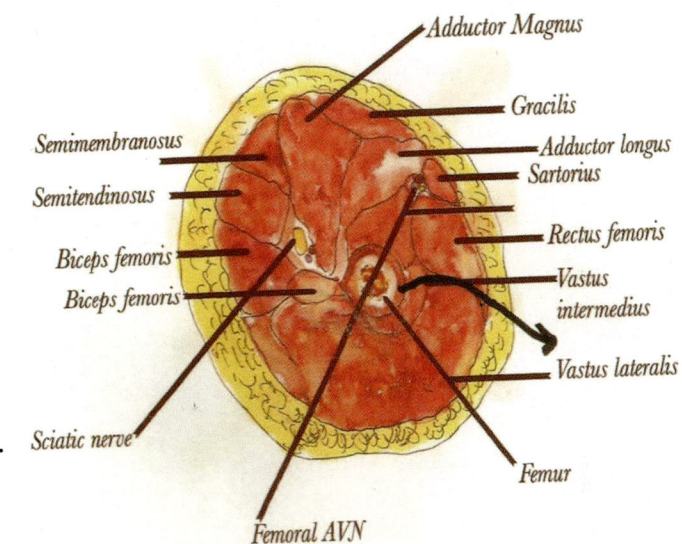

Adductor Magnus

Semimembranosus

Semitendinosus

Biceps femoris

Biceps femoris

Sciatic nerve

Gracilis

Adductor longus

Sartorius

Rectus femoris

Vastus intermedius

Vastus lateralis

Femur

Femoral AVN

Exposure: Beneath the skin and subcutaneous fat, the deep fascia is split in the direction of the shin incision to display the belly of rectus femoris and vastus lateralis. The two are separated from distal to proximal, and retracted to either side. Underneath we find the vastus inter-medius, which can be split in the direction of the incision to reach the femur directly.

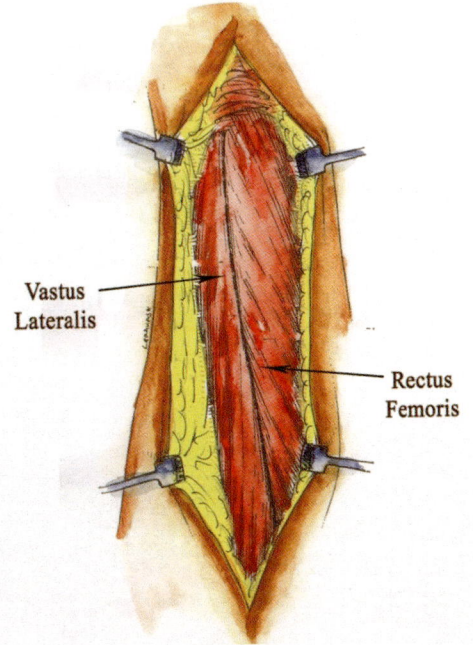

Vastus Lateralis

Rectus Femoris

In the upper part of the incision is the most impor-tant structure—the neuro-vascular leash to vastus lateralis—containing lateral femoral circumflex artery and nerve. This is to be protected at all costs and has to be identified, separated and retracted out of the way. The pressure on the retractors have to be periodically released to avoid neurological problems.

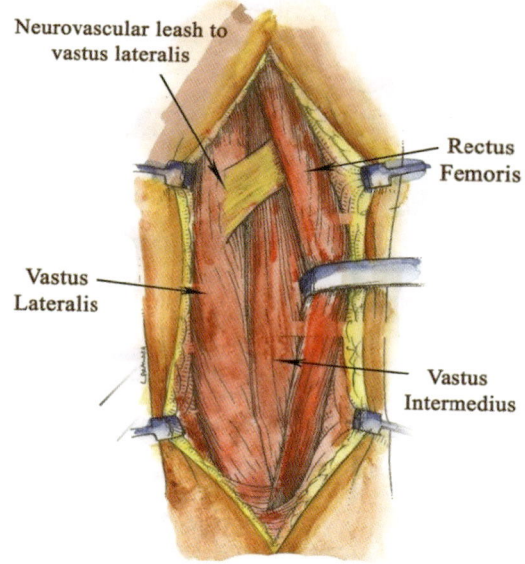

The periosteum is split in a linear fashion and the lower 80% of the femoral shaft is laid bare.

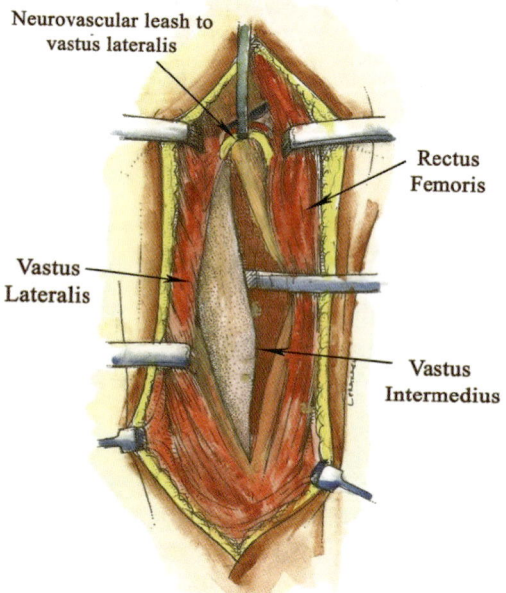

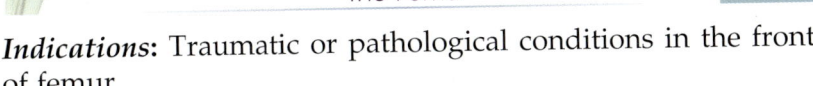

Indications: Traumatic or pathological conditions in the front of femur.

Advantages: Though it is an anterior approach, once the bone is reached, it can be identified and stripped almost circumferentially except for the most proximal parts.

Disadvantages: This is a transquadriceps approach and hence there is a real possibility of quadriceps fibrosis and adhesions producing flexion deficit.

The lateral circumflex femoral nerve and the artery to the vastus lateralis are at risk of damage in the proximal part of the incision.

The Lateral Approach to Femur

Access: This approach gives a complete exposure to the lateral and anterior aspects of femur, from the greater trochanter above to the lateral femoral condyle below.

Originally described by Henry, this incision can be extended proximaly to expose the hip and distally to expose the lateral aspect of the knee. This would thus be an extensile approach to femoral shaft.

Position: Lateral decubitus position with stands, clamps and sandbags to maintain a dead lateral position. The hip is draped up to the inguinal region and knee draped free to expose the area from buttock to knee. The knee is sometimes put under traction, either with an upper tibial or lower femoral skeletal pin traction.

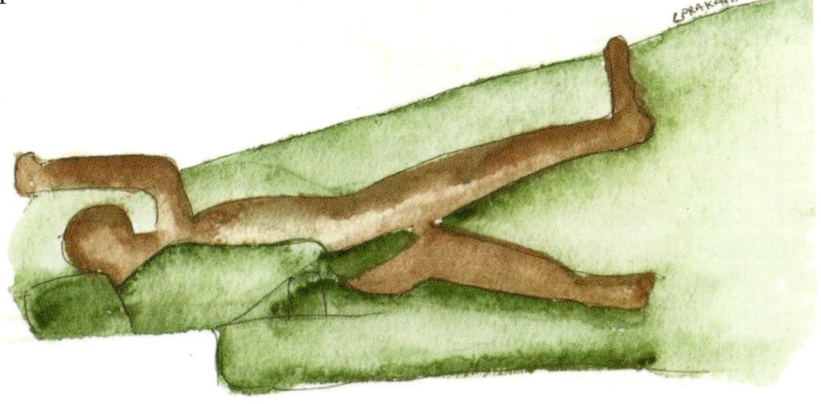

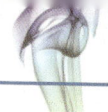

A distal femoral pin traction on an Ilizarov half ring or a Bohler's stirrup will allow traction to be applied when needed.

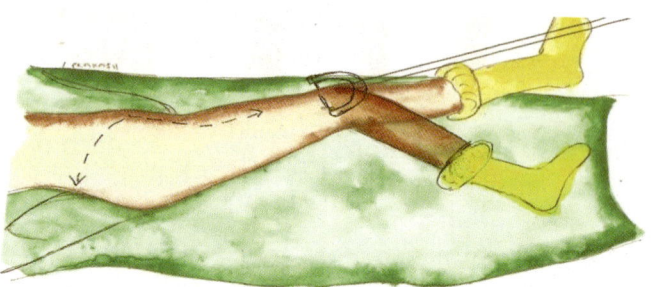

Plane: Transvastus approach. The fibres of vastus lateralis and vastus intermedius are split in the line of their fibres, and retracted on either side to expose the femur.

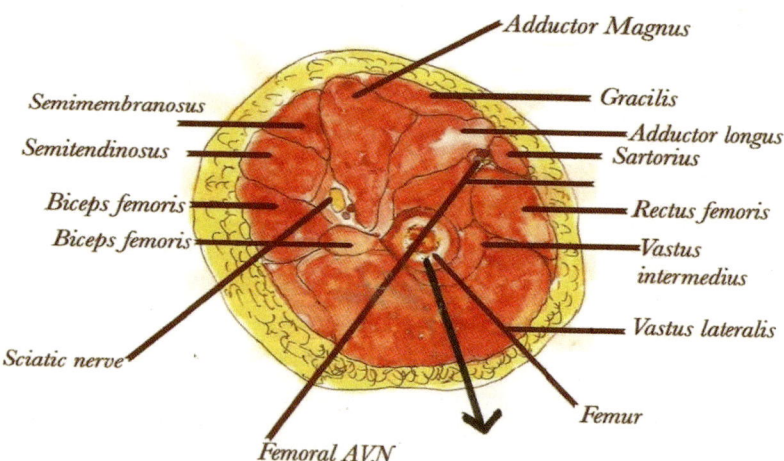

Incision: The line of incision is straight from the tip of the trochanter to the lateral epiconddyle of femur.

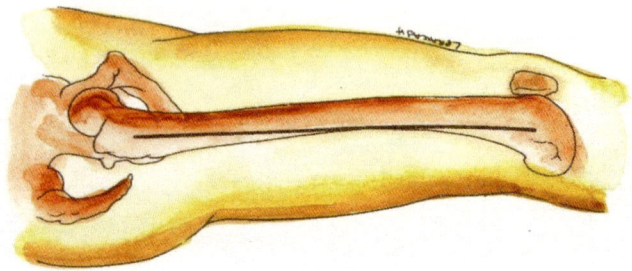

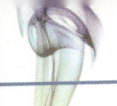

The length of the incision is dependant on the area of pathology and the requirements of exposure.

Dissections: Skin, subcutaneous fat and superficial fascia are incised in a straight line, to expose the glistening whitish tensor fascia lata underneath.

This is nicked in the line of the skin incision and cut both upwards and downwards. The important point is to ensure that the tensor fascia lata is cut along its anterior border.

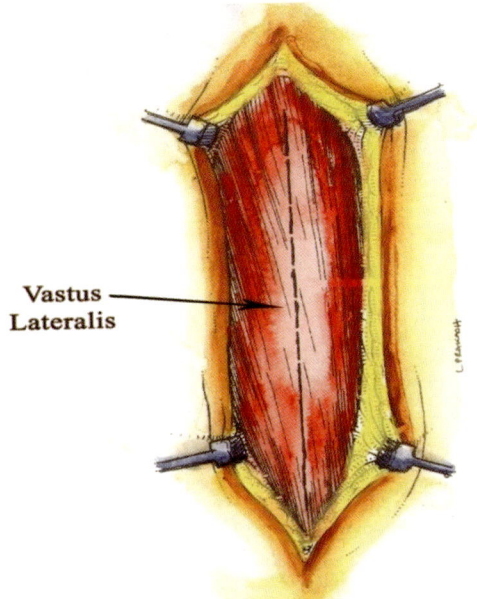

Vastus Lateralis

This now exposes the belly of the vastus lateralis throughout the length of the incision and it can be followed posteriorly along the intermuscular septum to the posterior border of femur.

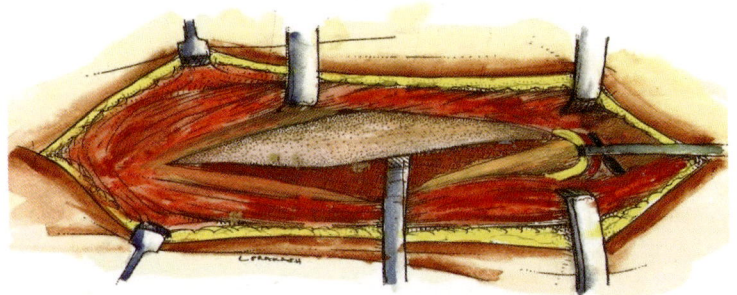

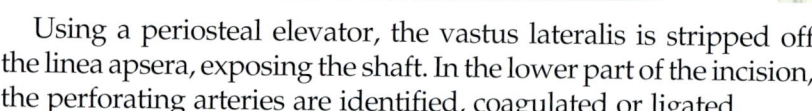

Using a periosteal elevator, the vastus lateralis is stripped off the linea apsera, exposing the shaft. In the lower part of the incision, the perforating arteries are identified, coagulated or ligated.

Properly positioned Hohmann retractors allow for visualization of the shaft of femur. One must be careful in positioning the points of the Hohmann retractors in the posterior part, and ensure that the lateral intermuscular septum is not perforated posteriorly (to ensure that the sciatic nerve and profunda femoris artery are not damaged).

Indications: This incision can be used for treating all fractures of femur from trochanteric to lateral femoral condyle.

It is also the approach of choice in tumours.

It can be extended proximally to expose the hip joint and distally to expose the knee joint.

Advantages: Minimal damage to quadriceps muscle.

Minimal scarring, leading to early return of full flexion.

Field is relatively bloodless, and approach is extremely easy.

Disadvantages: Improper positioning of spike retractors posteriorly might lead to injury to sciatic nerve or profunda femoris artery.

Posterolateral Approach

Access: This is a fairly versatile exposure, and routinely exposes the lateral aspect of the femoral shaft from the vastus lateralis origin proximally to the lateral epicondyle distally.

The incision can be extended both proximally and distally to expose the lateral aspects of both hip and knee.

Position: Supine with a sandbag under the ipsilateral hip.

The leg is draped free.

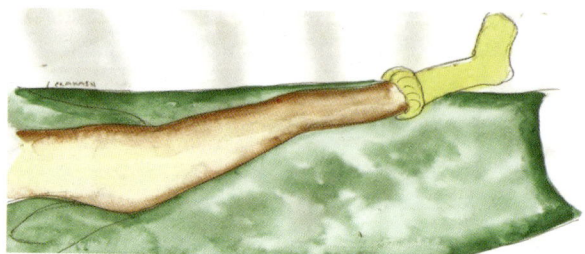

Plane: Between the vastus lateralis laterally and the two heads of biceps posteriorly.

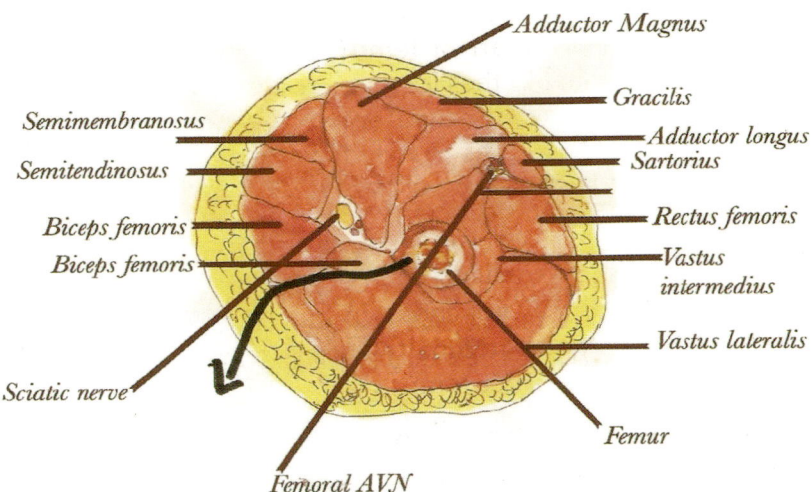

Incision: Straight line between greater trochanter and the lateral femoral epicondyle. It can be extended proximally or distally in a curved fashion depending on the needs.

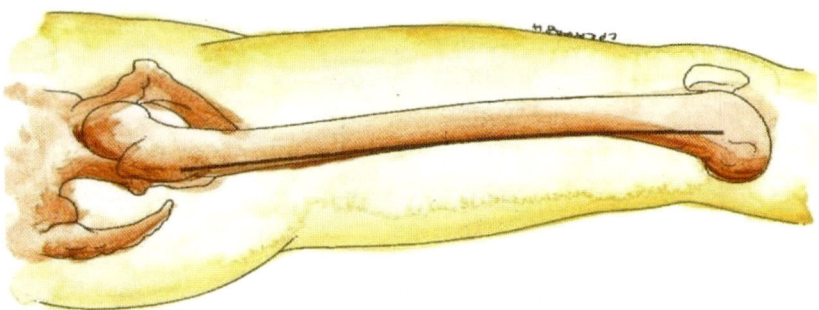

Dissections: The subcutaneous tissue, deep fascia, and tensor fascia lata are divided in line with the skin incision. The fascia lata is split along the anterior border of iliotibial band.

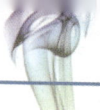

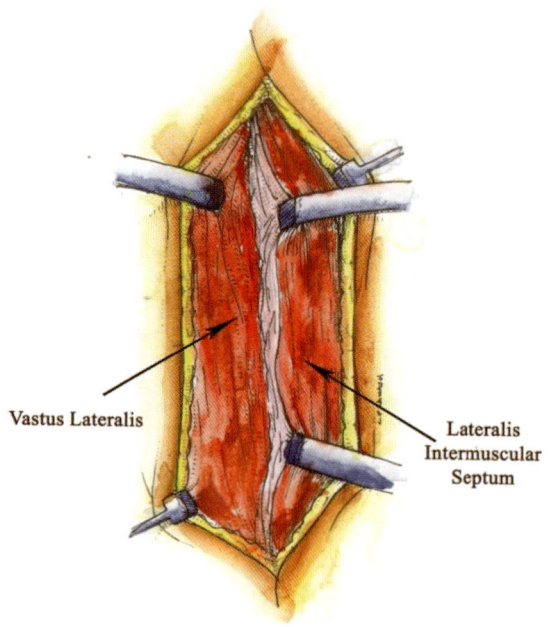

Vastus Lateralis

Lateralis
Intermuscular
Septum

The vastus lateralis is identified and retracted antreriorly to allow exposure of the lateral intermuscular septum posteriorly.

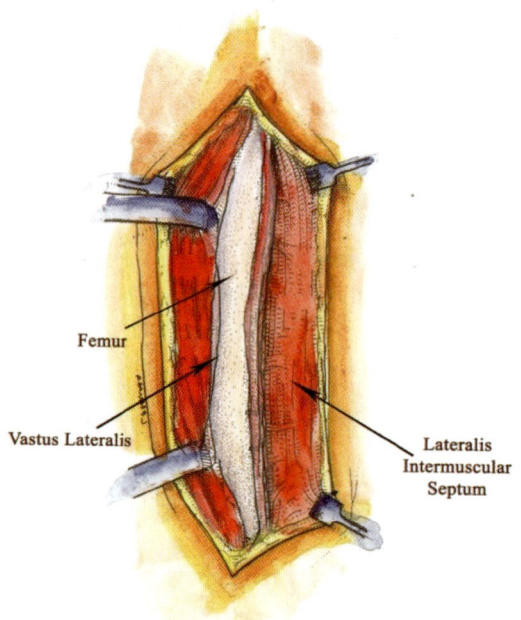

Femur

Vastus Lateralis

Lateralis
Intermuscular
Septum

The muscle belly is separated from the septum by blunt dissection; using a periosteal elevator, the periosteum is elevated off the linea aspera. Hohmann retractors allow visualization of the whole femur.

The perforating branches of the profunda femoris artery are identified in the distal part of the incision, caught and ligated or coagulated.

The vastus lateralis is now retractable anteriorly giving an excellent access to the femoral shaft.

Care must be taken with posterior Hohmann and the lateral intermuscular septum should not be perforated posteriorly. Here lies the sciatic nerve susceptible to injury by the Hohmann spikes.

Indications: Fractures of femur, including supracondylar fractures.

Tumours or other pathology of posterior and lateral femoral shaft.

Advantages: The quadriceps mechanism remains undisturbed. Less chances of muscle scarring and restricted knee flexion.

Gives a fairly extensive exposure from the hip to the knee and is useful in complex high velocity polytrauma.

No major structures are encountered during the exposure.

Disadvantages: Possibility of damage to sciatic nerve by Hohmann spike.

Posterior Approach

Access: Whole of the posterior surface of femoral diaphysis, giving an excellent exposure in the proximal and middle thirds.

Further inferior dissections are carried on along the medial aspect of the long head of biceps.

Position: The patient is positioned prone, with supports under iliac crests to ensure that abdomen moves freely. The leg is draped free to allow knee movements and also allow using the bent knee as a fulcrum for rotation of the shaft.

Plane: Initially between biceps and semitendinosus and then between biceps and adductor magnus.

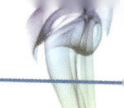

The shaft is reached posterior to sciatic nerve, behind the lateral intermuscular septum.

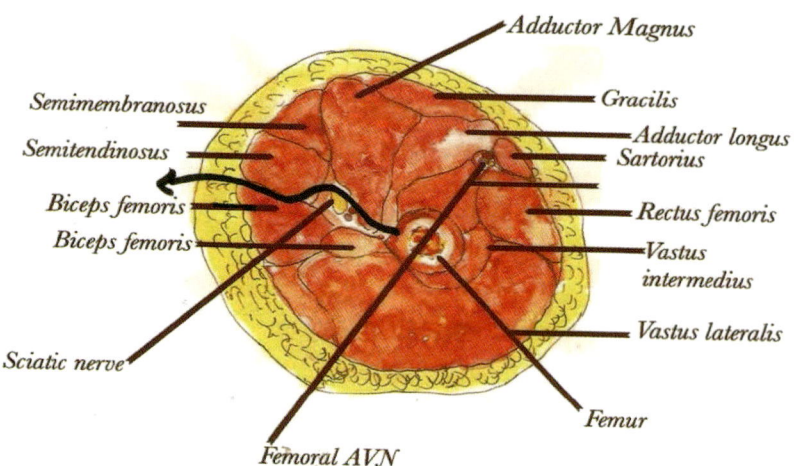

Incision: A straight incision from the midpoint of the gluteal fold to the midpoint of the popliteal fossa distally.

The posterior cutaneous nerve of the thigh should be identified and protected, as it lies quite superficially and close to skin incision.

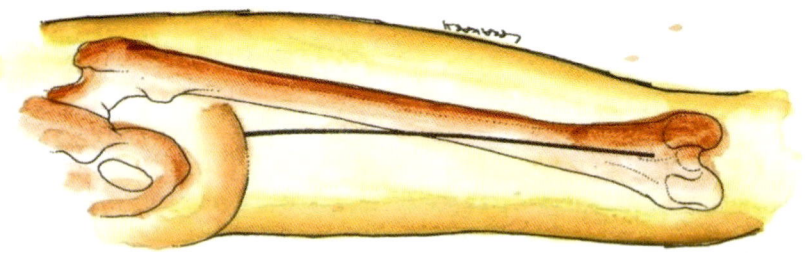

Dissections: The skin incision is deepened and care taken to identify, isolate, protect and retract the lateral cutaneous nerve of the thigh.

The long head of biceps is identified and the lateral border is the plane leading to the femoral shaft.

After retracting the long bicipital head medially, the interval between it and the short head is opened up by blunt gentle dissection.

Now is the most important step for this approach. The sciatic nerve is identified, as it lies deep to the long head of biceps. This should be carefully protected.

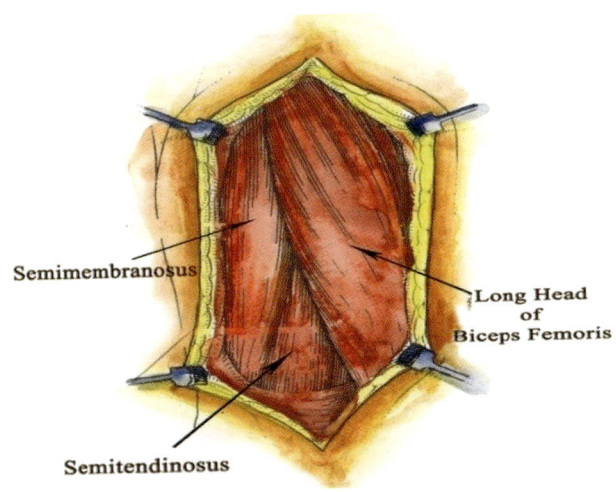

Semimembranosus

Long Head
of
Biceps Femoris

Semitendinosus

The proximal two-thirds of femur are exposed between biceps and vastus lateralis.

The middle and distal femurs are exposed between the medial side of long head of biceps and semitendinosus muscles.

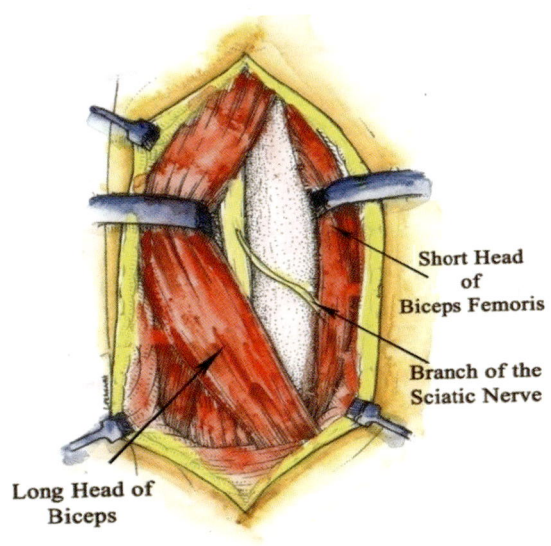

Short Head
of
Biceps Femoris

Branch of the
Sciatic Nerve

Long Head of
Biceps

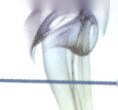

In the lower part of the incision, the popliteal artery and vein come from the medial side, and need identification and protection.

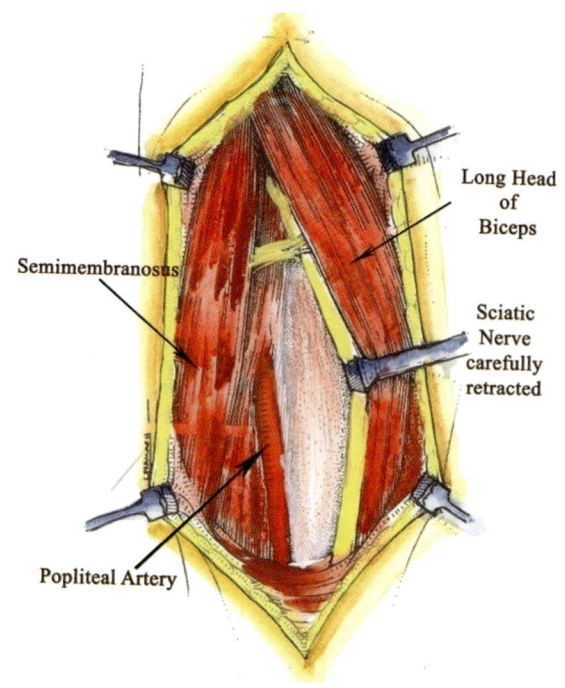

Indications: Lesions of sciatic nerve.

Tumours and other pathological conditions on the posterior aspect of femoral shaft.

Trauma to femur with injury to posterior structures.

Advantages: This is the only approach to expose the posterior aspect of femur and the whole length of sciatic nerve.

Disadvantages: Possibility of injury to sciatic nerve, and its branches to long head of biceps and semitendinosus.

Medial Approach to Proximal Femur including the Lesser Trochanter

This is essentially a Ludloff approach with an inferior extension.

Access: Proximal femur, medial aspect.

Lesser trochanter.

Medial aspect of femoral shaft in the adductor area.

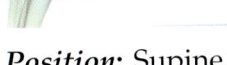

Position: Supine.

Leg draped free.

Hip is abducted and externally rotated to make adductors taut.

Perineum is well prepared. Scrotum is taped back in males.

Plane: Between adductor longus and brevis straight to medial aspect of femur. Division of iliopsoas facilitates exposure.

Incision: From pubic tubercle downwards over adductor longus as long inferiorly as required.

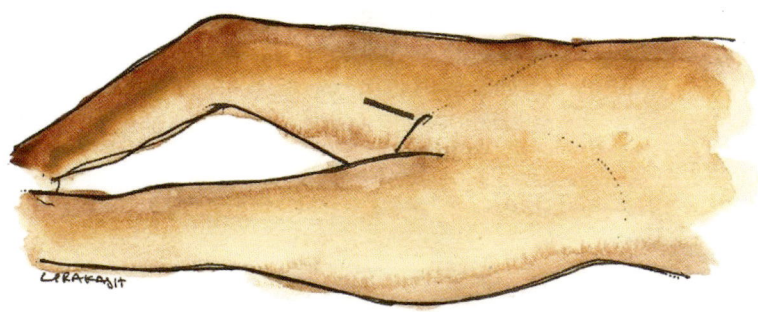

Dissections: Deep fascia is incised over adductor longus.

This muscle is detached from its insertion, if tight.

The plane between adductor longus and brevis is developed.

The obturator nerve is identified and protected. It lies in front of adductor brevis.

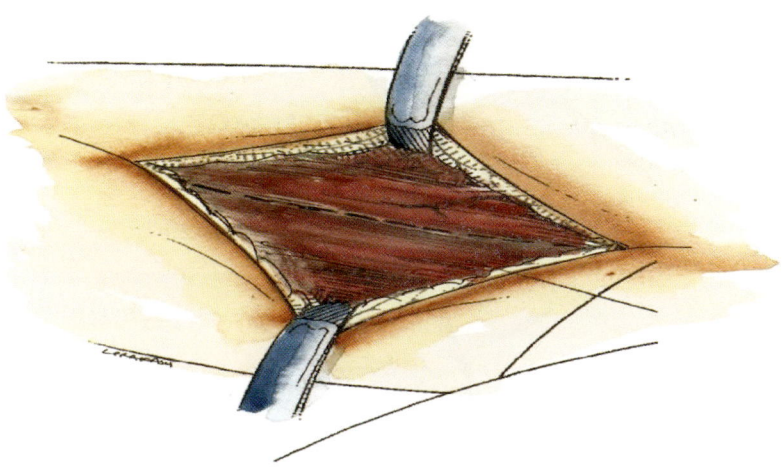

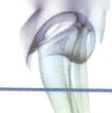

Indications: Approach of lesser trochanter, e.g. osteoid osteoma.

Advantages: Direct access to lesser trochanter.

Medial Approach to Posterior Femur

Access: This exposure provides a limited view of the posterior medial aspect of distal femur in the popliteal fossa.

Position: Supine with the leg draped free. Abduction of the hip allows approach to the medial side.

Plane: Between adductor magnus posteriorly and vastus lateralis anteriorly.

Incision: Straight incision, extending proximally from the adductor tubercle, along the course of the tendon of adductor magnus.

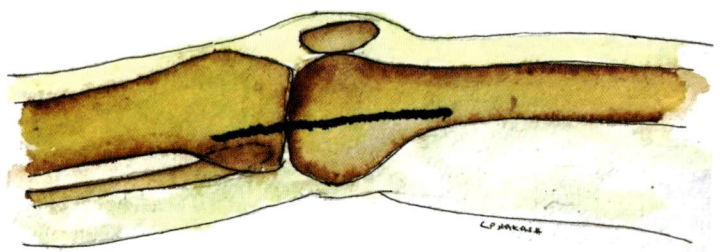

Dissections: The subcutaneous fat and deep fascia are incised in the line of the skin incision, and the sartorius muscle is identified.

The knee is flexed, and the sartorius falls backwards. Beneath this lies the adductor magnus.

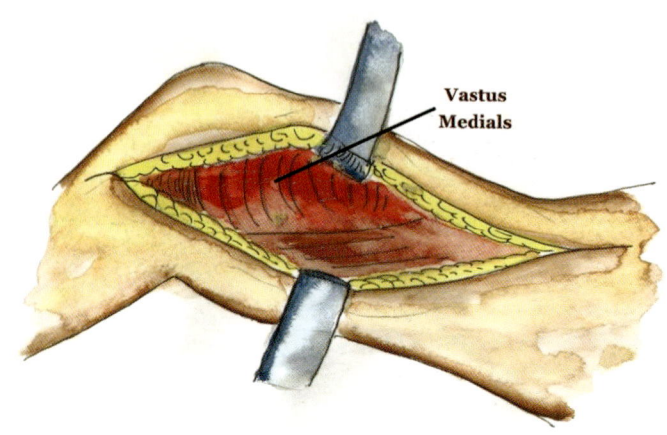

Vastus
Medials

Adductor magnus is retracted posteriorly and vastus lateralis anteriorly to expose the femoral shaft.

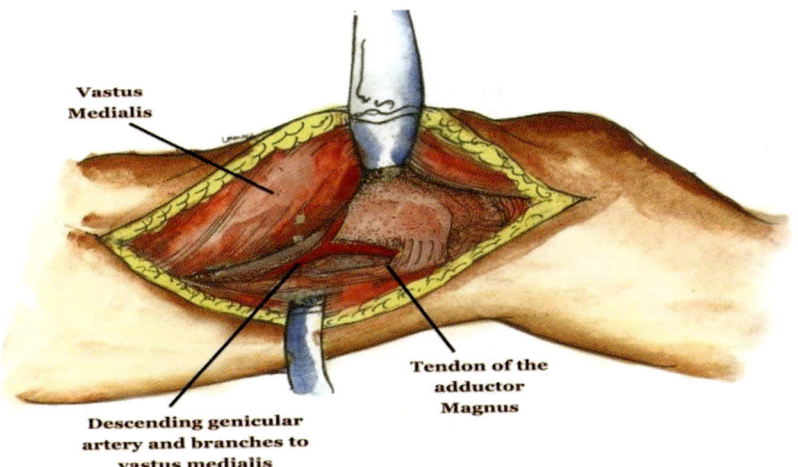

**Vastus
Medialis**

**Tendon of the
adductor
Magnus**

**Descending genicular
artery and branches to
vastus medialis**

The neurovascular bundle lies in the popliteal space exactly behind the femur and can be found behind the adductor magnus.

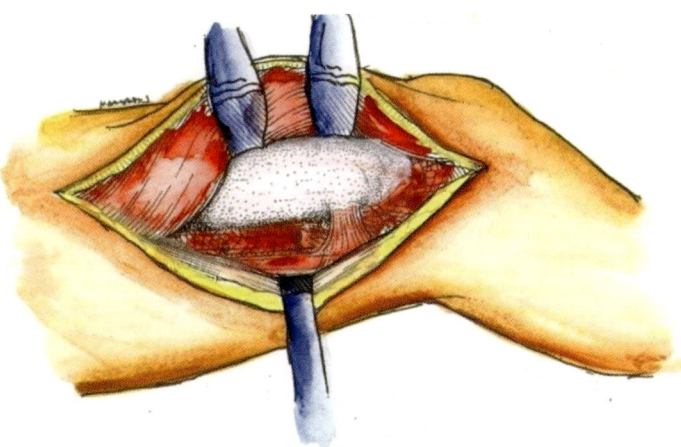

Indications: Tumours, including osteochondroma of the posteromedial aspect of distal femur.

Exposure of the neurovascular bundle, where vascular injury accompanies distal femoral fracture.

Posterior cruciate open surgery, though infrequently used these days.

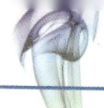

Lateral Approach to Posterior Femur

Access: Back of the knee and posterior surface of distal femur.

Position: Supine with a pillow and sandbag under the affected limb to give a slight lateral tril.
   Alternatively dead lateral.
   In both cases, the leg is draped free.

Plane: Between the iliotibial band anteriorly and the biceps posteriorly, following the lateral intermuscular septum.

Incision: Straight line parallel to the iliotibial band at the level of head of fibula.

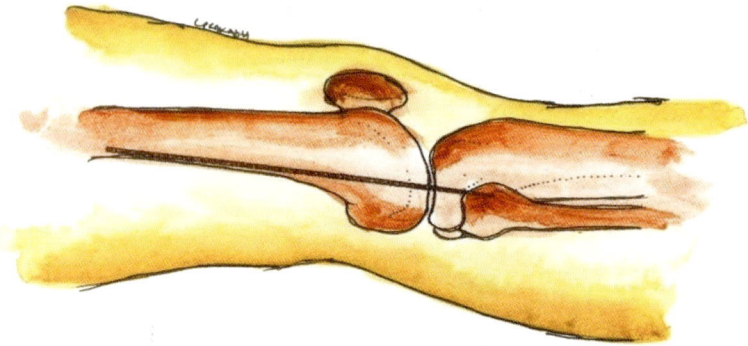

Dissections: Beneath the skin incision, the posterior border of the iliotibial band is identified and incised in the same line.

Iliotibual Tract

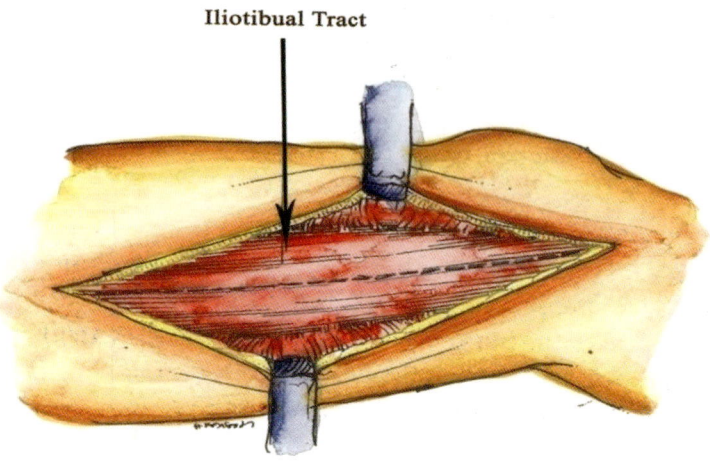

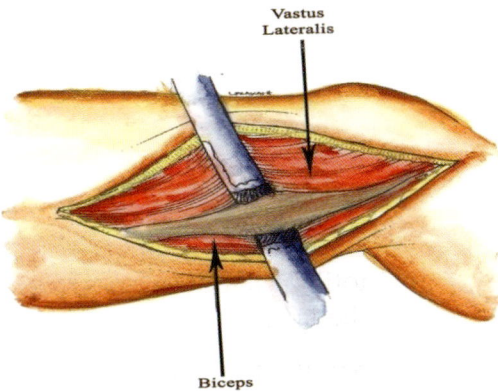

The iliotibial band is now separated from the short head of biceps. The biceps is retracted posteriorly and the iliotibial band anteriorly.

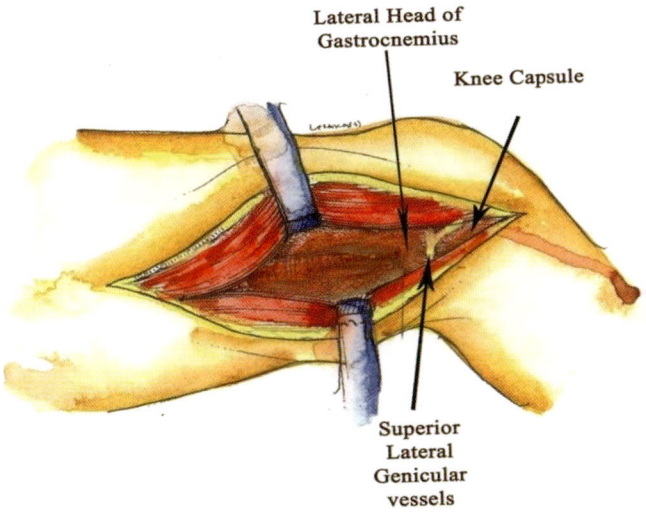

Both bicipital heads are retracted posteriorly, and the knee is flexed.

Posterior border of the distal femoral shaft is thus exposed.

The superior lateral genicular vessels will cross the incision in its distal part. These have to be identified, coagulated or ligated.

The common peroneal nerve lies along the medial edge of long head of biceps and should be protected.

Indications: Trauma to the distal part of femur.

Lateral instability repairs and reconstructions, including open repair of anterior cruciate ligament.

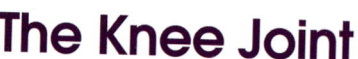

The Knee Joint

SURFACE LANDMARKS AND ANATOMY

The following structures are identifiable or palpable around the knee joint: Patella, medial epicondyle of femur, head of fibula, lateral femoral epicondyle, medial joint line, and lateral joint line.

Quadriceps, medial and lateral hamstrings.

Arteries

The femoral artery becomes the popliteal artery after it gives off the saphenous branch at the level of middle and distal thirds of femur. The popliteal artery enters through the adductor magnus and reaches posteriorly to the popliteal fossa.

Here it divides into anterior and posterior tibial arteries, and also gives off other large branches. The saphenous branch comes to the anteromedial aspect of the knee, which anastomoses with the genicular artery, and forms an anastomotic arch anteriorly.

The popliteal artery gives branches to adductor magnus and hamstrings. These then anastomose with the profunda femoris artery. Four genicular branches are given off, two medially and two laterally. A little below the two superior genicular arteries emerge the two sural arteries, one medial and the other lateral; and the whole lot anastomose with one another perfusing the knee with blood in all directions.

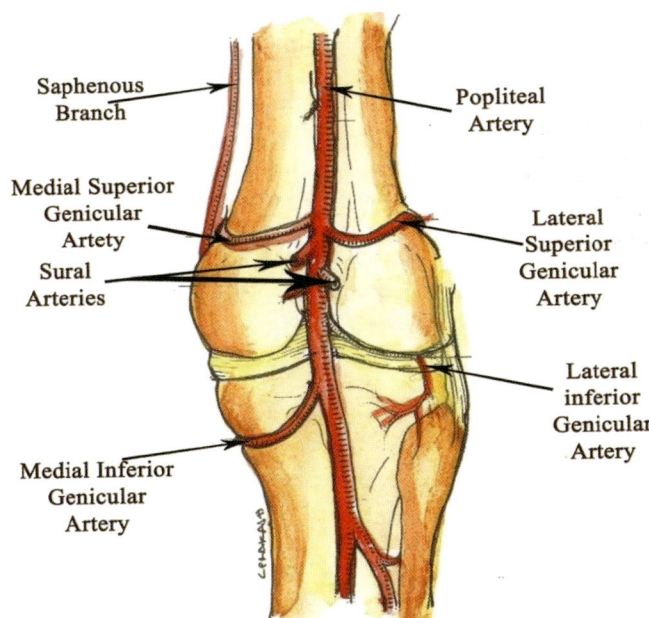

At the level of inferior border of popliteus, the popliteal artery divides into two: The anterior and posterior tibial arteries.

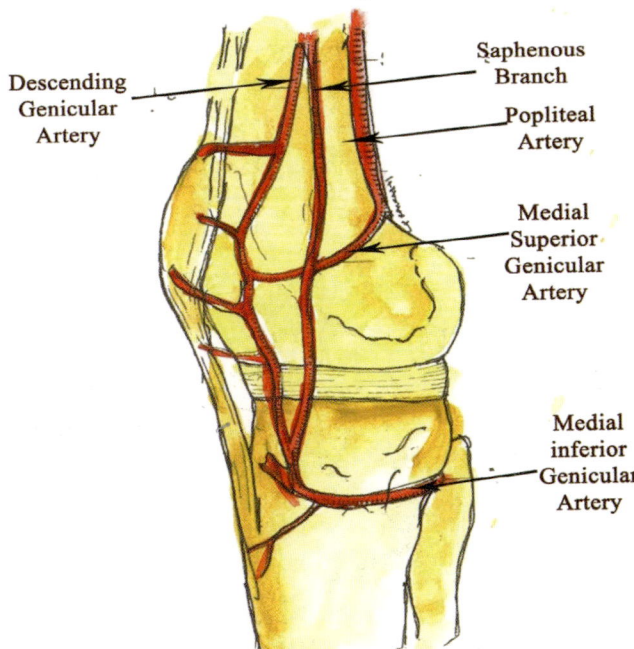

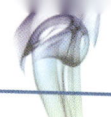

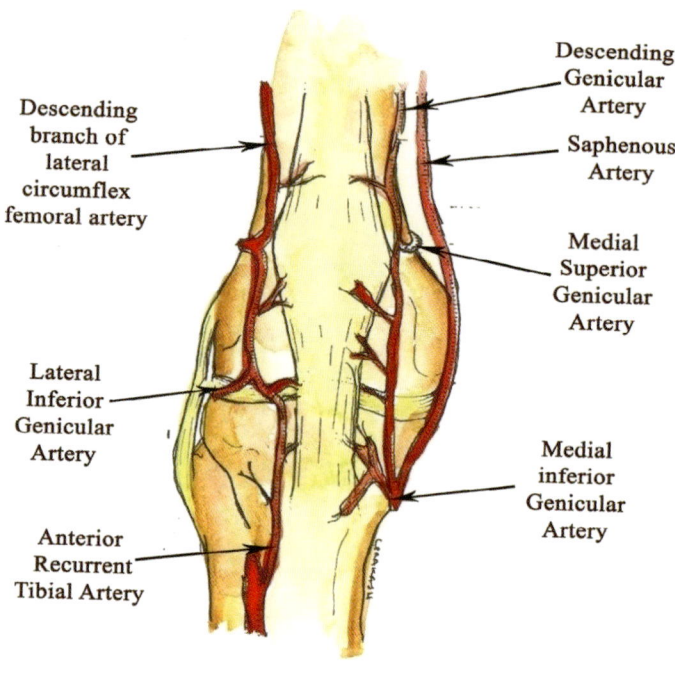

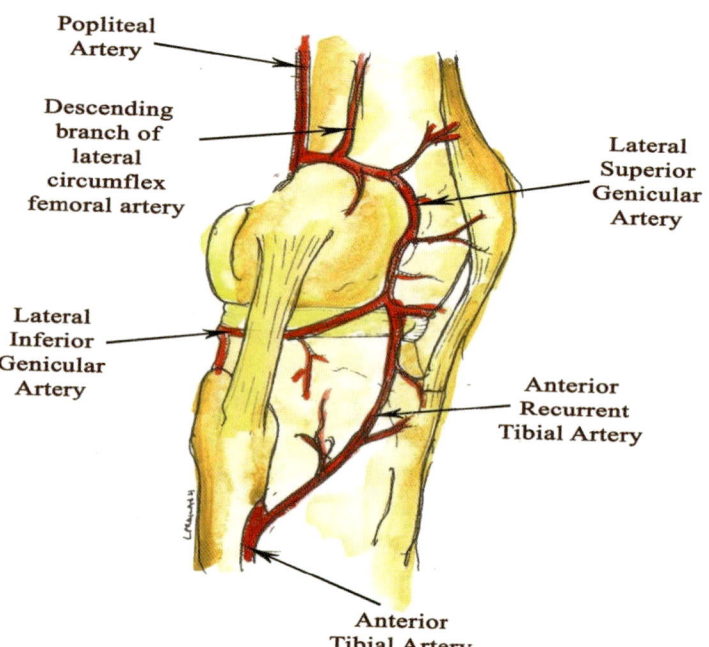

Veins

The deep veins accompany the arteries and their branches. They also bear the same names and follow the same course.

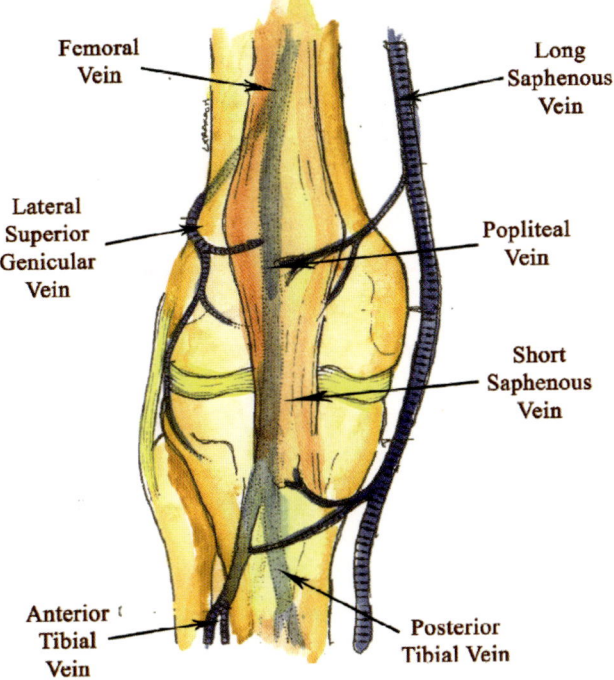

The popliteal vein is formed by the joining of the tibial veins at the lower border of popliteus. The short saphenous vein and its tributaries make up this vein which has venous branches corresponding to the arterial ones.

The long saphenous vein is the longest in the body. It crosses at the posteromedial aspect of the knee joint and is accompanied by the saphenous branch of the descending genicular artery.

Nerves

The long saphenous nerve is the longest cutaneous branch of the femoral nerve.

Crossing from the lateral to medial side of the femoral artery, it then accompanies the saphenous branch of the descending genicular artery, on the medial side of the knee between sartorius and gracilis.

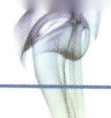

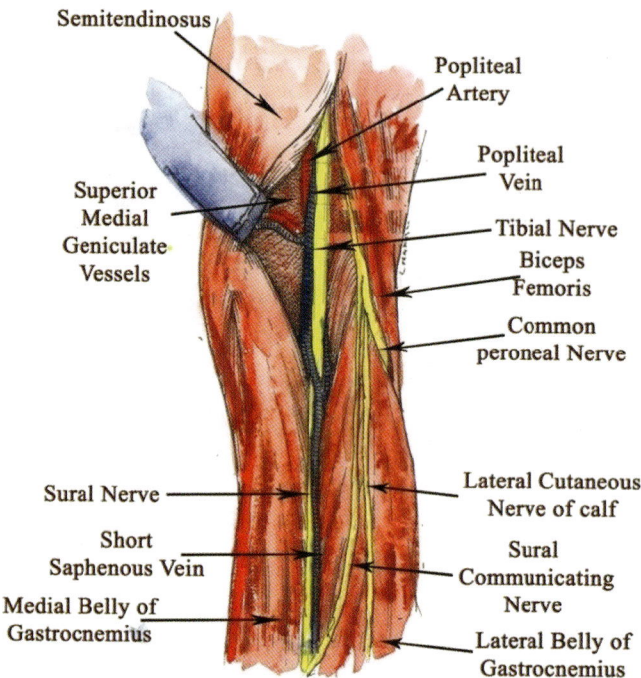

It then pierces the deep fascia and becomes superficial, branching into two and supplies the skin over anterior patella.

In the lower third of the thigh, the sciatic nerve divides into tibial and common peroneal nerves, a little above the knee.

The tibial nerve lies lateral to the vessels in the popliteal fossa; at the level of knee, it becomes superficial and then crosses the vessels to the medial side.

Throughout its course, the tibial nerve gives articular and muscular branches.

The common peroneal nerve is thinner than the tibial; it comes down obliquely in the upper popliteal fossa and spirals down over the neck of fibula as it descends. It gives off articular and muscular branches in its way.

It also gives off two cutaneous branches: lateral cutaneous nerve of the calf and the sural communicating branch.

History of Incisions around the Knee Joint

The knee joint is surrounded by important structures all around: Bones, tendons, muscles, ligaments and neurovascular structures.

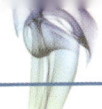

The rules of cutting, detaching, or mobilizing these structures are more or less straightforward and commonly followed, but a large variety of skin incisions have been tried in the past.

Not all incisions around the knee joint heal well and a number of approaches have been abandoned, both by their authors and others, because of skin necrosis and wound edge sloughing problems.

The changing disease patterns in the society and advances in surgical methods have altered the incisions around the knee, so that many of the original incisions are no longer used in their original form or have been abandoned altogether.

The advent of arthroscopy has rendered obsolete many incisions popular 50 years ago.

With the advent of arthroplasty and advancement in accurate repositioning of articular surfaces in complex trauma, the need for single incision offering an extensive approach has resulted in abandonment of the multiple small incisions for various joint compartments.

However, it is essential for an orthopaedic surgeon to not only know about our history, but also learn about the failed techniques of the past, so that it improves our fundamental knowledge of our fascinating subject.

I have thus described the abandoned and obsolete incisions and approaches initially, followed by a description of the approaches currently in fashion.

Medial Parapatellar Approach of Payr

Erwin Payr (1871–1946) was an Austrian-German surgeon born in Innsbruck.

Following graduation in 1894 at Innsbruck, he worked as an assistant at the first pathological anatomy institute in Vienna. He later became an assistant to Carl Nicoladoni at the University of Graz, where in 1899 he became trained in surgery.

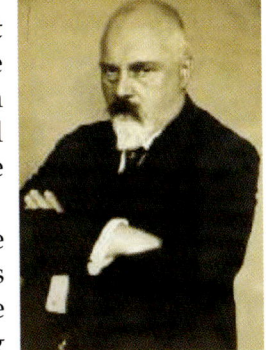

In 1907, he became chief surgeon at the University of Greifswald; in 1910, he was appointed professor of surgery at the University of Königsberg. The following

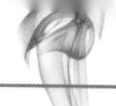

year he relocated to Leipzig, where he remained until his retirement in 1937.

Payr was regarded as an excellent physician known for his expertise in all facets of surgery. He was the first surgeon to use ozone treatments in order to control and kill bacteria, a practice he learned from Swiss therapist EA Fisch.

He also introduced the use of absorbable magnesium sutures in vascular and nerve surgery. He first reported animal experiments with reabsorbable magnesium tubular devices for vascular anastomosis, elegantly realizing intima-to-intima facing, however, just identifying in that first report its implicit mechanical limits.

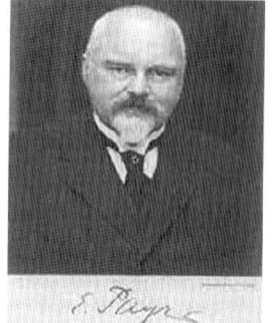

He used elderberry stems for capillary drainage of brain abscesses.

Splenic-flexure syndrome or "Payr's disease" is named after a condition he described.

A tool used in abdominal surgery, Payr pylorus clamp is also named after him, as is "Payr's sign", an indication of thrombophlebitis in which pain occurs when pressure is applied to the sole of the foot.

He described the S-shaped skin and capsular incision for the anterior approach to the knee in 1937. He was also the first to advice a medial parapatellar incision in the quadriceps mechanism to deflect the patella laterally to expose the whole interior of the knee.

However, the sharp curves in Payr's skin incision were not conducive to skin healing and were fraught with a great risk of sloughing of skin edges at the convexities.

The drawing below shows von Langenbeck's skin incision with Payr's incision for deeper structures.

However, Payr's incision of the quadriceps tendon by the medial parapatellar route least interfered with the dynamics of extensor mechanism and the patients were able to perform a straight leg raise in less than six weeks.

The current anterior Insall approach, used almost universally for most primary and revision knee replacements, is probably an amalgam of Langenbeck's skin incision (gentler curve) with

Payr's medial parapatellar incisions into the extensor mechanism and capsule.

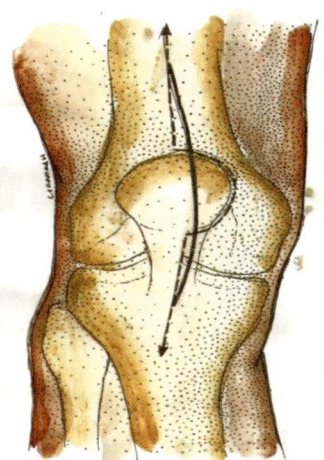

Oblique Parapatellar Incision

The subvastus approach as described by Erkes consists of a medial parapatellar arthrotomy and blunt dissection of the distal vastus medialis from the intermuscular septum and adductor magnus tendon, thereby exposing the subvastus region.

In contrast to standard surgical techniques, the subvastus approach preserves the integrity of the entire extensor mechanism.

Studies have demonstrated a quicker recovery of quadriceps muscle control, reduced postoperative pain and decreased scarring around the knee joint, should a revision become necessary.

The potential disadvantage, however, is inadequate exposure of the lateral patellofemoral compartment combined with increased tension on the patellar tendon insertion at the tibial tubercle accompanying retraction of the extensor mechanism.

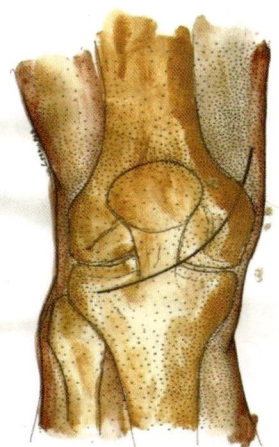

To decrease the tension at the tibial tubercle and to improve exposure of the knee joint, an extension of the mobilization of vastus medialis in the subvastus region might be helpful. The

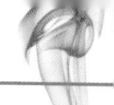

proximal border for a safe incision is controversial and might reflect the different exposure results achieved in various studies.

It is known that the subvastus technique interferes with the blood vessels and nerves in the region; the subvastus region contains the descending genicular artery and its branches, as well as the saphenous nerve. The descending genicular artery supplies vastus medialis, parts of the distal femur and the knee joint, while the saphenous nerve is sensory to the medial aspect of the lower leg.

This approach, described by Erkes in his classic paper (1929), is still used in select cases in some centres.

Transextensor Approaches

Textor in 1859, Ollier in 1891 and Putti in 1917 described approaches in which the extensor mechanism was transected to gain wide anterior access into the knee joint.

During closure, each devised methods to assure a secure closure of the divided extensor mechanism to ensure a decent quadriceps function.

However, all these incisions were plagued by either severe quadriceps lag or by skin dehiscence problems.

A short biography of these three great surgeons precedes the description of their exposures.

Cajetan von Textor (1782–1860) was a German surgeon born in the Ebersberg district of Upper Bavaria.

From 1804 to 1808, he studied at the University of Landshut, where he was a pupil of Philipp Franz von Walther.

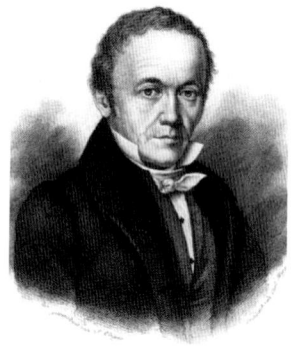

He spent the next few years on an extended educational journey throughout Europe, where he studied with Alexis Boyer in Paris, Antonio Scarpa in Pavia and Georg Joseph Beer in Vienna.

Afterwards he was second physician at the general hospital in Munich. In 1816, he was appointed professor of surgery and *Oberwundarzt* in the Juliusspital at the University of Würzburg. In 1832, he was relieved of his duties at Würzburg and banished

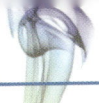

to the surgical school at Landshut because of suspicion of political ties to the July Revolution and the Hambach Festival.

In 1834, he was reinstated at Würzburg, where he remained for the rest of his career. One of his better known students was Bernhard Heine, inventor of the osteotome.

In the field of surgery, Cajetan von Textor was a specialist of bone and joint operations. Among his publications was a German translation of Alexis Boyer's surgical work titled Grundzüge zur Lehre der chirurgischen Operationen (1818–1827, 2nd edition 1834–1841).

He described an inverted U shaped incision shown by a dashed line in the illustration below.

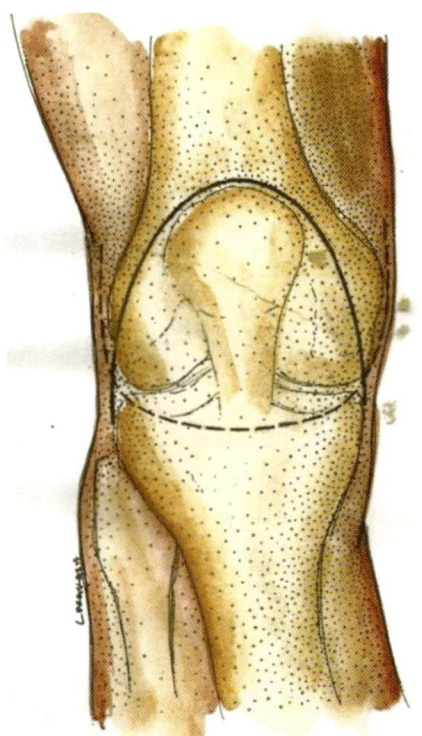

Putti of Italy described an almost similar approach, which was different only in placement of the skin incision. (It was a shallow U facing the direction opposite to the bold incision line above.)

Vittorio Putti (1880-1940): Vittorio Putti was professor in the University of Bologna, surgeon-in-chief of the Istituto Ortopedico Rizzoli, a founder of the Société Internationale de Chirurgie Orthopédique et de Traumatologie and president of its 1936 Congress, Honorary Member of the British Orthopaedic Association, the American Orthopaedic Association, Corresponding Member of the American Academy of 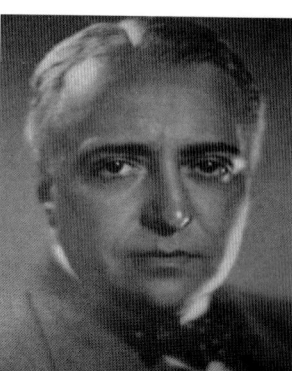 Orthopaedic Surgeons, and many other national organizations. He was a bibliographer, medical historian, orthopaedic investigator, and teacher of surgeons. He had been a foreign editor of The Journal of Bone and Joint Surgery since January 1928.

Bologna was a Roman city. The cathedral of San Pietro e San Paolo, built in part from Roman remains, was erected in the fourth century. The city has long been a seat of learning, and legends attribute the founding of the famous University of Bologna to Theodosius the Great in 425 AD.

The Istituto Ortopedico Rizzoli is situated on a hill on the outskirts of this fascinating old city and occupies the picturesque buildings of a Benedictine monastery known as San Michele in Bosco. The early years of this institute for crippled children were not noteworthy, until Alessandro Codivilla, modest and skillful master, became its director and surgeon-in-chief. This great general surgeon, after excelling in the surgery of the gastro-intestinal tract and the brain, devoted his talents to orthopaedic surgery, and the Istituto became world famous. Codivilla made original and important contributions to the surgery of fractures and the methods of tendon transfers, and to the development and standing of the specialty.

At his death in 1912, Codivilla was succeeded by Vittorio Putti, the son of a well-known surgeon who was for many years professor of surgery in the University of Bologna. Putti had first become identified with the Istituto Ortopedico Rizzoli in 1903, when Codivilla had appointed him as an assistant. Following two years of study in European clinics, he returned to the

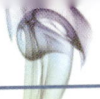

institution in 1909 as Vice-Director, and in 1914 became Director and Surgeon-in-Chief of the Istituto. He was also professor of orthopaedic surgery at the University of Bologna.

In 1922, Putti opened the country branch, which provided for the care of 100 cases of surgical tuberculosis, and as Director of this hospital (Istituto dio terapico Codivilla di Corona d'Ampezzo) in the Dolomites, he found frequent escape from his very strenuous city life.

A brilliant student, a wide reader, an able administrator, a resourceful and skilful surgeon with a mechanical bent, Putti enhanced the reputation of the Istituto Rizzoli, and like Codivilla, made lasting contributions to the history of medicine and to the technique of orthopaedic surgery.

In addition to being a tireless and exacting trainer of young surgeons, Putti encouraged his associates to become familiar with the history of medicine and the contributory sciences, to strive for exactitude in thought and action, and to appreciate beauty, not only of art and nature, but of character. His sanctum sanctorum, which he shared with his helpers, was the library (La Biblioteca Umberto I). On the walls of this dignified room are the same beautiful frescoes, executed by Canuti, that had given joy to the monks, and on its shelves are books and manuscripts covering a period of over 400 years.

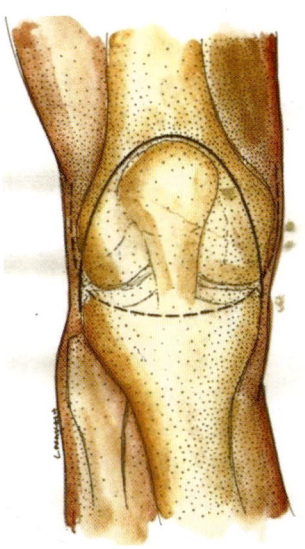

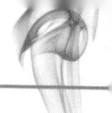

By his numerous original contributions, Putti became an international leader, a pioneer and an authority on bone and joint surgery, especially on congenital dislocation of the hip, its preluxation stage and its automatic reduction by the *divaricatore*, arthritis, arthroplasty, sciatica, the forcible manipulation of adult club feet, the open treatment of fractures and the use of skeletal traction and metal fixation, the equalization of leg lengths by bone lengthening, spinal anomalies, cineplastic amputations and artificial limbs, and the surgical treatment of the residual effects of poliomyelitis.

He published many monographs, not only on strictly medical and surgical subjects, but also on nonmedical subjects, as well as translations of old medical works. His large quarto "Berengario da Carpi", published in 1937, represents not only a profound and extensive piece of research, but the best biographical study of this great surgeon and anatomist who antedates Vesalius. This work alone places him among the great medical historians. His latest volume, pulished in 1940, is entitled "Cura operatoria delle fratture del collo del femore".

His titles are too numerous to mention, for he was a corresponding, honorary, or active member of most of the orthopaedic societies of the world. His honours included civilian, medical, surgical, military, and academic recognition. He received from the King the title of Grand Officiali of the Crown of Italy.

Louis Léopold Ollier: Louis Xavier Édouard Léopold Ollier (1830–1900) was a French surgeon born in Les Vans. His father and grandfather were also physicians.

Initially he studied natural sciences at Montpellier, and in 1851, began work as medical intern at Lyon Hospital. In 1857, he earned his medical doctorate in Paris, and in 1860, became chief surgeon at the Hôtel Dieu in Lyon. In 1877, he became a professor of clinical surgery.

Ollier is famous for his work in bone and joint surgery. He became internationally known for developing techniques involving bone resection, and is remembered for his extensive research of regeneration of bone by the periosteum following resection. A pioneer in the field of bone grafting, he also devised a surgical operation known as astragalectomy.

In 1872, he developed a split-thickness skin graft that was later improved upon by Karl Thiersch (Ollier-Thiersch graft).

His name is also associated with Ollier's disease, a bone disorder also known as multiple enchondromatosis. Furthermore, the cambium layer (inner layer of the periosteum where osteoblasts reside) is sometimes referred to as "Ollier's layer".

On 24 June 1894, Ollier was awarded commander of the Légion d'Honneur by French president Marie-François-Sadi Carnot.

Ironically, later that evening Carnot was stabbed by an assassin, and Ollier was summoned to tend to the dying president's wounds. Today, the museum of pathological anatomy at the University of Lyon is named in Ollier's honour.

He described an anterior approach in which the quadriceps tendon was cut in an H-shaped fashion to allow a complete exposure of the whole interior of the knee from the front. However, time proved that this was a bad approach and produced both skin problems and quadriceps function problems in most patients. These incisions of historical importance are only mentioned to bring awareness about the thought processes of the great scientists/surgeons before us.

The drawing on the next page shows the H-shaped incision in the extensor mechanism to facilitate the complete exposure of the interior of the knee.

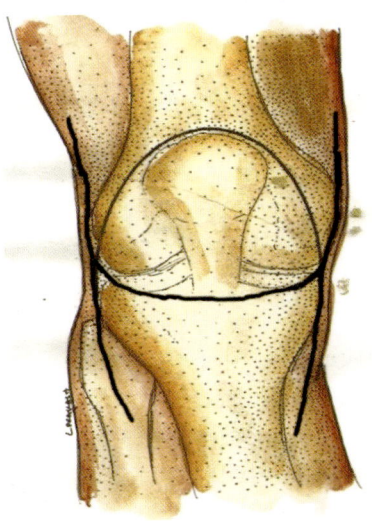

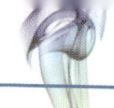

None of the three incisions is used currently, though modifications of these can be found in many of the modern approaches to the knee joint.

Between 1916 and 1977, many incisions were described for transpatellar approach.

Jones in 1916, and later Brackett and Hall in 1917 advocated a slightly curved anterior incision, which was transverse and followed the Ianger's line. The extensor mechanism was split and so was the patella, which was osteotomized transversely with a saw and later fixed with wires.

Devine in 1931 advocated a vertical splitting of patella in sagittal plane, while Von Volkman, as late as 1977 described an approach with a transverse splitting of the patella with a later fixation with screws and tension band wiring.

Similarly, a very popular incision of the past, the Mercedez Benz incision, has now been rather totally abandoned because of the associated skin problems, despite being given a wide exposure.

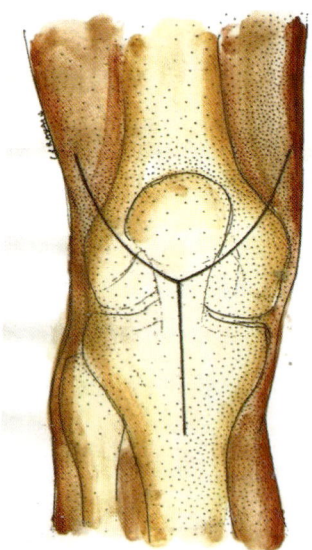

Menisectomy Incisions

Revolutions happen which change the face of history and our established practices are thrown away. In a similar manner, the advent of arthroscopy not only produced a new breed of surgeons, it also made numerous menisectomy incisions redundant.

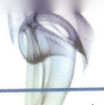

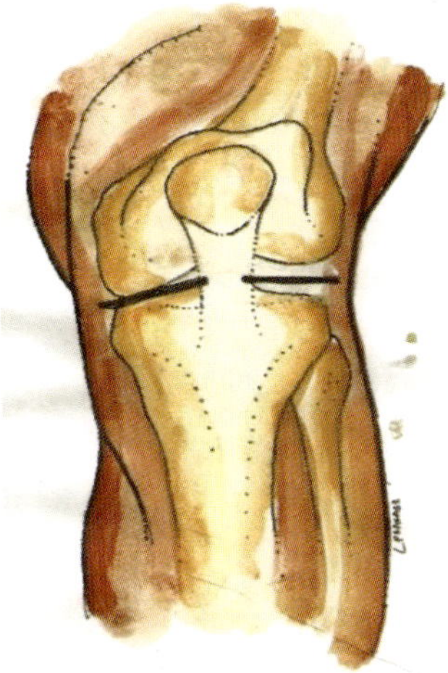

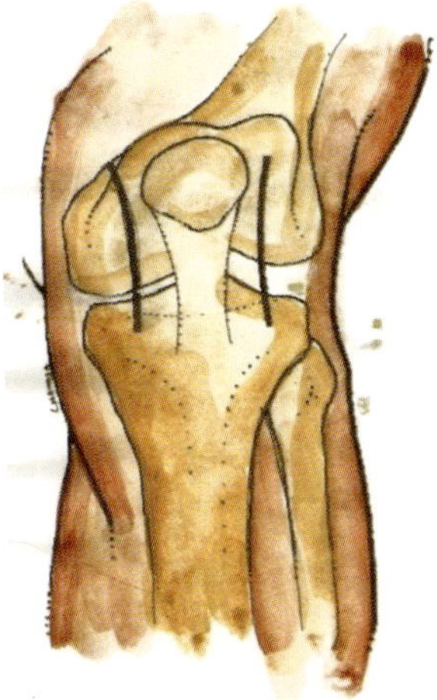

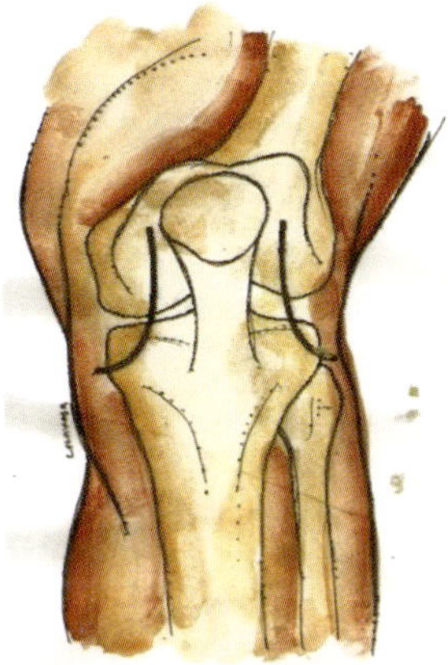

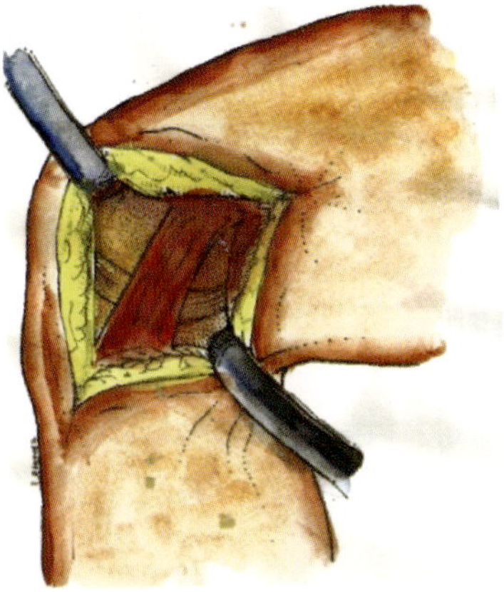

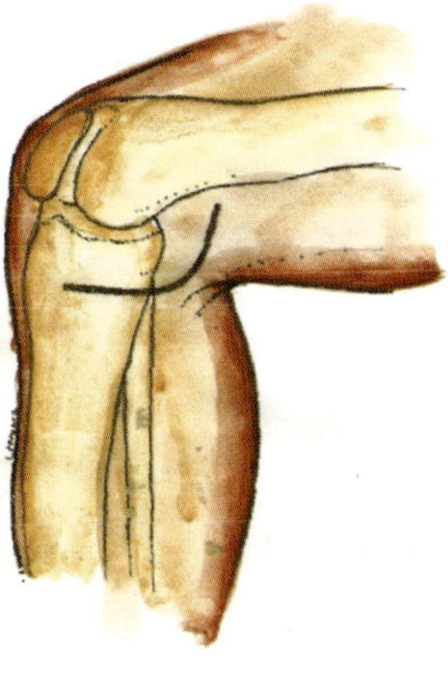

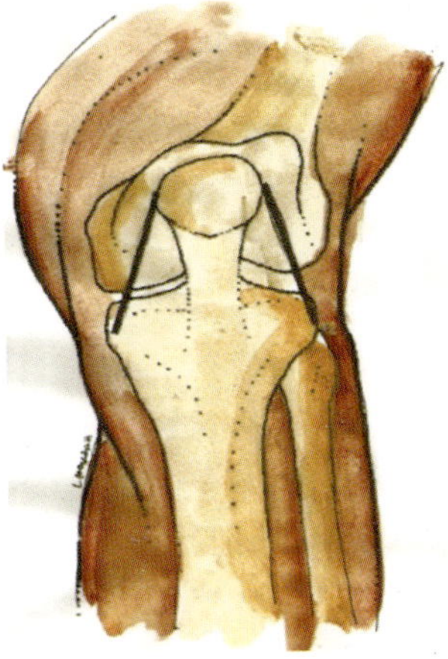

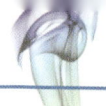

It would be an unnecessary detail to describe the layers and planes of these obsolete incisions, but I have drawn them all to give an idea about the types of incisions that have been described over the years. Almost all of them have been abandoned in modern times.

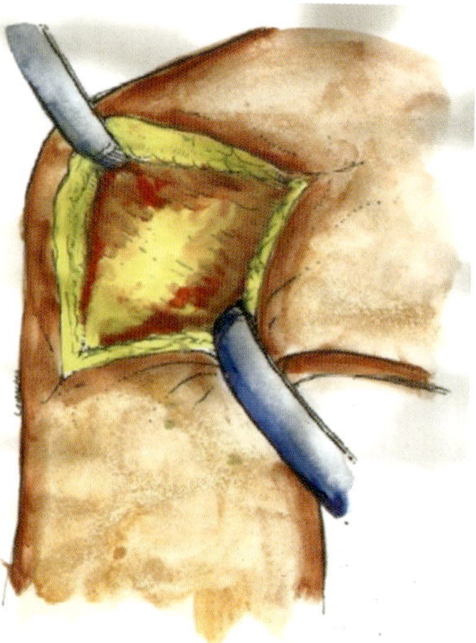

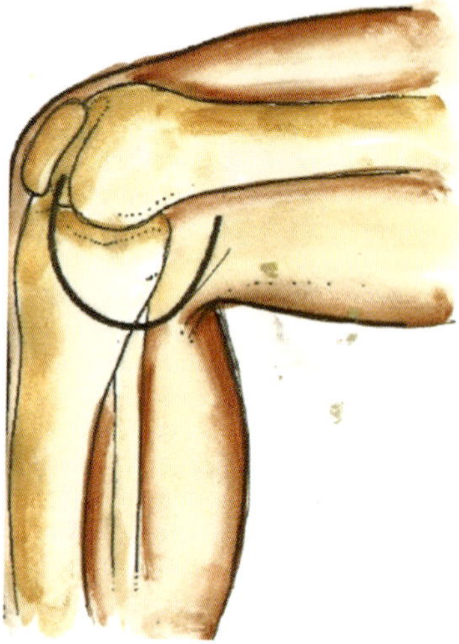

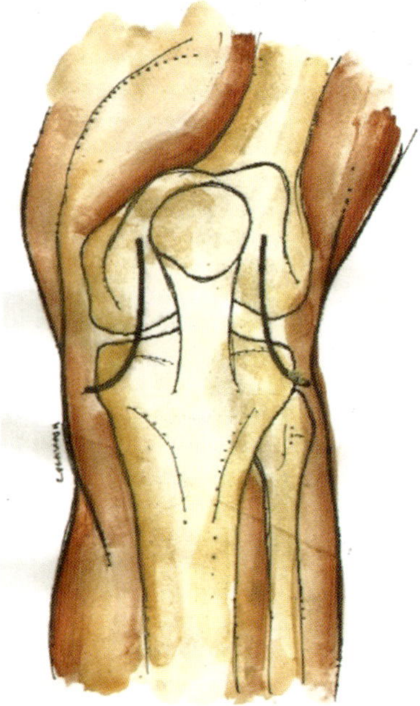

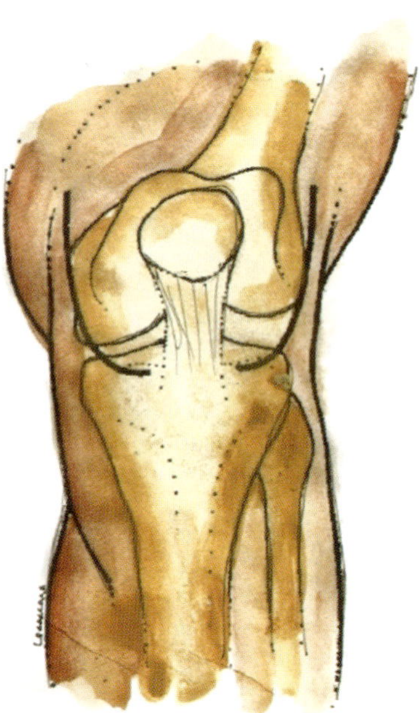

Other obsolete incisions for knee:

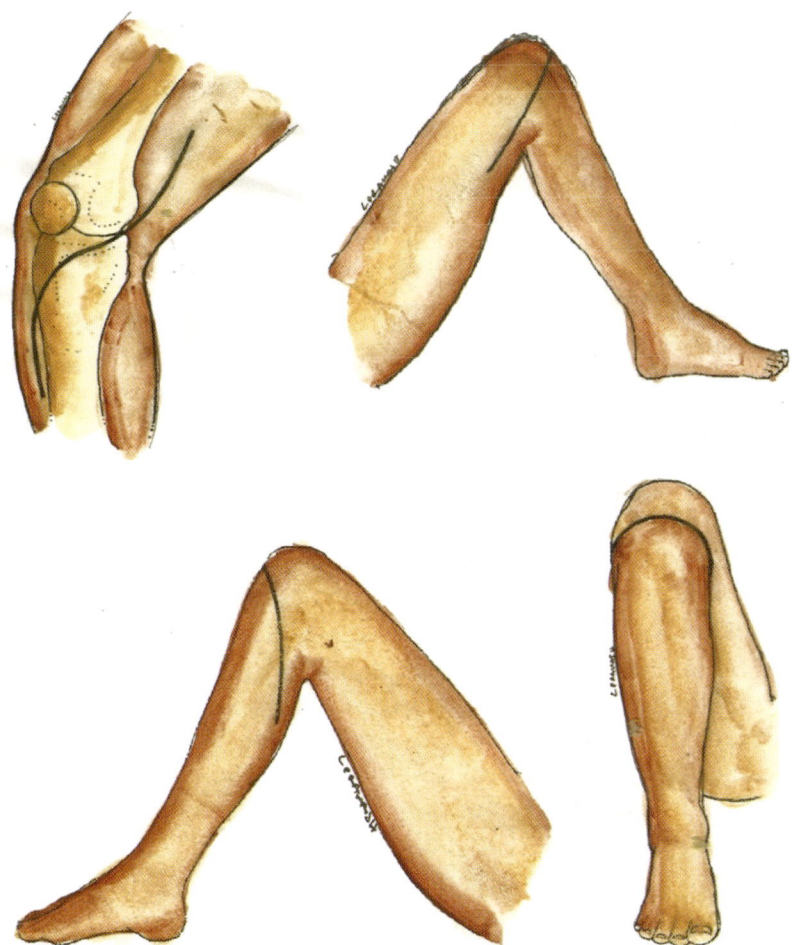

CURRENTLY FOLLOWED SURGICAL APPROACHES TO THE KNEE JOINT

The following are the currently used common approaches to the knee joint:

1. The classic anteromedial approach.
2. Insall's modificaion: The direct anterior approach.
3. Starr's Swashbuckler approach.
4. Posterior approaches:
   - Osgood and Brackett
   - Putti, Abbot

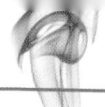

5. Lateral approach
- Bruser
- Ruedi, von Hoschletter and Schlumpf
6. Posterior Henderson approaches

The Anteromedial Approach

History

Bernhard Rudolf Konrad von Langenbeck (1810–1887): Von Langenbeck was a German surgeon known as the developer of Langenbeck's amputation and founder of *Langenbeck's Archives of Surgery.*

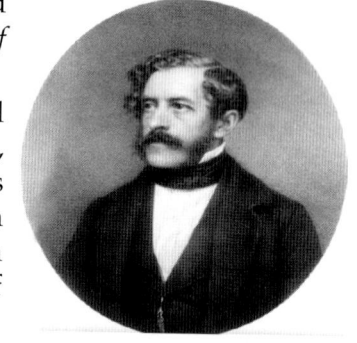

Born at Padingbüttel, he received his medical education at Göttingen, where one of his teachers was his uncle Konrad Johann Martin Langenbeck. He took his doctorate in 1835 with a thesis on the structure of the retina.

After a visit to France and England, he returned to Göttingen as *Privatdozent*, and in 1842 became Professor of Surgery and Director of the Friedrichs Hospital at Kiel. Six years later, he succeeded Johann Friedrich Dieffenbach (1794–1847) as director of the Clinical Institute for Surgery and Ophthalmology at the Charité in Berlin, and remained there till 1882, when failing health forced him to retire.

Langenbeck was a bold and skilful surgeon, but preferred not to operate while other means afforded a prospect of success. He specialized in military surgery and became an authority on the treatment of gunshot wounds. He served as general field-surgeon of the army in the First Schleswig War in 1848 and saw active service in the Second Schleswig War in 1864, being ennobled for his services.

He also served in the Austro-Prussian War in 1866, and the Franco-Prussian War of 1870–71. He was in Orléans at the end of 1870 after the city had been taken by the Prussians; in his capacity as surgeon or as consultant, he tended to the wounded men with whom every public building was packed.

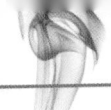
He also utilized the opportunities for instruction that thus arose, and the Militär-ärztliche Gesellschaft, which met twice a week for some months, and in the discussions of which every surgeon in the city, irrespective of nationality, was invited to take part, was mainly formed by his energy and enthusiasm. He died at Wiesbaden in September 1887.

von Langenbeck is perhaps best known today as the "father of the surgical residency". Under his tutelage at the Charite in Berlin, he conceived and developed a system whereby new medical graduates would live at the hospital as they gradually assumed a greater role in the day-to-day care and supervision of surgical patients. Among his most well-known "house staff" were such illustrious surgeons as Billroth and Emil Theodor Kocher. The great achievement of his house-staff model was acknowledged by no less than Sir William Osler and William Halsted, who quickly co-opted his concept into the teaching system of the Departments of Medicine and Surgery, respectively, at the John Hopkins University Hospital in the late 19th century.

In addition, he was the first to describe the medial parapatellar approach to the knee joint in 1878, which is described in more detail below.

This approach is the forerunner on which the modern anterior incision of the knee is based, and his slightly curved skin incision was modified by Insall and others to a straight midline incision to avoid skin problems at the apex of the convexity and to minimize the area of paraesthesia left by cutting the superficial cutaneous patellar branch.

Access
- Patella and subpatellar fat pad
- Suprapatellar pouch
- Medial compartment
- Lateral compartment
- With division of cruciates, the whole of the knee interior can be visualized.

Positioning: Supine on the operating table with a sandbag under the buttock to keep the hip in neutral rotation.

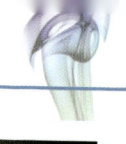

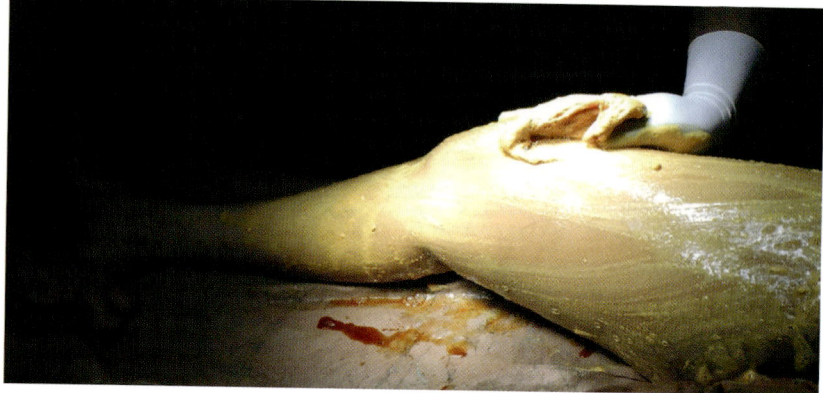

If a tourniquet is used, it should be applied high up and one should ensure that this does not interfere with full flexion and extension of the knee.

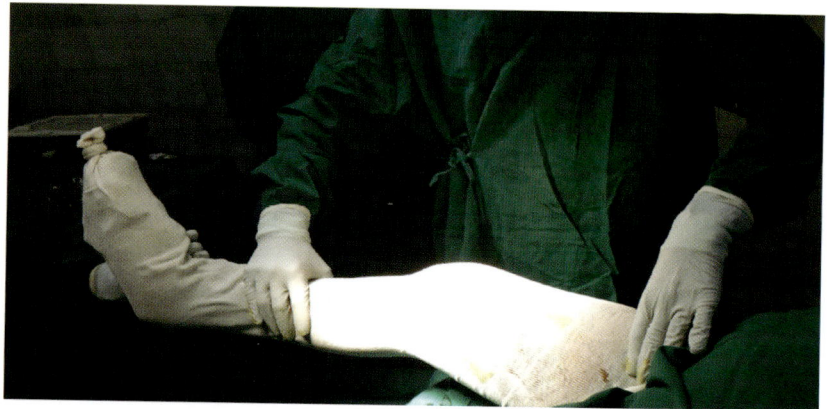

Limb is prepared from groin to ankle.

The upper drapes are as high as the pathology requires, stopping at the tourniquet level if it is used.

The foot and ankle are covered with thin drapes, to allow identification of all toes under the drape.

As the knee is usually flexed and extended repeatedly during the course of surgery, the drapes should be secure and the operating area should be isolated with an adhesive opsite.

A stockinette can be rolled from the foot right up to the tourniquet. This is cut in the midline anteriorly, spread to both sides of patella and anchored with an adhesive steri drape.

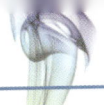

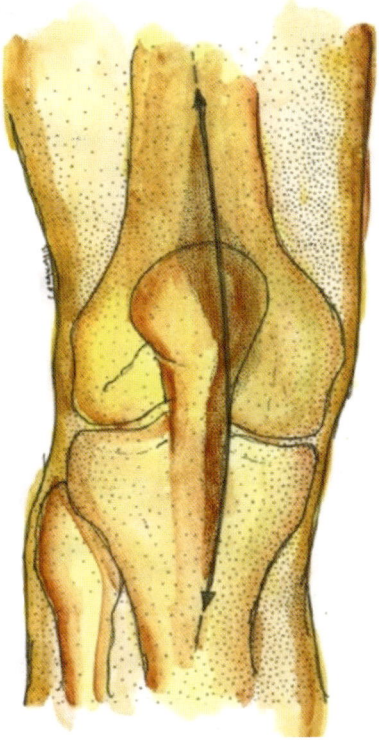

The incision: Anteromedial skin incision, starting 5 cm above patella, curving medially and ending 2.5 cm below the tibial tuberosity.

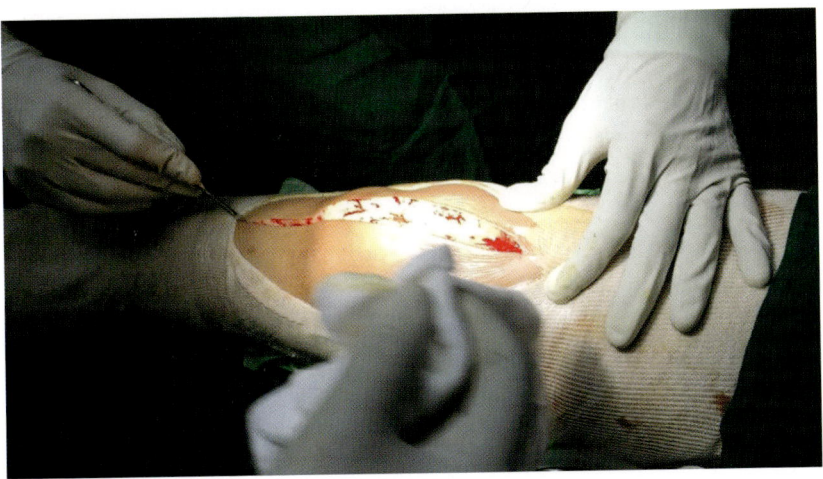

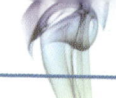

The deep exposure and approach: The subcutaneous fat and deep fascia are incised in line with the skin.

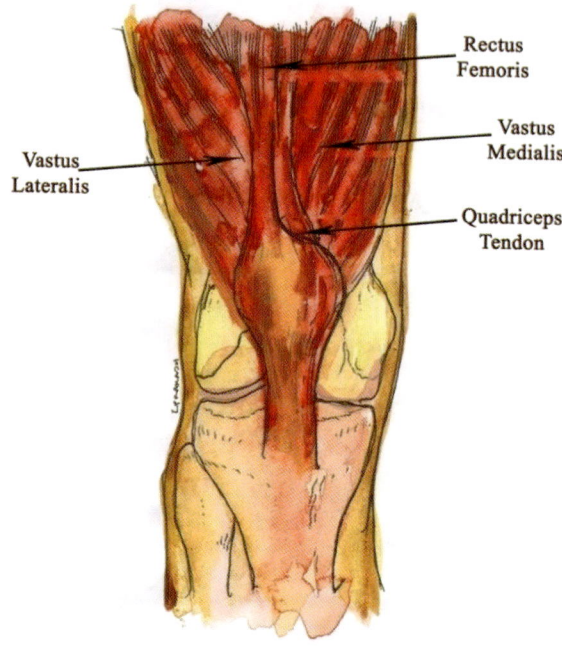

The belly of quadriceps muscle and its attachment to patella is identified.

A linear cut is made in the middle of the quadriceps tendon and the same is brought down right up to the upper border of patella.

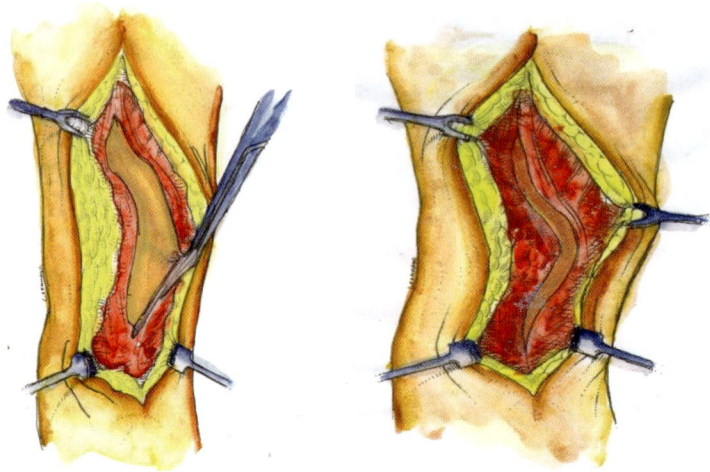

This cut is now skirted around the medial border of patella, leaving a decent strip to the bone for subsequent reattachment.

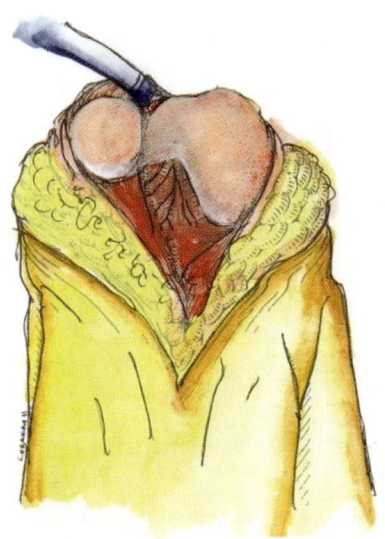

This is then brought to the level of the tibial tuberosity by curving it inwards.

The patella is everted laterally as the knee is slowly flexed.

Everted and dislocated patella

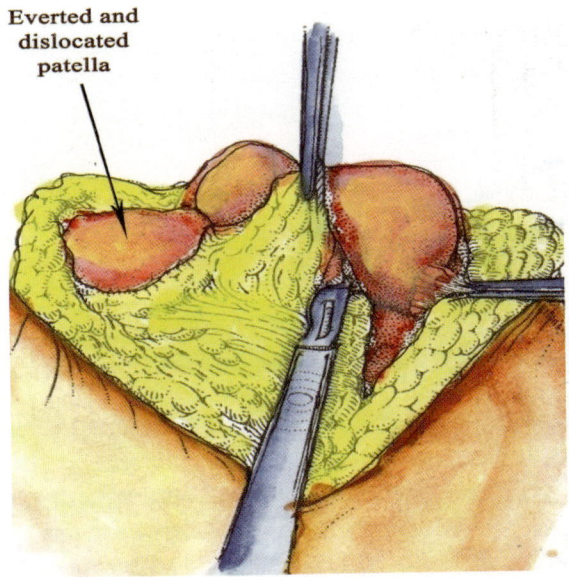

The infrapatellar fat pad can now be excised, to improve visualization of the lateral compartment of the knee.

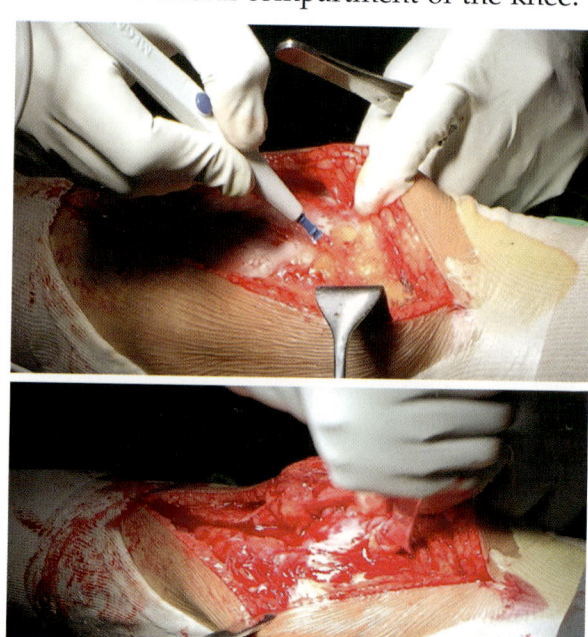

Flexion beyond 90° with lateral translation of the patella brings the whole of the interior of the knee into view.

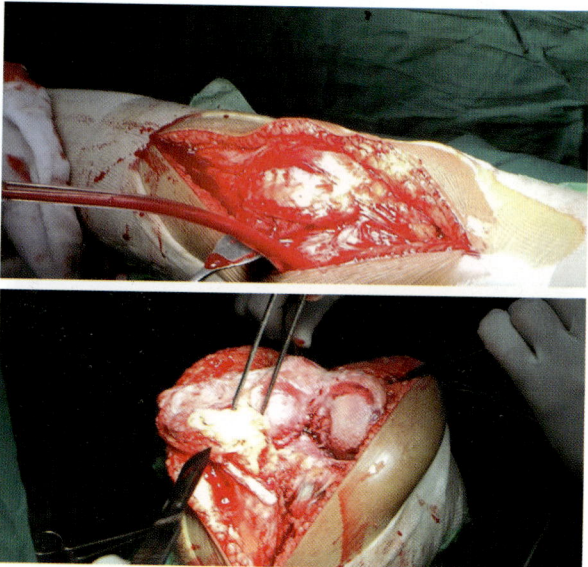

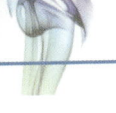
A cutting diathermy is often used to cut the quadriceps belly, skirting around the medial border of patella.

Excision of the infrapatellar fat pad facilitates full visualization of knee interior.

In arthroplasties, either anterior or both cruciates are excised, which allows an almost complete anterior translation of the tibia to enable us to visualize its posterior aspect.

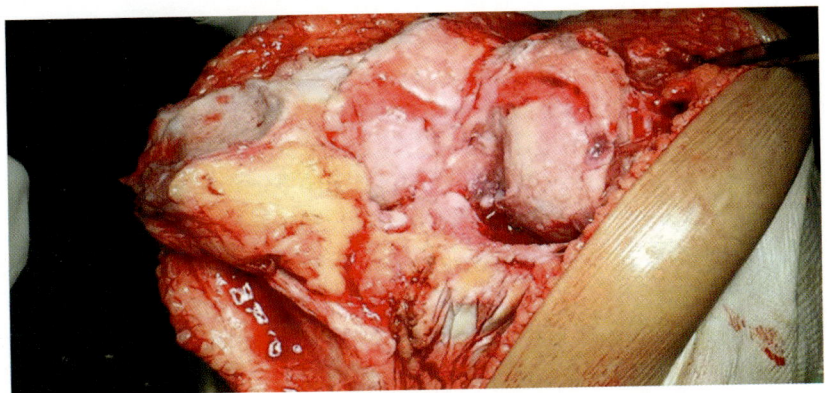

Both cruciates and the anterior two-thirds of menisci are now clearly visible and so is most of the anterior synovium.

The infrapatellar fat pad excision, followed by a judicious placement of Hohmann retractors, allows us to visualize the lateral aspect of the knee joint.

Indications for the anteromedial approach to the knee:

1. Traumatic pathology of the knee joint, especially intra-articular fractures needing accurate reconstruction.
2. Anterior synovectomy.
3. Primary total knee replacement.
4. Revision total knee replacement.
5. Replacement by megaprosthesis for tumorous conditions.
6. Arthrodesis of the knee.

Anterior Approach

History: This incision and approach was described by John Insall.

John Nevil Insall (1930-2000) was a pioneering English orthopaedic surgeon who contributed extensively to the advancement of total knee replacement surgery. He designed four models of widely used systems.

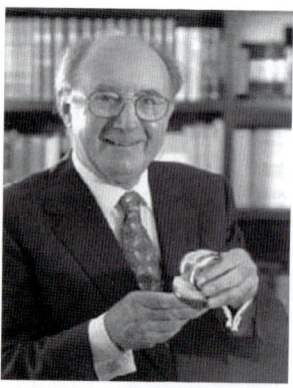

Born in Bournemouth, England, he attended Corpus Christi College, Cambridge, graduating in 1953. He worked as a physician and orthopaedic surgeon in England and Canada before joining the Hospital for Special Surgery in New York City. He founded the Insall Scott Kelly Institute for Orthopaedics and Sports Medicine at Beth Israel and the Knee Society.

In addition to his preeminent knee textbook "Surgery of the Knee" (Churchill-Livingstone, 2000), Dr Insall wrote approximately 150 peer-reviewed articles, 41 book chapters and 5 books. He has also trained over 200 orthopaedic residents and 100 national and international knee fellows throughout his academic career.

His publications were "Current Concepts in Primary and Revision Total Knee Arthroplasty" and "Surgery of the Knee, Volume I".

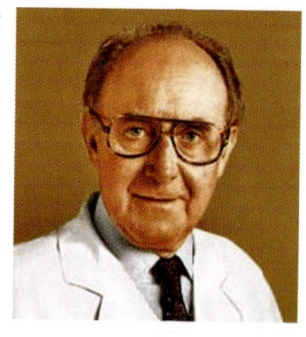

Dr Insall was a founding member of the Knee Society in 1983 and became its president in 1987. He was instrumental in the development of the Knee Society scoring system.

John Insall's contributions to orthopaedic surgery are legendary. His articles appeared in The Journal of Bone and Joint Surgery over four decades, beginning with reports on his experience with valgus tibial osteotomy for the treatment of osteoarthritis of the knee. Subsequent articles dealt with techniques for the treatment of patellar chondromalacia and malalignment as well as iliotibial band transfer for the treatment of knees with anterior cruciate ligament deficiency. His most

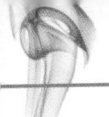

outstanding publication is the classic book Surgery of the Knee (now in its third edition), coedited by his colleague and dear friend Dr Norman Scott.

Dr Insall will be most remembered for his numerous contributions to knee arthroplasty. His work with the total condylar knee prosthesis began in 1974 at the Hospital for Special Surgery, and, with Albert Burstein, he designed the Insall-Burstein knee prosthesis, first implanted in 1978. With Michael Freeman, he pioneered the philosophy of excision of the cruciate ligaments and soft tissue releases during knee arthroplasty. Among his special talents was his ability to devise arthroplasty techniques that were forgiving yet effective, allowing countless otherwise crippled patients throughout the world to resume normal lives. His most recent design innovations involved mobile-bearing inserts and fixed bearings that allowed high degrees of flexion.

Dr Insall also developed exposure techniques (e.g. the "quadriceps snip"), quadricepsplasty, for the treatment of patellar instability, ligament releases for the treatment of angular deformity, and intraoperative guidelines for femoral component rotation. He was a pioneer in the two-stage revision for septic knee arthroplasty. In addition, he was responsible for the design of many instruments used intraoperatively to facilitate the accurate implantation of prosthetic components.

His long-term follow-up studies of clinical results in various populations of patients, such as those who are young, elderly, or obese and those who have diabetes, psoriasis, or poliomyelitis, are the gold standard against which all future results will be compared.

John Insall was an acknowledged master surgeon. His clinical skills were complemented by his equally strong ability to teach others by both word and example. Some 60 surgeons, many now world-renowned themselves, served as his fellows. They formed the Insall Club in his honour and meet annually to share experiences and promote research in knee arthroplasty techniques.

His lectures were classics, and he served frequently as the keynote speaker at national meetings. He was an annual fixture,

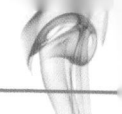

for example, at Seth Greenwald's Current Concepts Meeting in Orlando, Larry Dorr's Master Techniques in Los Angeles, and, of course, the ISK meeting in New York City. He adopted Leo Whiteside's technique of video presentation in lieu of slides, delivering messages that were clear, precise, and, when appropriate, entertaining.

The Insall award was established to honour Dr Insall's achievements and contributions to orthopaedics. This award recognizes outstanding papers concerning clinical results and techniques. The John N. Insall Travelling Fellowship, awarded to four candidates internationally, allows those individuals to travel to prominent knee surgery centres.

He died of lung cancer on December 30, 2000, at Beth Israel Medical Centre in Manhattan.

Insall essentially modified the anteromedial approach to avoid the skin and healing problems that plagued his initial knee replacements. In addition, by the conventional anteromedial approach, a significant percentage of his patients complained of a large area of denervation in the skin area over patella. By shifting the skin and subcutaneous tissue incisions to midline, he reduced this area of paraesthesia considerably.

Access: Excellent exposure to anterior knee joint. By excising one or both cruciates, the tibia can be translated fully forward, exposing the whole of the knee.

It must be remembered that in extension, the neurovascular bundle is stretched and close to the posterior femur and tibia. On the contrary, in flexion, the vessels fall back considerably. Bone cuts should thus be only done with the knee in flexion.

As this incision is primarily used for total knee replacements and has been originally described for this procedure, the steps for the same have been described.

Positioning: Supine on the operating table with a sandbag under the buttock to keep the hip in neutral rotation.

If a tourniquet is used, it should be applied high up and one should ensure that this does not interfere with full flexion and extension of the knee.

Limb is prepared from groin to ankle.

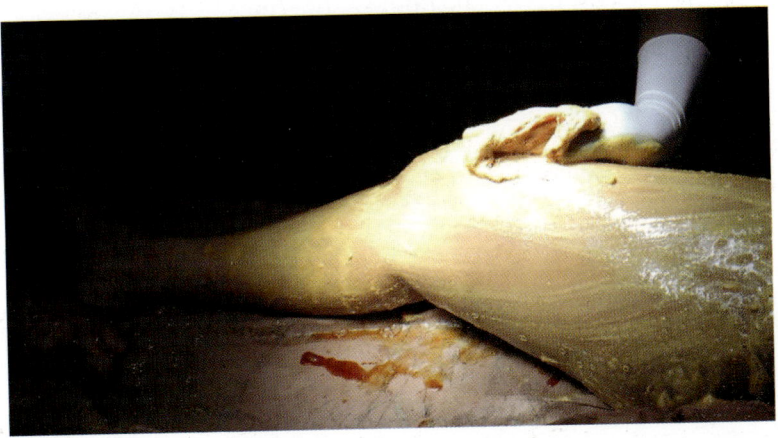

The upper drapes are as high as the pathology requires, stopping at the tourniquet level, if it is used.

The foot and ankle are covered with thin drapes, to allow identification of all toes under the drape.

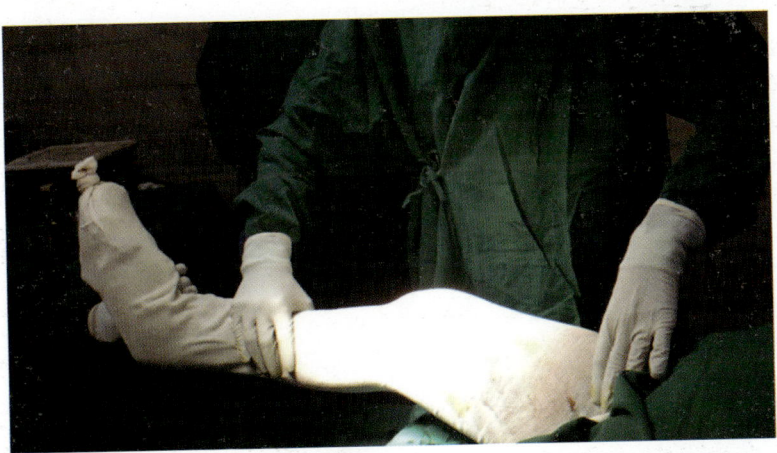

As the knee is usually flexed and extended repeatedly during the course of surgery, the drapes should be secure and the operating area should be isolated with an adhesive opsite.

A stockinette can be rolled from the foot right up to the tourniquet. This is cut in the midline anteriorly, spread to both sides of patella and anchored with an adhesive steri drape.

The incision: Straight midline incision centred over patella extending 7.5 cm above and below patella.

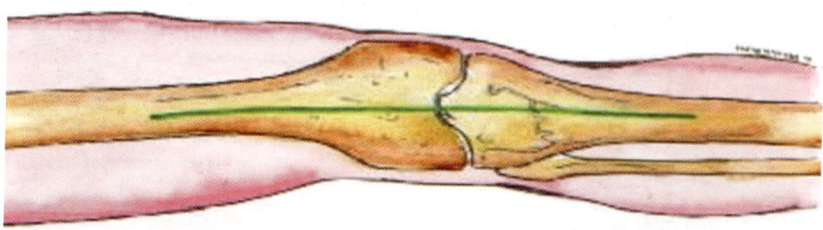

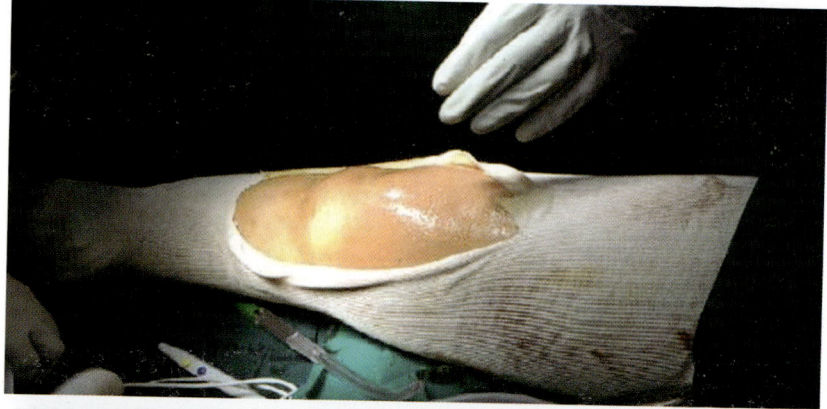

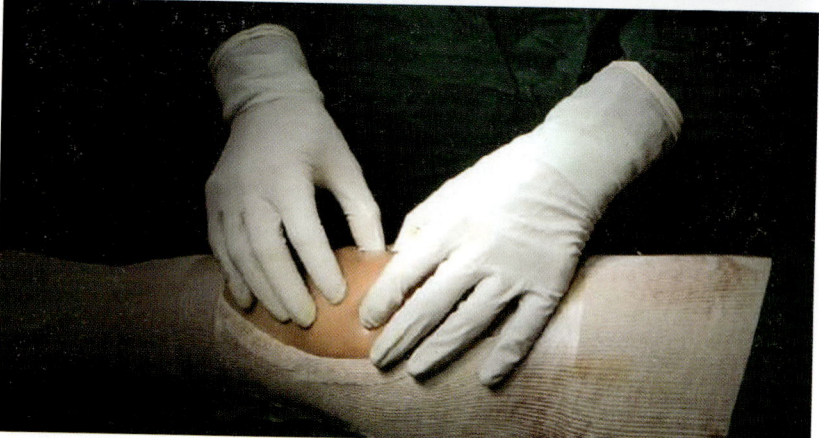

Patella is the landmark over which the incision is centred.

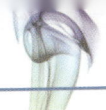

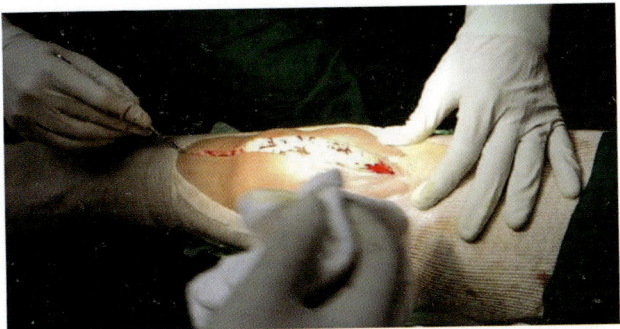

Straight midline skin incision over patella up to the tibial tuberosity.

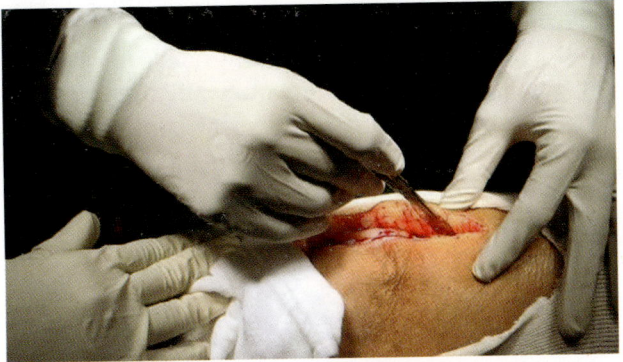

The incision can be extended superiorly or inferiorly as needed in each case.

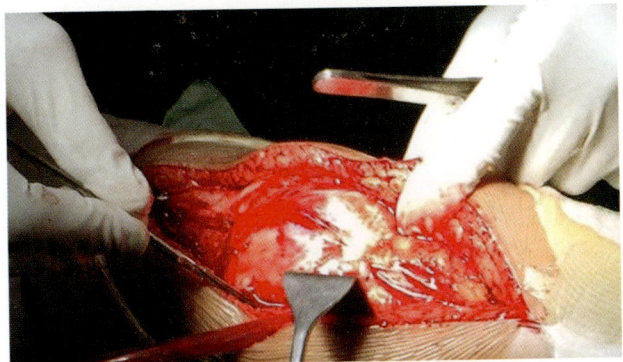

Quadriceps tendon is incised in the line of its fibres, and the deep incision skirts around the medial patellar border straightening down below it, up to the tibial tuberosity.

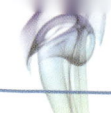

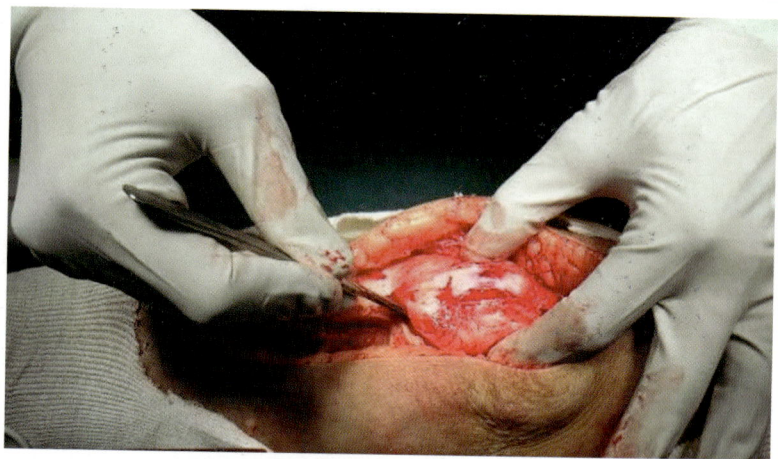

It is usual to make two deep linear incisions, one above and one below the patella and then curve it around the medial patellar border, leaving enough soft tissue for subsequent suturing.

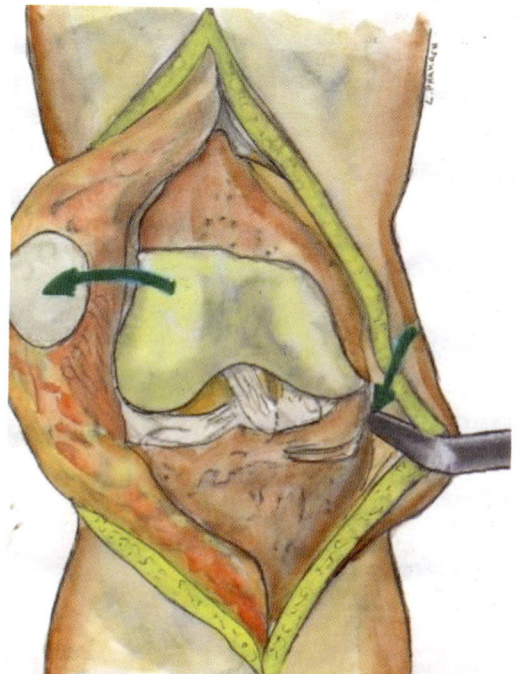

The patella is deflected laterally exposing the knee.

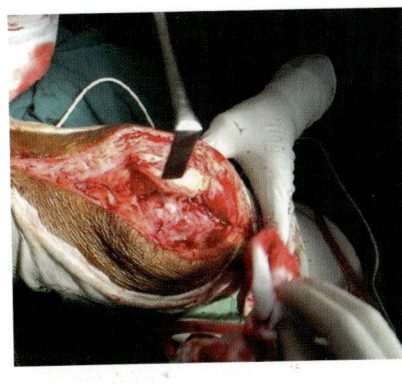

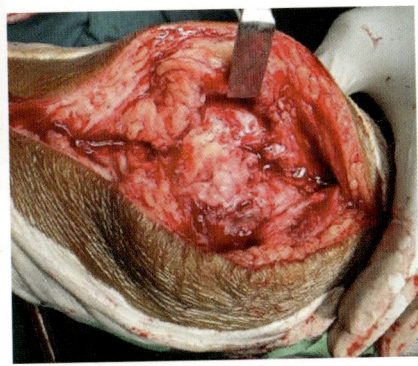

The interior of the knee is now visualized.

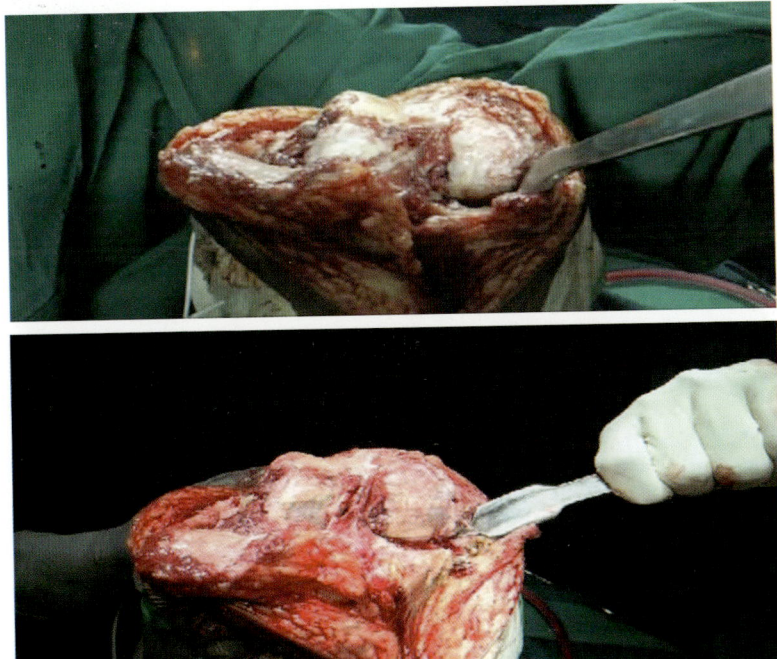

Flexion of the knee shifts the patella further laterally and gives a decent exposure.

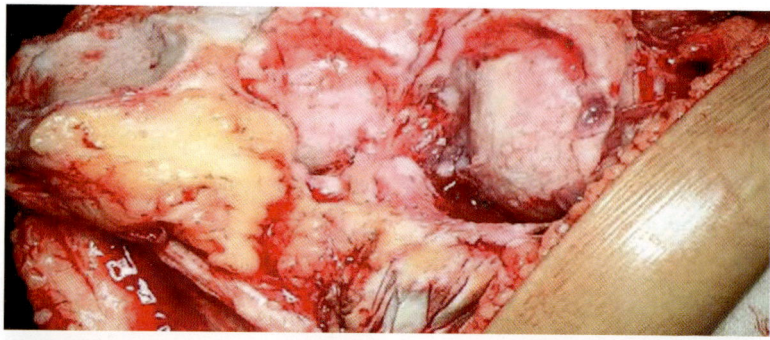

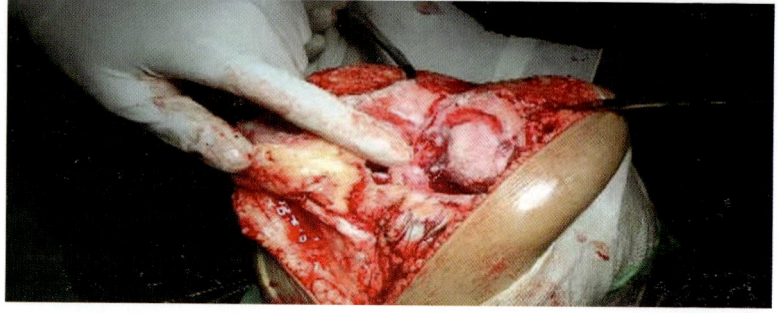

The anterior cruciate is invariably present even in the most damaged osteoarthritic knees, while they are damaged and frayed in rheumatoids.

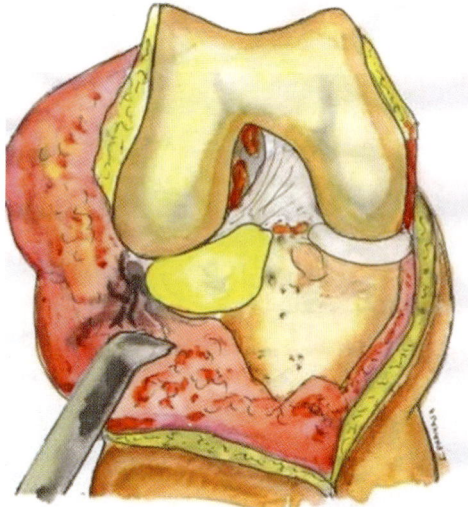

Anterior translation of tibia stretches the ACL.

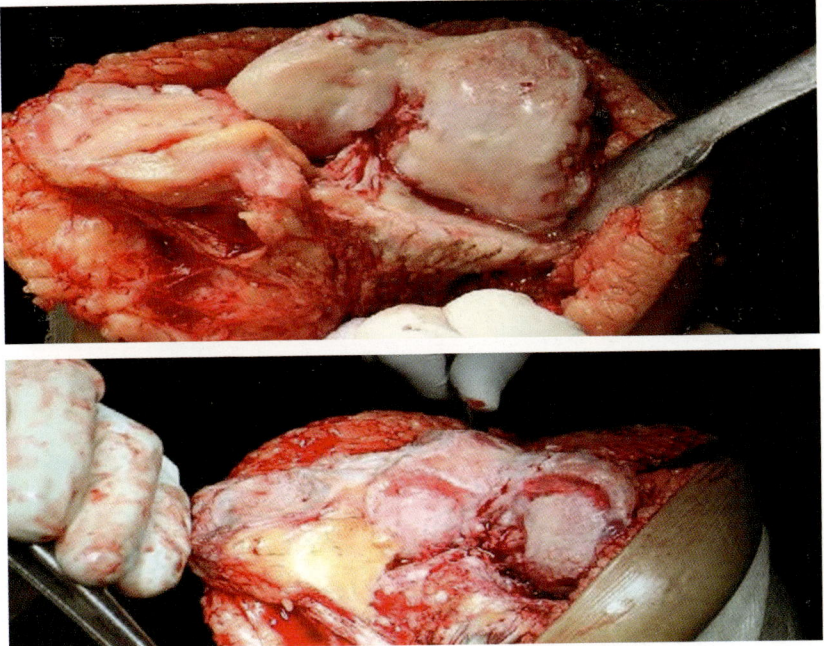

Judicious placement of Hohmann retractors allows good visualization of knee interior.

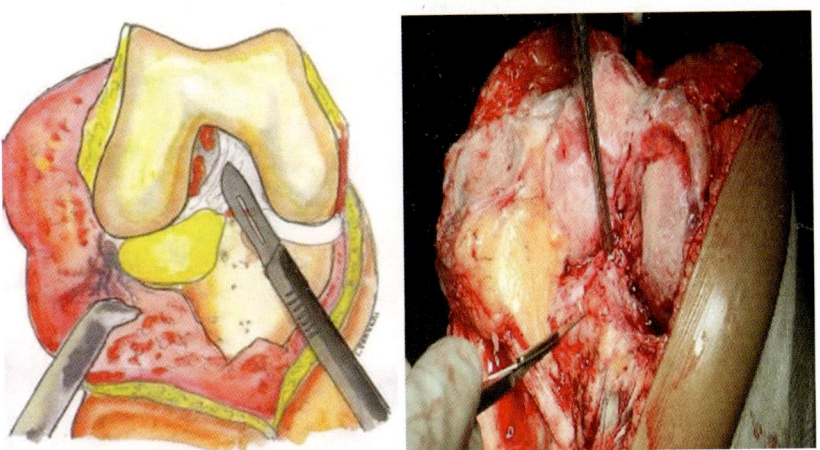

The anterior cruciate is excised.

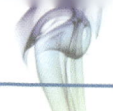

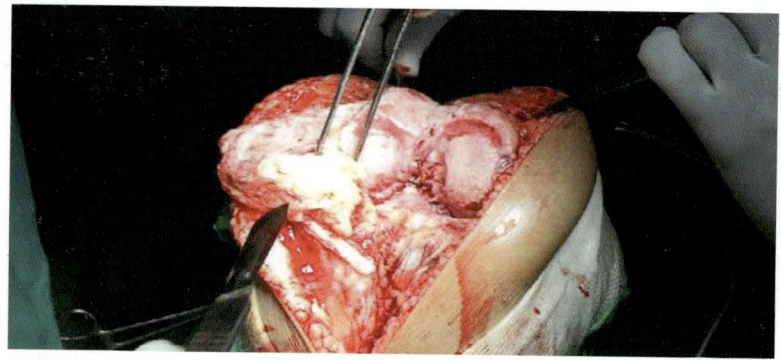

Excision of anterior cruciate and infrapatellar fat pad facilitates full anterior translation of tibia, essential for proper instrumentation.

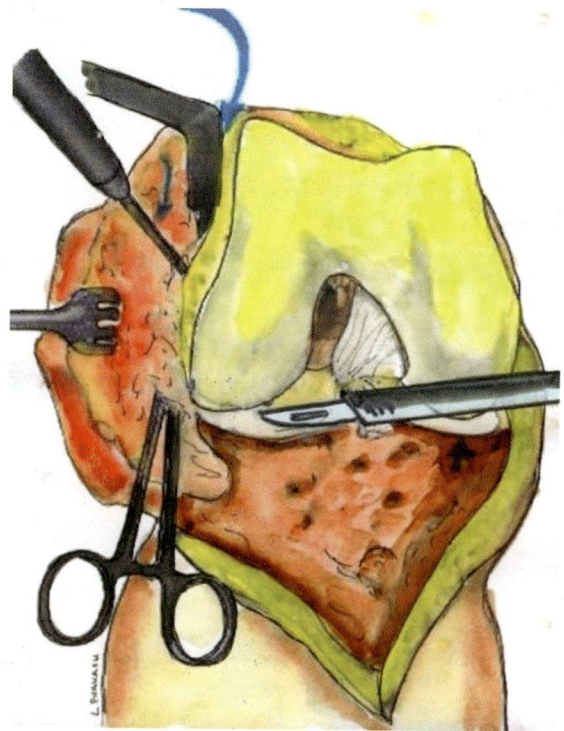

Both menisci are excised.

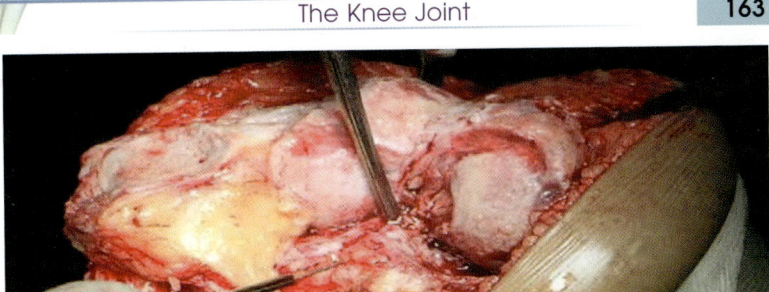

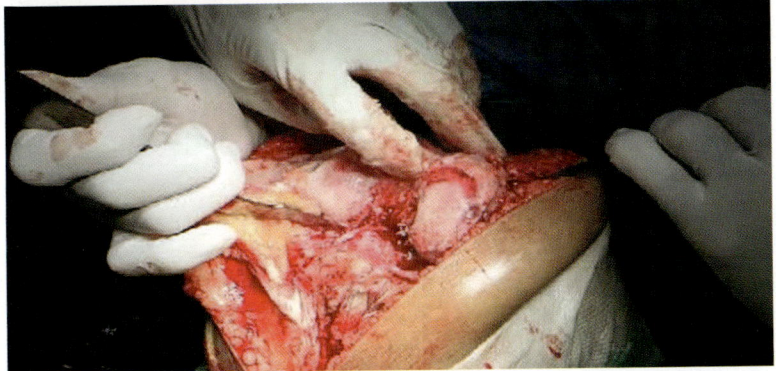

Depending on the compartment involved, meniscus on one side is usually more damaged than the other.

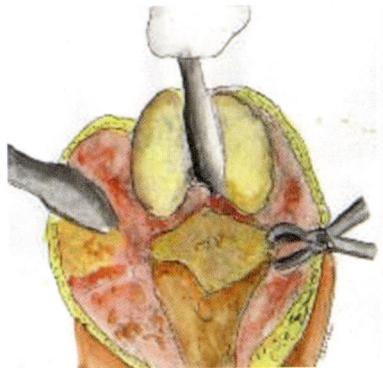

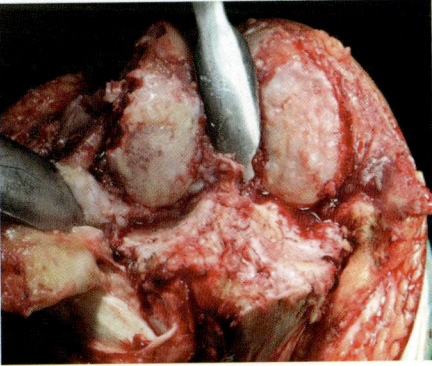

A Hohmann retractor in the intercondylar area pulls the tibia well forward, providing a decent view of the knee interior.

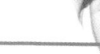

Indications:
- Primary knee replacement.
- Revision knee replacement.
- Replacement for tumours by custom prosthesis.
- Joint debridement.
- Anterior synovectomy.

The Swashbuckler's Approach

This is a modified anterolateral approach to the distal femur. This is actually nothing but a minor modification of the Ruedi approach, described earlier.

This approach was also used for TKR in severe valgus knees in the early stages by Freeman, Goodellow, and others, but was later abandoned in favour of Insall's direct anterior approach.

The trick of this incision is developing full thickness skin flaps from the lateral edge of the tibial tubercle, to the superolateral corner of the patella. Flaps are developed to visualise the lateral patellar retinaculum.

The approach allows surgical exposure of the entire articular surface of the distal femur.

The quadriceps muscle bellies are spared during the approach.

The skin incision used does not interfere with subsequent total knee arthroplasty, if post-traumatic arthritis develops and arthroplasty is necessary.

This approach was first described by Starr, and later modified by Beltran *et al*, who shortened the incision restricting it to the knee joint, and called it a Modified Swashbuckler's approach.

Access: Provides an almost complete view of the lower femur including both condyles, the under surface of patella, the menisci and the upper surface of tibia.

Positioning: Supine on the operating table with a sandbag under the buttock to keep the hip in neutral rotation.

If a tourniquet is used, it should be applied high up and one should ensure that this does not interfere with full flexion and extension of the knee.

Limb is prepared from groin to ankle. A high triangular sandbag is kept under the knee to place it in thirty degrees of flexion.

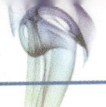

The upper drapers are as high as the pathology requires, stopping at the tourniquet level, if it is used.

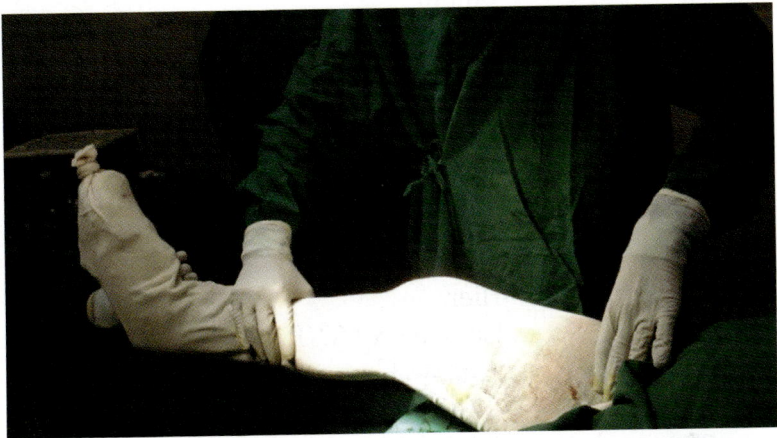

The foot and ankle are covered with thin drapes, to allow identification of al toes under the drape.

As the knee is usually repeatedly flexed and extended during the course of surgery, the drapes should be secure and the operating area should be isolated with an adhesive opsite.

A stockinette can be rolled from the foot right up to the tourniquet. This is cut in the midline anteriorly, spread to both sides of patella and anchored with an adhesive steri drape.

The incision: I will first describe a mini-Swashbuckler approach which can then be extended to a full blown Swashbuckler's approach, if situations necessitate it.

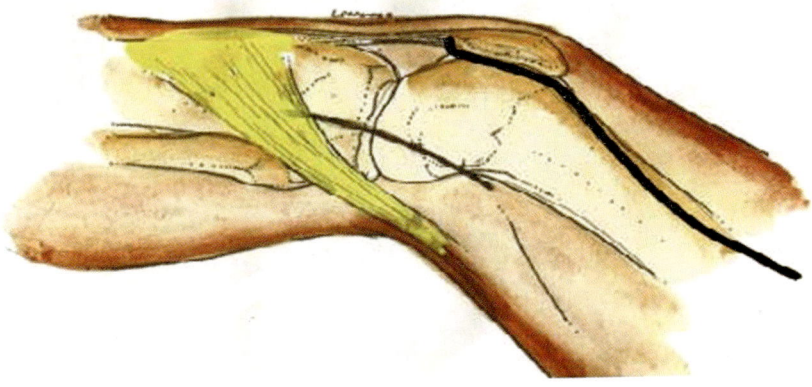

In mini-Swashbuckler approach, a 12 cm incision is made extending from the lateral edge of the tibial tubercle to the superolateral corner of the patella.

Sharp dissection is then used to develop full thickness skin flaps. Flaps are developed only enough to visualise the underlying lateral patellar retinaculum.

A trapezoidal shaped incision through the retinaculum is then used to gain access to the knee joint.

This incision begins distally at the lateral edge of the patellar tendon, and extends proximal along the lateral margin of the patella before being carried laterally across the retinaculum at the distal end of the vastus lateralis muscle belly.

Four sequential steps are then utilised to gain improved access to the distal femur.

First, the patellar tendon is bluntly swept off the retropatellar fat pad with finger dissection, and an Army-Navy retractor placed to protect the tendon.

Second, the entire fat pad and synovial reflection is excised en bloc to the level of the intermeniscal ligament, taking care to protect the menisci and the intermeniscal ligament.

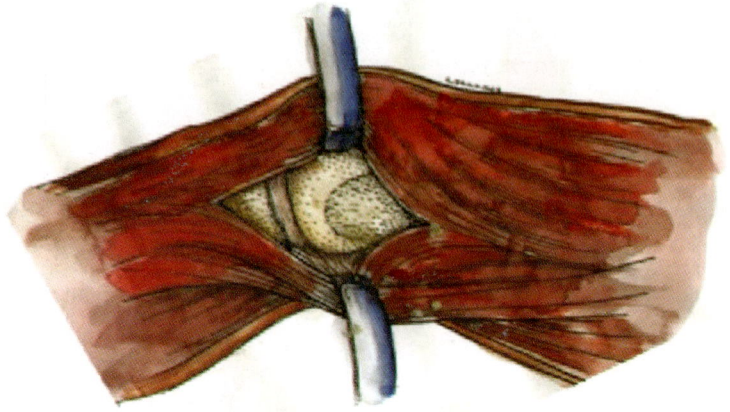

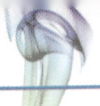
The third step involves ensuring complete release of the retinaculum distally to the tibial tubercle.

Finally, the superior retinaculum is released proximally enough to gain access to the suprapatellar pouch.

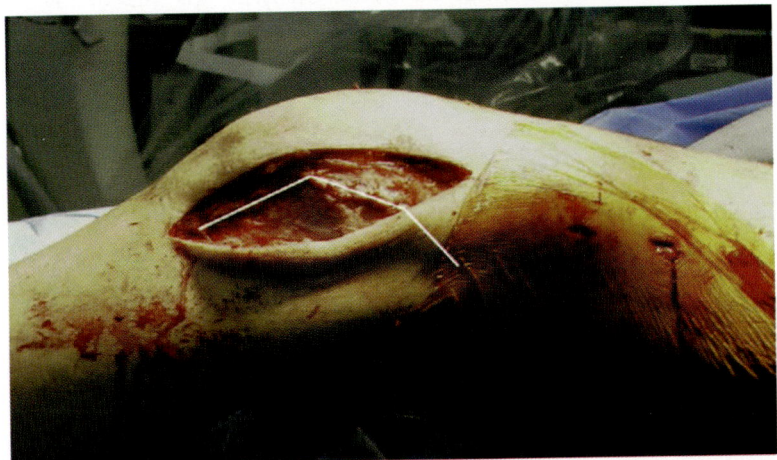

Two sharp Hohmann retractors are then placed to improve exposure. The first Hohmann retractor is placed through the medial capsule, just over the medial meniscus on to the medial proximal tibia and aids in retraction of the patella. The second Hohmann retractor is placed across the suprapatellar pouch.

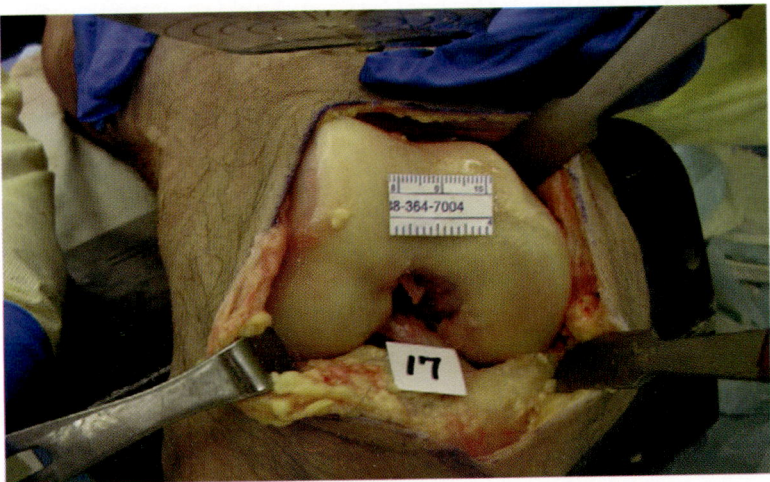

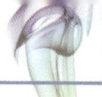

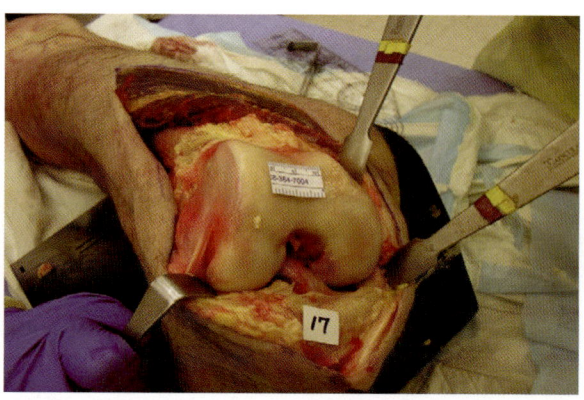

At this point, the mini-Swashbuckler exposure is complete.

The traditional extensile Swashbuckler approach is performed by extending the incision proximally in a longitudinal fashion to a length of 30 cm or more.

The length of the femoral incision depends upon the pathology.

For the deep dissection, the vastus fascia is incised in line with the skin incision and elevated off the underlying vastus lateralis until the intermuscular septum.

Using a Cobb elevator, the vastus lateralis muscle belly is elevated off the intermuscular septum.

Two additional Hohmann retractors are then placed across the femoral shaft and the muscle belly is retracted medially.

If an accessory genu articularis muscle is present, this is mobilised off the distal femoral shaft and also retracted medially.

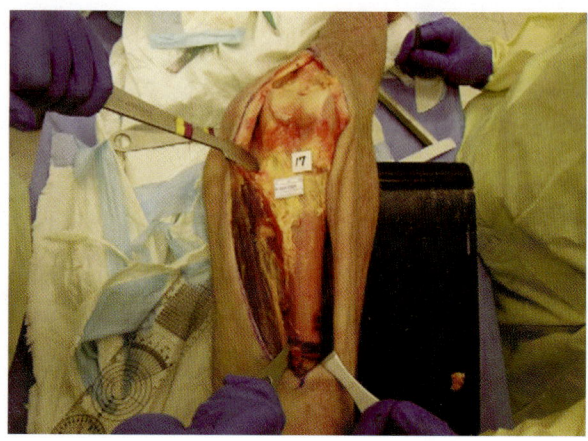

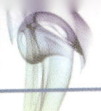

The following intraoperative pictures show the sequence in a patient in whom a comminuted supracondylar femoral fracture is being fixed.

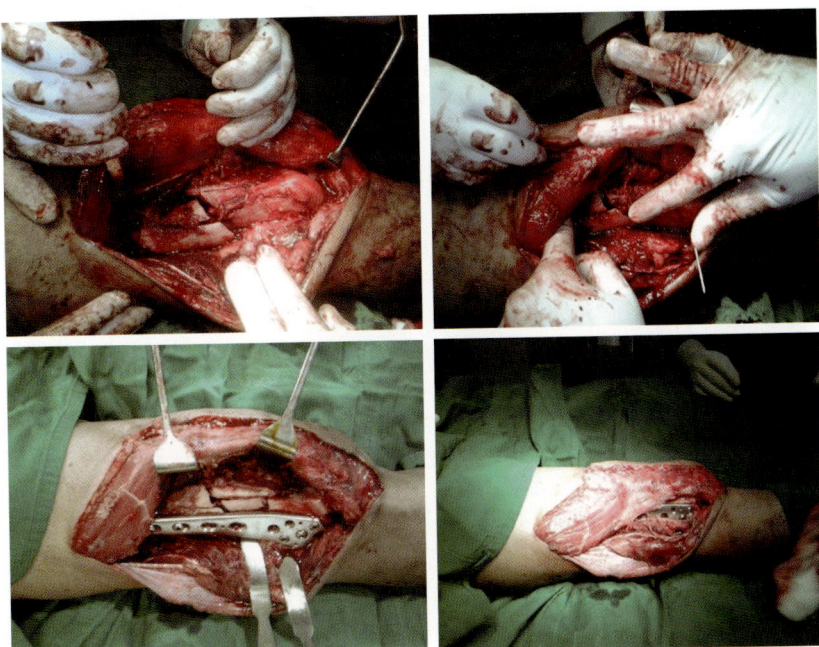

Indications:
- Intra-articular fractures of the distal femoral condyle.
- Supracondylar and associated shaft fractures.

Posterior Approach to the Knee Joint

This approach has been described by Brackett and Osgood, Putti, and Abbot.

Before we discuss the approach, it would be appropriate to learn something about the greats who have contributed to the posterior approaches to the knee joint.

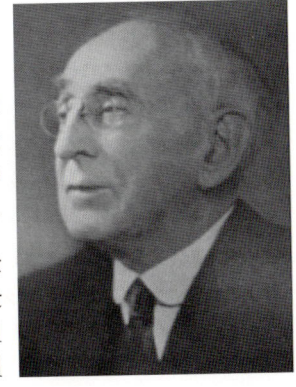

Elliott Gray Brackett (1860–1942): Whilst still in medical school, young Brackett was afflicted with Pott's spine and confined to bed for a year, at Harvard

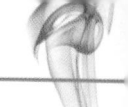

Medical School, where Dr Edward H. Bradford took care of him through this illness. This probably made him decide to be an orthopaedic surgeon.

Even while in the hospital, he completed his medical course in time, by asking his classmates to bring the lecture notes to his hospital bed. In 1886, he received an internship at the Boston City Hospital, and although he was on crutches, he did not miss a day of service. These facts have a bearing on the way he handled his patients and dealt with many difficult situations. He never gave up.

Dr Brackett was elected editor of *The Journal of Orthopaedic Surgery* in 1921, which later became *The Journal of Bone and Joint Surgery*.

When he took over the editorship, the *Journal* had not progressed very far beyond the early stage of its development. In those times, it was the convention that all papers read at scientific sessions of the Association be published. It often happened that under this rule, papers that were not worthy of the journal were also published.

Early in his administration, Brackett initiated the appointment of a group of local and foreign editors who added to the national and international character of the *Journal*, a matter that was always very much in Dr Brackett's mind, for he believed that such a publication could be a real factor in the development of better understanding and closer cooperation between nations.

When Dr Brackett became editor, the total list of subscribers numbered 797. At the time of his death, the number of paid subscriptions was over 3,500. During the 20 years of his editorship, the budget of the *Journal* was increased eightfold.

For the first five years that Dr Brackett had charge of the *Journal*, he provided office space in his own house. He never received salary for his work; when the Association members made the first attempt to show their appreciation of his services in the form of an honorarium, he persuaded the Executive Committee to put the sum into a fund to be used at the discretion of the editor to defray the expense of illustrations.

At the end of the Spanish–American War in July 1898, he was sent to Cuba as representative of the Massachusetts Volunteer Aid Association. His assignment was to receive supplies sent on hospital ships and to determine the needs of the men. His first concern was for the sick among the troops ready to be evacuated to the United States and he made provision for their care on transports. Then, at the request of General Wood, he took charge of a hospital in Santiago and also organized work for the care of the sick in the city, where serious epidemics had developed.

He also visited China and Russia on many occasions as a representative of the orthopaedic community of the western world. He was one of the earliest to desribe the posterior approach to the knee joint.

Vittorio Putti (1880–1940): Vittorio Putti was professor in the University of Bologna, surgeon-in-chief of the Istituto Ortopedico Rizzoli, a founder of the Société Internationale de Chirurgie Orthopédique et de Traumatologie and president of its 1936 Congress, Honorary Member of the British Orthopaedic Association, the American Orthopaedic Association, Corresponding Member of the American Academy of Orthopaedic Surgeons, and many other 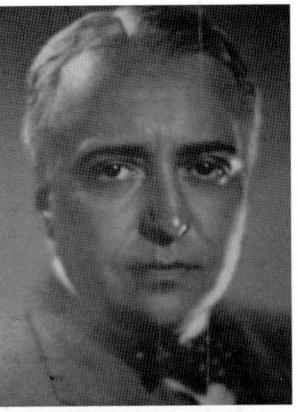 national organizations. He was a bibliographer, medical historian, orthopaedic investigator, and teacher of surgeons. He had been a foreign editor of The Journal of Bone and Joint Surgery since January 1928.

Bologna was a Roman city. The Cathedral of San Pietro e San Paolo, built in part from the Roman remains, was erected in the fourth century. The city has long been a seat of learning, and legends attribute the founding of the famous University of Bologna to Theodosius the Great in 425 AD.

The Istituto Ortopedico Rizzoli is situated on a hill on the outskirts of this fascinating old city and occupies the picturesque buildings of a Benedictine monastery known as San Michele in Bosco. The early years of this institute for crippled children were not noteworthy, until Alessandro Codivilla, modest and skillful master, became its director and surgeon-in-chief. This great

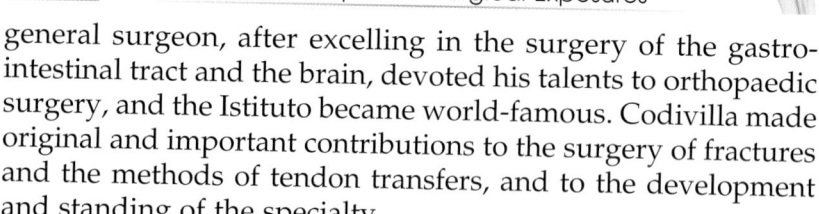

general surgeon, after excelling in the surgery of the gastro-intestinal tract and the brain, devoted his talents to orthopaedic surgery, and the Istituto became world-famous. Codivilla made original and important contributions to the surgery of fractures and the methods of tendon transfers, and to the development and standing of the specialty.

At his death in 1912, Codivilla was succeeded by Vittorio Putti, the son of a well-known surgeon who was for many years professor of surgery in the University of Bologna. Putti had first become identified with the Istituto Ortopedico Rizzoli in 1903, when Codivilla had appointed him as an assistant. Following two years of study in European clinics, he returned to the institution in 1909 as Vice-Director, and in 1914 became director and surgeon-in-chief of the Istituto. He was also professor of orthopaedic surgery at the University of Bologna.

In 1922, Putti opened the country branch, which provided for the care of 100 cases of surgical tuberculosis, and as director of this hospital (Istituto dio terapico Codivilla di Corona d'Ampezzo) in the Dolomites, he found frequent escape from his very strenuous city life.

A brilliant student, a wide reader, an able administrator, a resourceful and skilful surgeon with a mechanical bent, he enhanced the reputation of the Istituto Rizzoli, and like Codivilla, made lasting contributions to the history of medicine and to the technique of orthopaedic surgery.

In addition to being a tireless and exacting trainer of young surgeons, Putti encouraged his associates to become familiar with the history of medicine and the contributory sciences, to strive for exactitude in thought and action, and to appreciate beauty, not only of art and nature, but of character. His sanctum sanctorum, which he shared with his helpers, was the library (La Biblioteca Umberto I). On the walls of this dignified room are the same beautiful frescoes, executed by Canuti, that had given joy to the monks, and on its shelves are books and manuscripts covering a period of over 400 years.

By his numerous original contributions he became an international leader, a pioneer and an authority on bone and joint surgery, especially on congenital dislocation of the hip, its preluxation stage and its automatic reduction by the divaricatore,

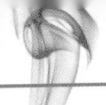

arthritis, arthroplasty, "sciatica", the forcible manipulation of adult club feet, the open treatment of fractures and the use of skeletal traction and metal fixation, the equalization of leg lengths by bone lengthening, spinal anomalies, cineplastic amputations and artificial limbs, and the surgical treatment of the residual effects of poliomyelitis.

He published many monographs, not only on strictly medical and surgical subjects, but also on nonmedical subjects; as well as translations of old medical works. His large quarto, "Berengario da Carpi," published in 1937, represents not only a profound and extensive piece of research, but the best biographical study of this great surgeon and anatomist, who antedates Vesalius. This work alone places him among the great medical historians. His latest volume, pulished in 1940, is entitled "Cura operatoria delle fratture del collo del femore."

His titles were too numerous to mention, for he was a corresponding, honorary, or active member of most of the orthopaedic societies of the world. His honours included civilian, medical, surgical, military, and academic recognition. He received from the King the title of Grand Officiali of the Crown of Italy.

He was one of the earliest to describe the posterior approach to the knee joint.

Robert Bayley Osgood (1873–1956): Robert Osgood was born in Salem, Massachusetts, July 6, 1873, the son of John Christopher and Martha Ellen (Whipple) Osgood. Following an education in the public schools of Salem, Robert Osgood was admitted to Amherst College, from which he was graduated in 1895 after the usual classical training in Greek, Latin, and English literature.

Osgood was granted his degree from Harvard Medical School in 1899. During his last year in medical school, he served as a student intern at the House of the Good Samaritan. This institution was devoted to the care of patients with chronic diseases; at that time, it was to a large extent filled with

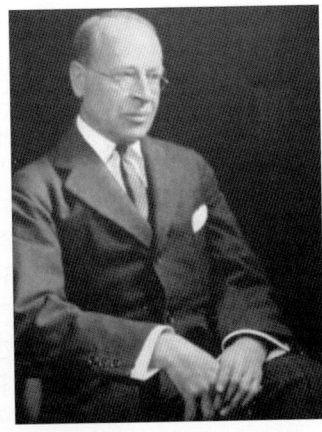

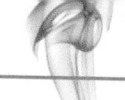

tubercular patients, of which many had tuberculous joint disease. Undoubtedly, it was from assisting such orthopaedic surgeons as Edward Bradford, Elliott Brackett, and Joel E. Goldthwait in the care of these patients that he became interested in orthopaedic surgery. Following graduation, he served a surgical internship at the Massachusetts General Hospital.

At that time, the first machines for clinical roentgenographic study were introduced, following Roentgen's great discovery of X-rays in 1895. After finishing his internship, Osgood's first hospital appointment was that of a radiologist at the Boston Children's Hospital in 1902 and 1903. It was while working there that he made the observations on the growth and traumatic disturbances of the tibial tubercle during adolescence, which were published in a paper on January 29, 1903. These lesions have since become known as Osgood-Schlatter disease, Schlatter having at a later date also described the condition.

In 1903, Robert Osgood went to study in Germany, France, and England; in England, he made the acquaintance of Hugh Owen Thomas and his nephew Robert Jones, whose work made a deep impression on him.

With the development of an orthopaedic inpatient service at the Massachusetts General Hospital in 1911, following the successful efforts of Dr Goldthwait in raising funds to build Ward I, Bob Osgood's clinical work was centred in the Massachusetts General Hospital. At about this time, he became instructor of surgery at the Harvard Medical School.

Upon returning to Boston and upon the retirement of Dr Elliott Brackett, Bob Osgood was promoted to head of the orthopaedic service of the Massachusetts General Hospital. His weekly orthopaedic rounds were stellar performances, not so much because of what he said, but because of the opportunity he offered to all staff members for full discussion.

In 1922, Bob Osgood left the Massachusetts General Hospital and became Chief of the Orthopaedic Service at the Boston Children's Hospital; this carried with it the title of Professor of Orthopaedic Surgery at the Harvard Medical School.

His former pupils and associates combined on the occasion of his 70th birthday to publish in the Archives of Surgery, a special number dedicated to him; in the following year another

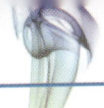
group of pupils and associates united to arrange for the painting of his portrait by Mr Samuel Hopkinson. This excellent work now hangs in the Massachusetts General Hospital.

Robert Bayley Osgood died on October 2, 1956, in Boston, at the age of 83.

He was one of the early pioneers to describe the posterior approach to the knee joint.

Access
- Posterior capsule of knee joint
- Posterior aspects of femoral condyles
- Posterior aspect of tibial condyles
- Posterior compartment of knee
- Posterior half of menisci
- Posterior cruciate ligament
- Pusterior neurovascular bundle

Position
- Prone position
- Sandbag under iliac spines
- Cushion to allow free abdomen
- Tourniquet is applied as high as possible.

Incision: The incision begins posteromedially about 7.5 cm above the knee joint over the belly of semitendinosus muscle.

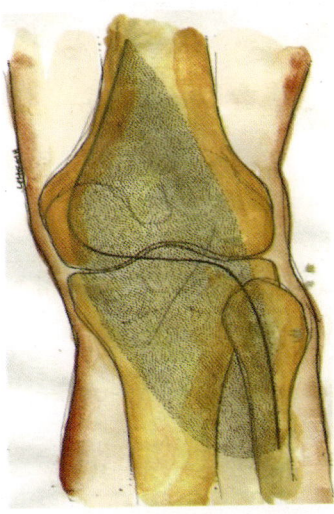

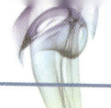

The incision is brought down straight over the tendon of semitendinosus right up to the knee joint level.

It then traverses laterally at the level of the joint line up to the lateral gastrocnemius.

The incision then descends down laterally over the lateral belly of gastrocnemius for another 7.5 to 10 cm, as shown in the drawings.

Deep incisions and approach: The skin and superficial fascia are cut in the line of the incision.

The deep fascia is split in a linear fashion to expose the popliteal fossa.

The short saphenous vein and the sural nerve are identified, as they exit between the two heads of gastrocnemius.

The sural nerve is delicately followed upwards as it emerges from the tibial nerve.

Once the tibial nerve has been identified, it is gently dissected to expose its branches to soleus, plantaris, and the two heads of gastrocnemius muscle.

The vessels accompanying these branches are also carefully identified and protected. All dissections at this stage should be blunt and the neurovascular structures must be handled extremely delicately.

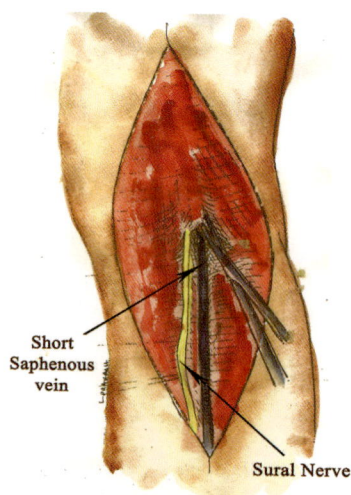

Short Saphenous vein

Sural Nerve

The tibial nerve is followed up gently till it joins the common peroneal nerve and begins ascending as the sciatic nerve.

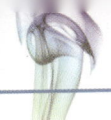

The common peroneal nerve is now exposed and followed down along the medial border of biceps. Care should be taken to avoid damage to the lateral cutaneous nerve of the calf.

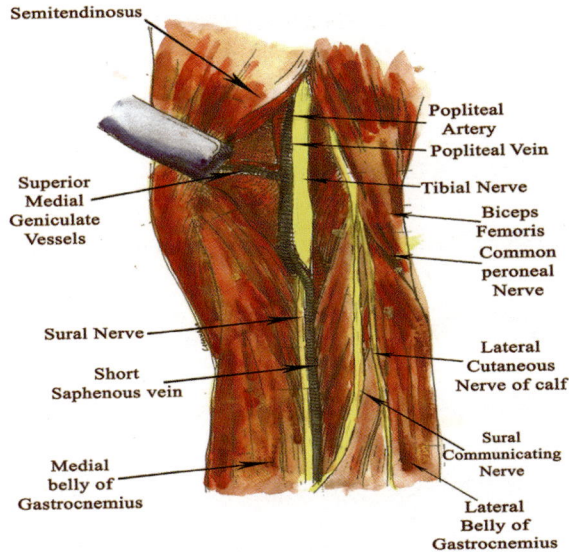

At this stage, it is possible to identify the popliteal artery and vein.

The neurovascular bundle is gently retracted to locate the superior genicular vessels. They pass beneath the hamstrings.

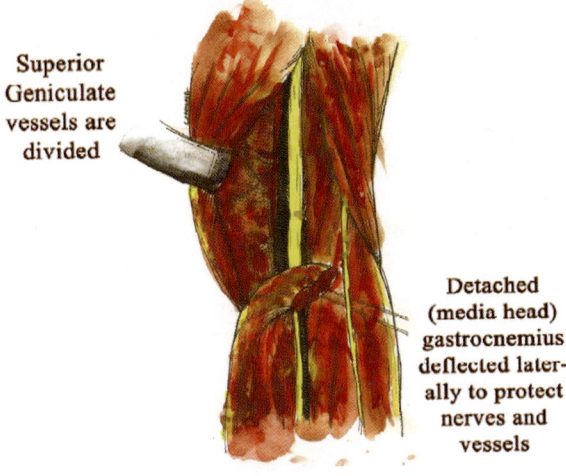

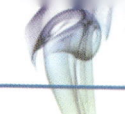

The next step is detaching the medial head of gastrocnemius, close to its origin, leaving a decent amount of tissue for re-attachment.

The medial head of gastrocnemius is now deflected laterally to protect and retract the vessels and nerves.

Now most of the posterior aspect of knee joint can be visualized, and if additional lateral exposure is required, the lateral head of gastrocnemius too is detached.

Care must be taken to protect the lateral popliteal nerve.

Indications

1. Trauma and fractures to the posterior aspect of lower femur or upper tibia.
2. Tibial spine fractures including avulsion of posterior cruciate ligament.
3. Tumours or tumorous conditions of this area.
4. Pathologies of posterior knee capsule.

Anteromedial and Posteromedial Approaches

Access

1. Medial ligament
2. Posteromedial capsule
3. Posterior oblique ligament
4. Posterior cruciate ligament

The approaches allow for exposure of both popliteal fossa and anterior knee joint by the anteromedial approach and to the popliteal fossa alone in the posteromedial approach.

Position and draping: The patient is placed supine with a sand-bag under the buttock.

A high tourniquet is applied.

The leg is draped free and bulky drapes are avoided to allow feeling of the foot direction under the drapes.

One must be able to freely flex and extend the knee after draping.

Incision: With the leg in full external rotation, the knee is flexed to about 50°.

The surgeon operates from the opposite side so that the medial aspect of posteromedial knee is in view.

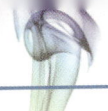
The anteromedial incision is made in front of the level of long saphenous vein.

The curved incision has its apex about 2.5 cm medial to the patella, and the incision extends about 8.0 cm proximally and distally.

This incision will not only expose the popliteal fossa, but will also allow anterior arthrotomy.

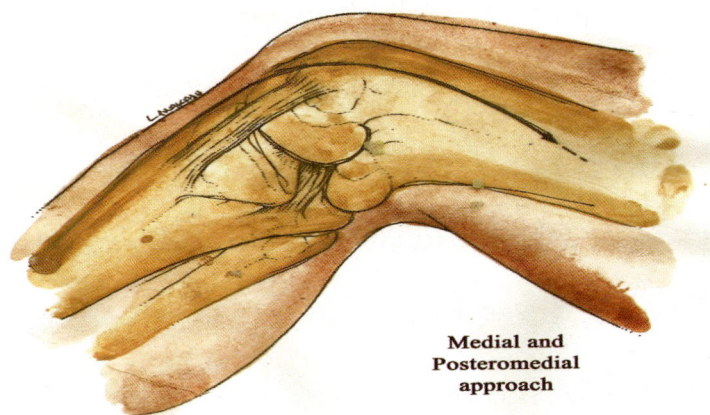

**Medial and
Posteromedial
approach**

The posteromedial incision is similar in length but is well posterior to the saphenous vein and nerve.

The apex of this incision's curvature will lie at the posterior border of medial femoral condyle.

**Medial tibial
collateral
ligament**

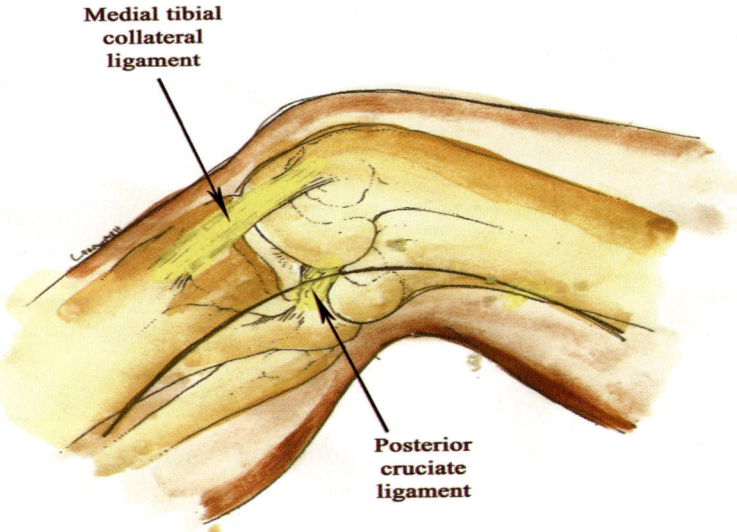

**Posterior
cruciate
ligament**

Proximally the incision is over the semimembranosus, while distally it is posterior to the medial border of tibia as shown in the diagram below.

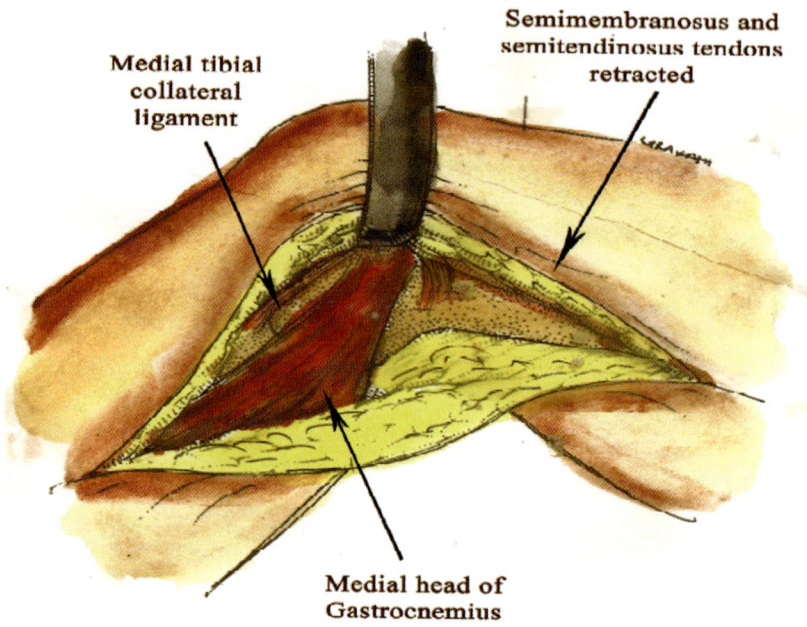

Medial tibial collateral ligament

Semimembranosus and semitendinosus tendons retracted

Medial head of Gastrocnemius

Approach: The incision is deepened to the deep fascia; over the upper tibia, it is deepened to the bone.

In case an anterior incision is used, a thick flap of soft tissues containing the saphenous nerve and vein is retracted posteriorly as a single flap.

Once the medial tibia is reached, the tendons of semi-membranosus and semitendinosus are identified. Anterior retraction of both of these will bring the fascia into view over the medial head of gastrocnemius.

The fascia is incised in line of the muscle fibres, and the muscle is traced superiorly till its femoral attachment.

The medial head of gastrocnemius is detached close to its origin, in case exposure of the posterior cruciate ligament is needed.

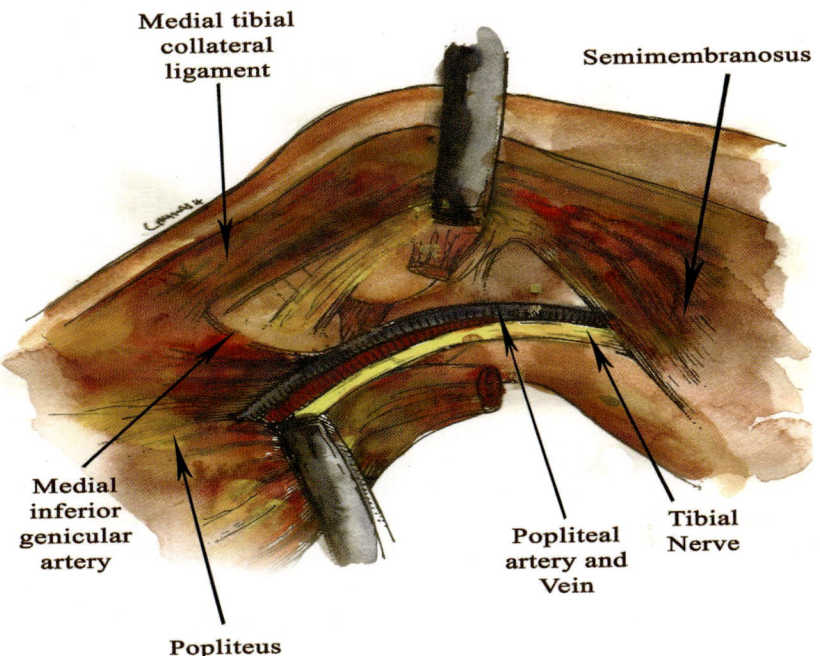

The insertion of popliteus into the tibia is now identified. At the upper border of this muscle, deep to the medial collateral ligament, the medial inferior genicular artery is located, identified and ligated.

Popliteus is now detached from the tibia, leaving sufficient tissue for reattachment, and its retraction posteriorly brings to view the plane between it and the posterior capsule of the knee joint.

The retracted popliteus protects the popliteal vessels and medial popliteal nerve.

Posterior cruciate and the posteromedial border of the upper tibia are now exposed. The posterior aspect of medial femoral condyle too is brought into view.

If the anterior curved incision is used, an anterior arthrotomy can be performed at this stage.

The medial colleteral ligament can be inspected and repaired with this exposure.

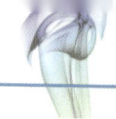

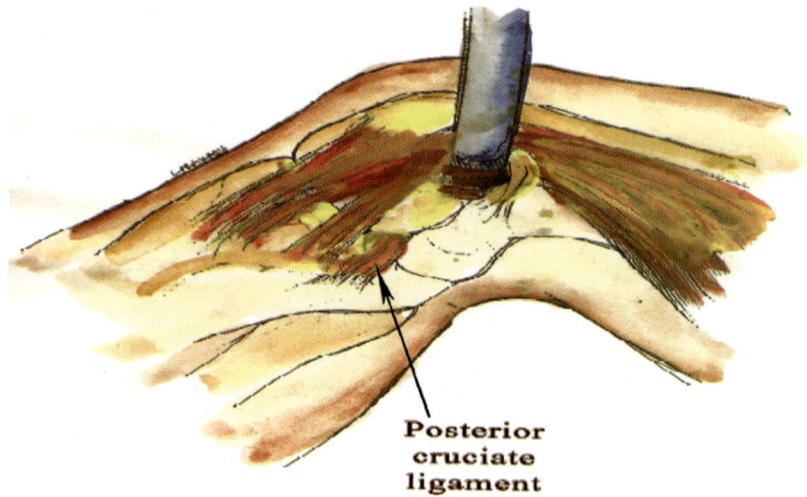

Posterior
cruciate
ligament

Indications

With the advent of arthroscopic procedures, this incision is infrequently used, but when used, its chief indications are:

1. Posterior cruciate repair or reconstruction.
2. Posterior oblique ligament repair or reconstruction.
3. Medial collateral ligament repair or reconstruction.

Lateral Approach to the Knee

History: This approach was first described by Bruser.

David M Bruser: Dr David M Bruser was born May 11, 1911, in Humboldt, SK, the son of Calman and Hinda Bruser. He completed high school at St Johns College in Winnipeg and earned a BA at the University of Manitoba. Bruser received his MD from the university in 1936, and served as a junior and senior intern in general surgery at Winnipeg General Hospital.

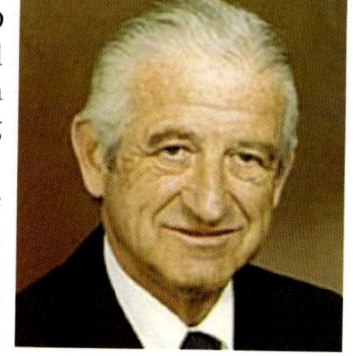

After a six-month stint in the pathology department at Stanford University in California, he returned to Winnipeg General as senior resident in surgery. Bruser received

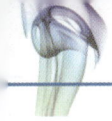
a Master of Surgery degree in 1939 and was certified by the Royal College of Physicians and Surgeons of Canada.

When the Second World War broke out, Bruser joined the Royal Canadian Air Force and served as Medical Officer at training stations in Penhold, AB and at Fort MacLeod.

He continued serving with the RCAF combined services at Deer Lodge Veterans Hospital.

Bruser was discharged in 1945 with the rank of Squadron Leader. In 1950, he took the examinations of the Royal College of Surgeons in Montreal, where he received his Fellowship in Orthopaedics. He then began practice in Winnipeg at the Mall Medical Group, which he and a group of friends and colleagues founded.

At the same time, Bruser began lecturing in orthopaedic surgery at the University of Manitoba. He held orthopaedic appointments at Winnipeg General Hospital, Misericordia General, Deer Lodge Veterans Hospital and later at the Manitoba Rehabilitation Centre. He also served as chief of orthopaedics at Misericordia General and Deer Lodge.

Bruser retired from the University of Manitoba faculty in 1978 as Associate Professor of Medicine and was elevated to the Honourary Medical Staff at the Health Sciences Centre.

He retired completely from practice in 1987. Bruser specialized in knee surgery and his article on the approach to the lateral miniscus of the knee joint, which he originated, was published in the British Journal of Orthopaedics and the definitive text book Campbell's Operative Orthopaedics.

Bruser's Lateral Approach

Access

1. Lateral compartment of the knee.
2. Complete exposure of the lateral meniscus.

The advantage of this approach is that the lateral collateral is preserved fully.

Position and draping: The patient is placed supine with a sand-bag under the buttock.

A high tourniquet is applied.

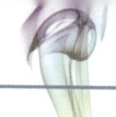

The leg is draped free and bulky drapes are avoided to allow feeling of the foot direction under the drapes.

One must be able to freely flex and extend the knee after draping.

Approach: The knee is flexed to 110°, allowing the sole to rest on the operating table.

The surgeon operates from the same side.

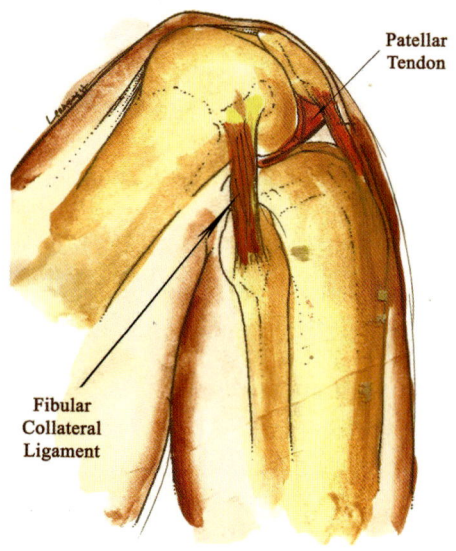

Patellar Tendon

Fibular Collateral Ligament

The incision is transverse, parallel to the knee joint line exactly at the level of the knee joint.

Beginning anteriorly at the patellar tendon, it stops just short of fibular collateral ligament posteriorly.

The subcutaneous tissue is divided in the line of the skin incision to expose the iliotibial band.

The knee is hyperflexed till the fibres of iliotibial band become parallel to the skin incision. This is the most important step of this approach.

The iliotibial band is split as far back as possible posteriorly, without damage to the lateral collateral ligament.

This brings to view the synovium and also the lateral inferior genicular artery, which lies in the plane between lateral collateral ligament and the synovium.

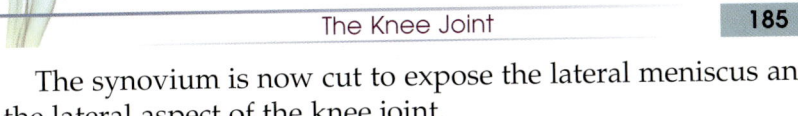

The synovium is now cut to expose the lateral meniscus and the lateral aspect of the knee joint.

Indications: Exposure of the lateral knee joint for isolated pathologies.

Lateral meniscus pathologies and their repair.

Lateral Approaches to Distal Femur and Proximal Tibia

These approaches have been described by Ruedi, von Hochsetter and Schlumpf.

These approaches are extremely useful for intra-articular and periarticular fractures around the knee. These are specially useful for bad tibial plateau fractures and lower femoral condylar injuries.

Surgeons confronted with acute trauma are frequently under great pressure to act quickly. Only a few have an infallible three-dimensional memory as regards the different approaches necessary for treating fractures by internal fixation. Thus there is a real need for a reference book on the approaches to the extremities.

This is true both for the emergency situation and for the "evening before" preoperative planning. Thomas Ruedi was one of the early AO teachers, founder members and a gifted trauma surgeon. He is also a wonderful artist and an unusual illustrator.

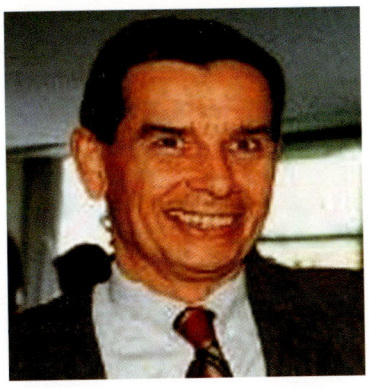

His classic book Surgical Exposures for Internal Fixation was the first to describe these approaches.

The access: The lower femoral shaft including the femoral condyles.

Detaching tibial tubercle gives a wide access to the lateral aspect of knee joint.

An extended incision allows the complete visualization of the knee joint.

Position and draping: The patient is placed supine with a sand-bag under the buttock.

A high tourniquet is applied.

The leg is draped free and bulky drapes are avoided to allow feeling of the foot direction under the drapes.

One must be able to freely flex and extend the knee after draping.

Approach: The knee is flexed to 20°, allowing the back of the heel to rest on the operating table.

The surgeon operates from the same side.

Incision: The incision is along an imaginary line beginning from the middle of trochanteric flare, decending down straight to the lateral femoral condyle, and then curving to tibial tuberosity, continuing down straight towards second toe.

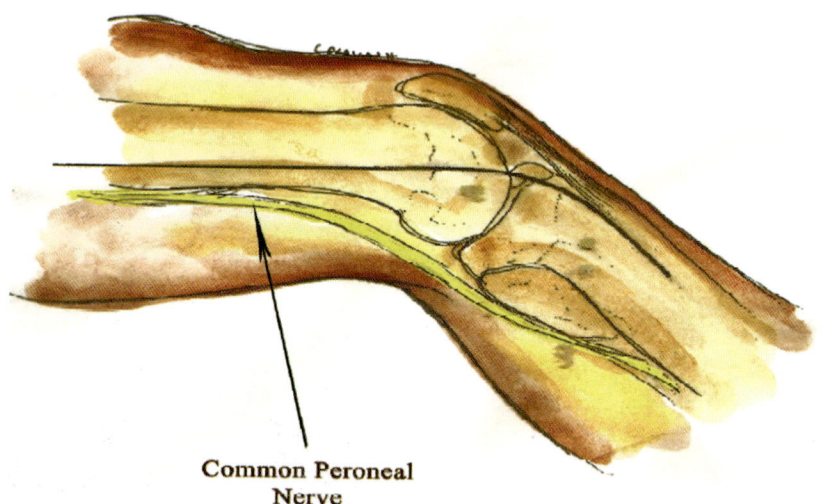

Common Peroneal Nerve

Lateral approach to Distal Femur

The exposure: Skin incision is over the line from greater trochanter to lateral epicondyle of femur and then reaching tibial tubercle.

The tensor fascia lata is split in the line of skin incision.

The vastus lateralis is identified and followed to the intermuscular septum and its attachment to the femur.

Using a periosteal elevator, the lateral intermuscular septum is erased from the femur and the vastus lateralis is deflected anteriorly.

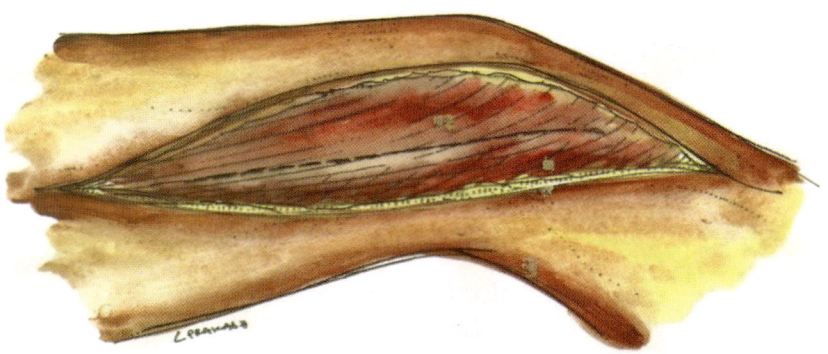

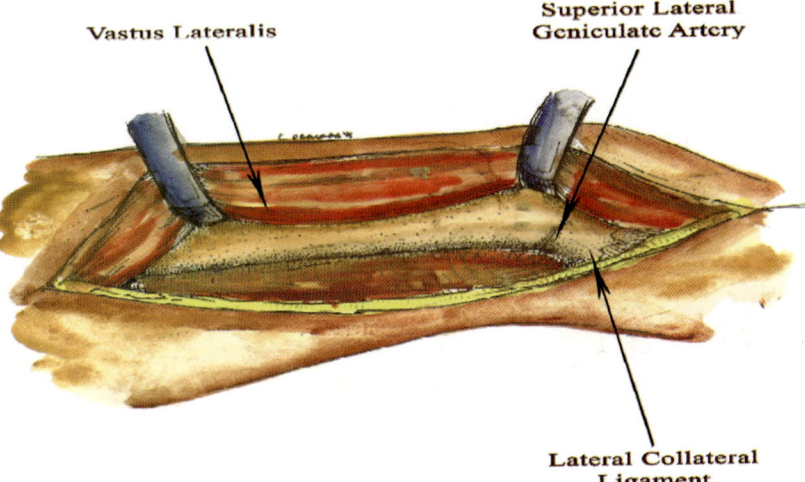

Vastus Lateralis

**Superior Lateral
Geniculate Artery**

**Lateral Collateral
Ligament**

In front of the superior attachment of lateral collateral ligament, the capsule is cut in the line of skin incision.

If the incision is to be extended proximally, then the superior lateral genicular artery and perforating vessels to the vastus lateralis are identified, and ligated.

If further exposure is needed, the incision into the capsule is continued up to the tibial tuberosity, lateral to the patellar tendon.

The tuberosity may be detached with sufficient bone for later reattachment, allowing the mobilization of patella supero-medially and bringing the infrapatellar fat pad into view.

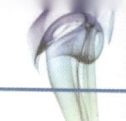

Patella Reflected

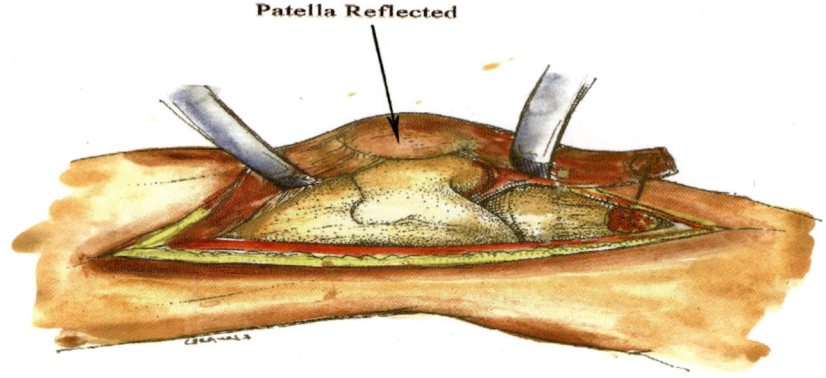

The infrapatellar fat pad is now excised to expose almost whole interior of the knee from the lateral side.

Indications

- Supracondylar femoral fractures
- Intra articular fractures
- Tibial plateau fractures
- Tumours of lower femoral shaft.

Lateral Parapatellar Approach

Ruedi, von Hochstetter and Schlumpf.

Access

- Lateral aspect of the knee
- Lateral femoral condyle
- Lateral tibial condyle and upper part of tibia
- On detachment of tibial tuberosity, this gives an almost complete exposure to the interior of the knee.

Position and draping: The patient is placed supine with a sandbag under the buttock.

A high tourniquet is applied.

The leg is draped free and bulky drapes are avoided to allow feeling of the foot direction under the drapes.

One must be able to freely flex and extend the knee after draping.

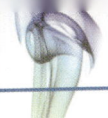

Skin incision: Straight incision about 10 to 12 cm above the patella, over the belly of vastus lateralis, continuing down to the lateral border of patella up to the tibial tuberosity.

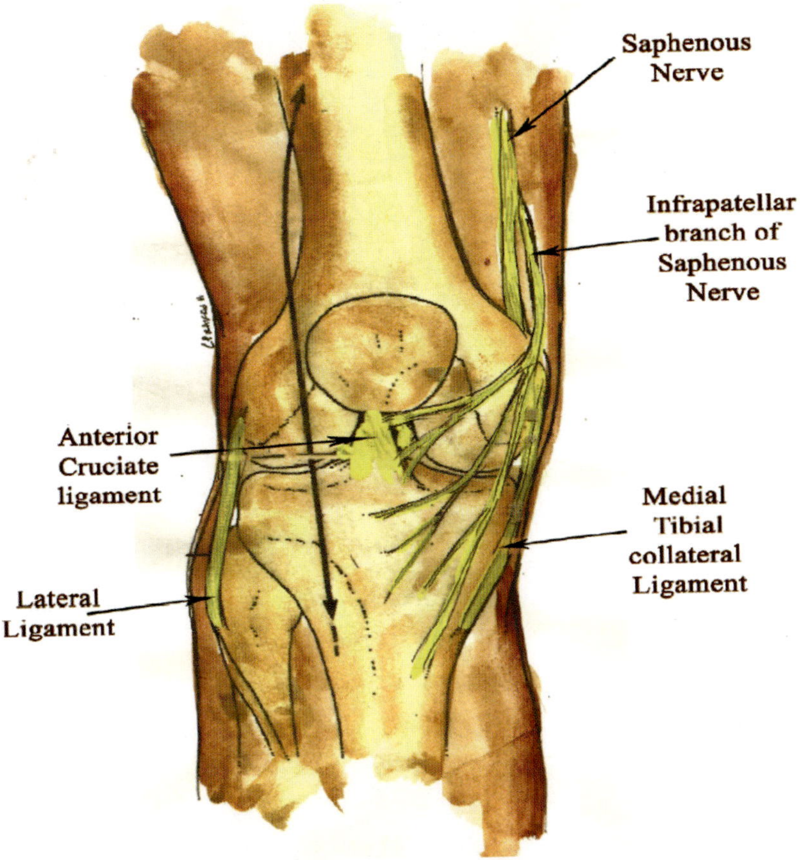

Saphenous
Nerve

Infrapatellar
branch of
Saphenous
Nerve

Anterior
Cruciate
ligament

Medial
Tibial
collateral
Ligament

Lateral
Ligament

Approach: The joint is entered from the lateral border of the patella.

Joint capsule is incised in the line of skin incision.

A sharp lateral subperiosteal dissection allows us to raise the lateral joint capsule, iliotibial band, and the tibial extensor muscles as a single flap.

The Girdy's tubercle is now detached with a sharp osteotome, and the lateral dissection to be carried posteriorly to the lateral collateral ligament.

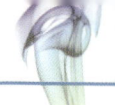

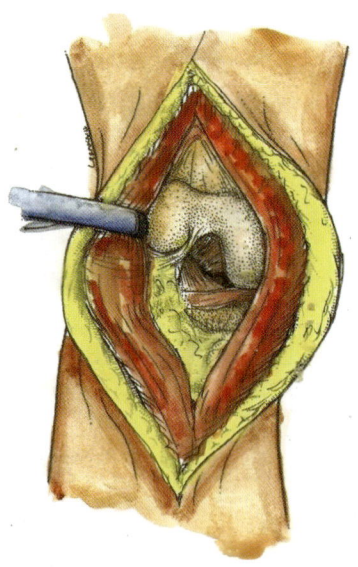

The medial aspect of the joint is now tackled. The skin flap is seperated using blunt finger dissection to expose the medial belly of quadriceps.

A medial parapatellar incision is now made, and the patella is dislocated laterally to visualize the interior of almost the whole knee joint.

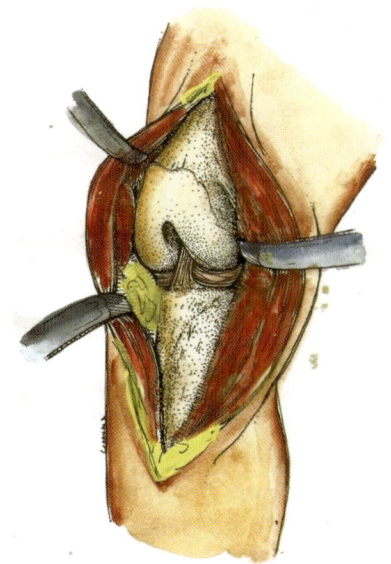

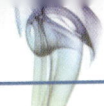

The medial capsule is now freed from the upper tibia by sharp dissection.

In case there is a need for exposure of proximal third of tibia, the pes anserinus tendon is detached with a thin sliver of bone, to facilitate reattachment during closure.

Indications

- Trauma to upper tibia, especially complex intra-articular fractures.
- Cruciate and collateral repairs.
- Tumours and other pathology of proximal tibia.

Posterior Approaches to the Knee

Both the posteromedial and posterolateral approaches to the knee have been described by Melvin Starkey Henderson.

Melvin Starkey Henderson (1883–1954): Dr Melvin Starkey Henderson was born in St Paul, Minnesota in 1883. He received his early schooling in St Paul and later in Winnipeg, Manitoba. He received the degree of MB from the University of Toronto in 1906, and the degree of MD from the same institution in 1914.

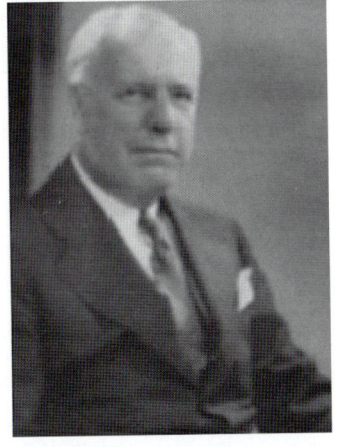

He went to Rochester to work as clinical assistant to the Mayo brothers. His interest in their work and the development of the Mayo Clinic never lagged from that time until his death.

During 1909–1911, Dr Henderson worked as a surgical assistant to Dr William J Mayo and his colleagues.

In 1910, Dr Henderson felt that a section devoted to this specialty should be formed in the rapidly growing group. His idea found approval soon.

Recognizing the developing specialty of orthopaedic surgery, the Mayo brothers sent Dr Henderson to Liverpool to work under Sir Robert Jones and to visit Sir Harold Stiles in Edinburgh during 1911.

He returned to Rochester and resumed charge of organizing and directing the section of orthopaedic surgery at the Mayo Clinic.

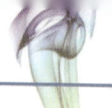

Dr Henderson contributed much to the growing specialty of orthopaedic surgery. His outstanding efforts were in the treatment of fractures, particularly bone-grafting procedures for un-united fractures and for fractures of the neck of the femur. He also developed an operation for the treatment of recurrent dislocation of the shoulder, which became widely recognized. He wrote many papers on internal derangements of the knee joint and other orthopaedic subjects.

His creed might be quoted from his own Presidential Address to the American Orthopaedic Association in 1934: "We as specialists must ever be on the alert to acquire knowledge pertaining to our specialty, and to assimilate, digest, and make use of new facts, thus acquiring that elusive something called wisdom."

Dr Henderson died on June 17, 1954.

Posteromedial Approach

Access: Limited access to the posteromedial compartment of the knee.

Position and draping: The patient is placed supine with a sandbag under the buttock.

A high tourniquet is applied.

The leg is draped free and bulky drapes are avoided to allow feeling of the foot direction under the drapes.

One must be able to freely flex and extend the knee after draping.

Approach: The knee is flexed to 90°, allowing the back of the heel to rest on the operating table.

The surgeon operates from the opposite side.

Incision: From the adductor tubercle to the tibial attachment of the medial collateral ligament.

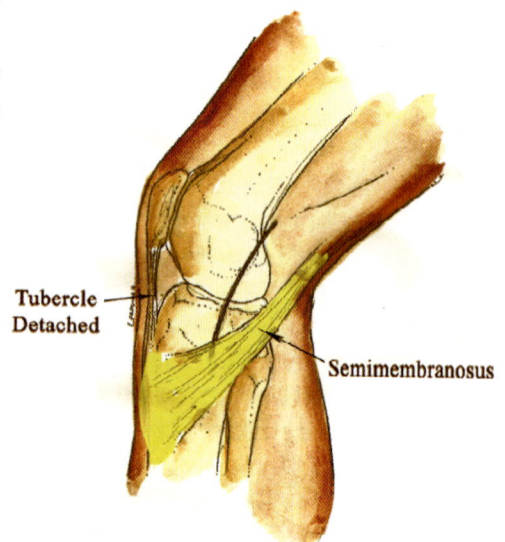

Tubercle Detached

Semimembranosus

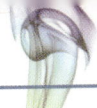

The incision is slightly curved, the convexity anteriorly.

The incision follows the posterior margin of the medial collateral ligament relaxed in 90° of flexion.

The medial hamstrings are relaxed and fall out of the way.

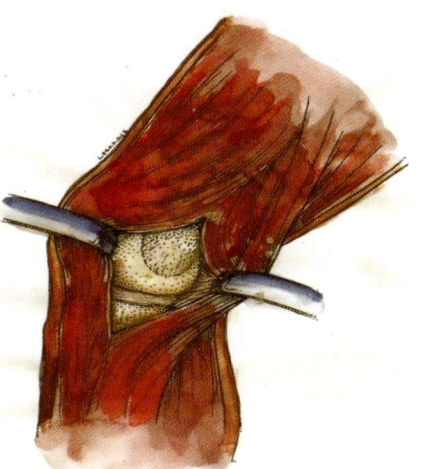

Approach: The fibres of medial collateral ligaments are identified running more or less parallel to the skin incision.

The ligament is incised in line of the skin incision parallel to its fibres, to expose the capsule.

Opening up of the capsule exposes the posteromedial aspect of the knee joint.

Indications

- Repair of the posterior horn of medial meniscus.
- Removal of loose bodies.
- Drainage of the knee, if this is the affected area.

Posterolateral Approach

Access

- Posterior half of lateral meniscus.
- Lateral femoral condyle.
- Posterolateral aspect of the knee joint.

Position and draping: The patient is placed supine with a sand-bag under the buttock.

A high tourniquet is applied.

The leg is draped free and bulky drapes are avoided to allow feeling of the foot direction under the drapes.

One must be able to freely flex and extend the knee after draping.

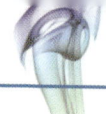

Approach: The knee is flexed to 90°, allowing the back of the heel to rest on the operating table.

The surgeon operates from the same side.

Incision: Curved incision with the convexity anteriorly.

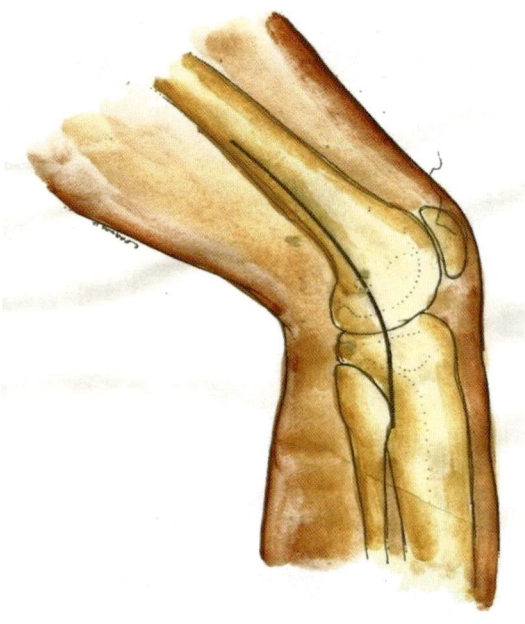

The incision is along the biceps up to the fibular head, lying anterior to the common peroneal nerve.

The dissections: The biceps belly is followed down to the intermuscular septum at the linea aspera, and the femoral shaft is exposed in the superior part of the incision.

This is followed downwards to the lateral femoral condyle, and the attachment of fibular colleteral ligament is exposed.

The popliteus tendon is retracted posteriorly to expose the joint capsule.

The synovium is excised to expose the posterior aspect of the knee.

Additional exposure is achieved by mobilizing the lateral head of gastrocnemius posteriorly.

A vertical capsular incision exposes the posterior part of lateral femoral condyle.

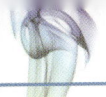

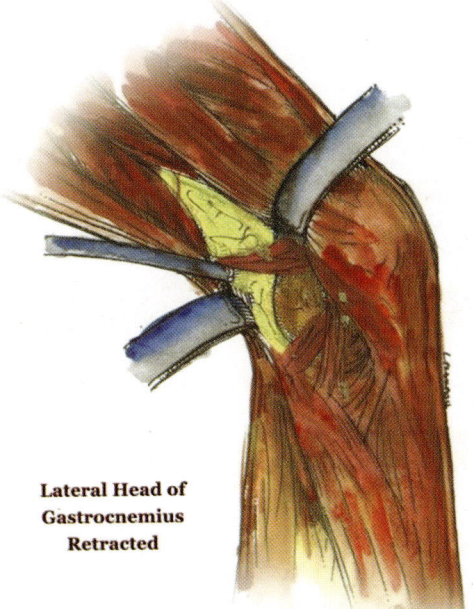

**Lateral Head of
Gastrocnemius
Retracted**

Indications:
- Chondral fractures and loose bodies in the posterolateral aspect of the knee joint.
- Posterolateral drainage of the knee joint.

5

The Tibia and Fibula

ANATOMY OF THE TIBIA

Superficial Nerves

Superficial Peroneal Nerve

The superficial peroneal nerve is a terminal branch of the common peroneal nerve. After passing around the neck of the fibula, it pierces the deep fibres of the peroneus longus and divides into superficial and deep branches.

The superficial peroneal nerve descends in the belly of the peroneus longus until it reaches the proximal end of peroneus brevis, after which it runs distally between extensor digitorum and peroneus brevis (anterior intermuscular septum).

In the lower third of the leg, the nerve pierces the deep fascia and descends into the foot as two branches: the medial and intermediate dorsal cutaneous nerves of the foot.

Saphenous Nerve

The saphenous nerve is the longest branch of the femoral nerve, arising in the femoral triangle; it accompanies the femoral artery through the subsartorial canal. It leaves the artery at this point and pierces the deep fascia at the posteromedial side of the knee, descending distally closely to the great saphenous vein.

It crosses the distal third of the tibia along with the great saphenous vein, descending in front of the medial malleolus to end on the medial side of the foot.

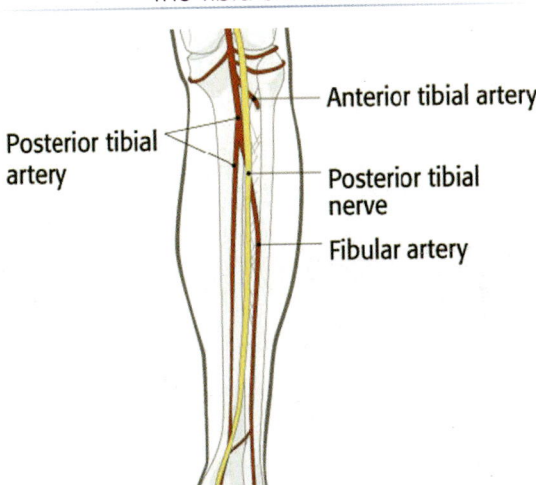

Anterior tibial artery

Posterior tibial artery

Posterior tibial nerve

Fibular artery

Sural Nerve

The sural nerve arises in the popliteal fossa as a terminal branch of the tibial nerve. It descends between the medial and lateral heads of gastrocnemius, under the deep fascia.

Half-way down the leg, it pierces the deep fascia and accompanies the short saphenous vein to the back of the lateral malleolus. It supplies sensation to the lateral side of the foot and small toe.

Superficial Veins

Long Saphenous Vein

The long saphenous vein begins along the medial side of the foot and ascends in front of the medial malleolus, passing obliquely across the distal third of the medial border of the tibia. At the level of the knee, it is found posteromedially.

Short Saphenous Vein

The short saphenous vein begins in the foot and runs behind the lateral malleolus, ascending the leg first lateral to the Achilles tendon and then in the midline of the gastrocnemius. As it ascends through the leg, it is superficial to the deep fascia until it reaches the popliteal space, where it pierces the fascia to enter the popliteal vein. In the lower half of the leg, it is accompanied by the sural nerve.

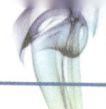

Deep Nerves and Vessels

Anterior Tibial Artery and Deep Peroneal Neve

The anterior tibial artery arises as a terminal branch of the popliteal artery at the lower border of the popliteus muscle.

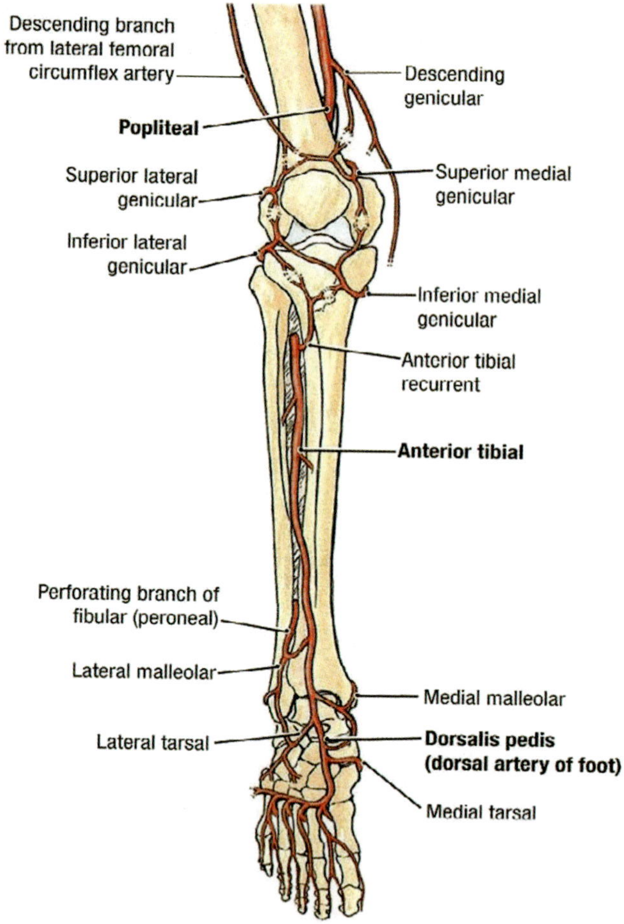

Descending branch from lateral femoral circumflex artery

Popliteal

Superior lateral genicular

Inferior lateral genicular

Descending genicular

Superior medial genicular

Inferior medial genicular

Anterior tibial recurrent

Anterior tibial

Perforating branch of fibular (peroneal)

Lateral malleolar

Lateral tarsal

Medial malleolar

Dorsalis pedis (dorsal artery of foot)

Medial tarsal

Here it passes forwards through the interosseous membrane and then descends distally on the front of the membrane.

The deep peroneal nerve, arising as a terminal branch of the common peroneal nerve, pierces the anterior intermuscular septum and the extensor digitorum longus to approach the anterior tibial artery from its lateral side.

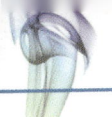
Sciatic nerve

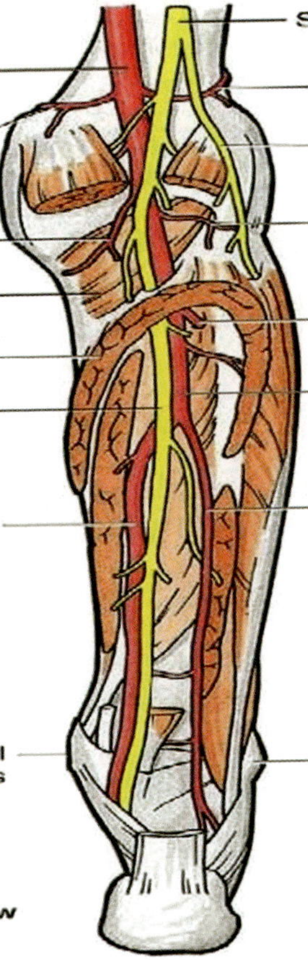

Popliteal artery

Superior lateral
genicular artery

Superior medial
genicular artery

Common fibular
nerve

Inferior medial
genicular artery

Inferior lateral
genicular artery

Popliteus

Anterior tibial
artery

Soleus

Posterior tibial
artery

Tibial nerve

Posterior tibial
artery

Fibular artery

Medial
malleolus

Lateral
malleolus

A Posterior view

The anterior tibial artery and the deep peroneal nerve descend together in the interval between tibialis anterior and extensor digitorum longus. They are initially deep in the leg, being close to the interosseus membrane, but become more superficial distally.

Near the ankle, they are crossed by the tendon of the extensor hallucis longus and enter the foot between extensor hallucis longus and extensor digitorum longus.

The anterior tibial artery gives off three branches: Anterior tibial recurrent, lateral and medial malleolar branches. These may be injured through the anterior approach to the tibia, if the incision is carried across the ankle joint.

The deep peroneal nerve continues lateral to the artery and ends midway between the malleoli by dividing into lateral and medial terminal branches.

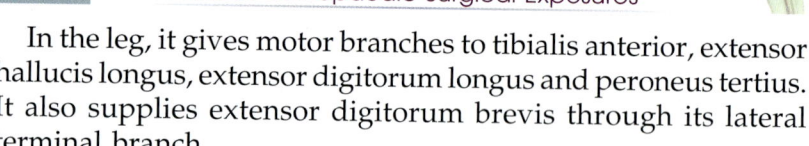

In the leg, it gives motor branches to tibialis anterior, extensor hallucis longus, extensor digitorum longus and peroneus tertius. It also supplies extensor digitorum brevis through its lateral terminal branch.

Posterior Tibial Artery and Tibial Nerve

The posterior tibial artery, a branch of the popliteal artery, begins at the lower border of the popliteus muscle.

The artery descends distally in the leg, under the soleus, lying on the fascia over tibialis posterior, below the flexor hallucis longus.

The tibial nerve is the terminal branch of the sciatic nerve, and descends with the posterior tibial artery. In the upper leg, both lie on the posterior surface of popliteus, the nerve being medial to the artery, but then crossing behind the artery to run on its lateral side in the leg.

In the middle of the leg, these two structures are found posteromedial to the tibialis posterior muscle; in the distal third of the leg, they lie between the Achilles tendon and the medial border of the tibia before passing behind the medial malleolus to enter the foot.

The posterior tibial nerve gives motor branches to tibialis posterior as well as to flexor digitorum longus, flexor hallucis longus and soleus.

Along with the posterior tibial artery, these structures may be injured through a posterolateral approach (Harmon) to the tibia if the surgeon fails to get deep to the tibialis posterior. The posterior tibial artery, in its distal third, gives off an anastomotic branch from its lateral side, which communicates directly with the peroneal artery. This branch is commonly divided during a posterolateral approach.

Peroneal Artery

The peroneal artery arises from the posterior tibial artery, approximately 2 or 3 cm below popliteus. The artery descends laterally crossing tibialis posterior in front of the soleus to reach the fibula. It runs alongside the fibula distally on the interosseus membrane in front of flexor hallucis longus. Once again, injury to this artery is prone to occur through the posterolateral approach to the tibia, particularly in the middle and distal thirds.

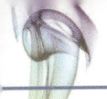

SURGICAL APPROACHES TO THE TIBIA

- Anterior
- Medial
- Posterolateral (Harmon)
- Posterior (Banks and Laufman)

Anterior Approach

Access: Exposure of lateral or medial border of the tibia.

Incision: The skin incision begins 3 cm behind the crest of the tibia (just behind Gerdy's tubercle) and extends distally in a straight line.

The incision should be 1 cm lateral to the crest of the tibia.

Distally, the incision curves medially along the lateral edge of the tibialis anterior tendon.

Great care should be taken in making this incision to ensure that the skin and subcutaneous tissues along with the deep fascia are incorporated one single thick flap.

Approach: The skin and subcutaneous tissue are cut right up to the subcutaneous anteromedial surface of the tibia. The flap should be of full thickness incorporating all the structures.

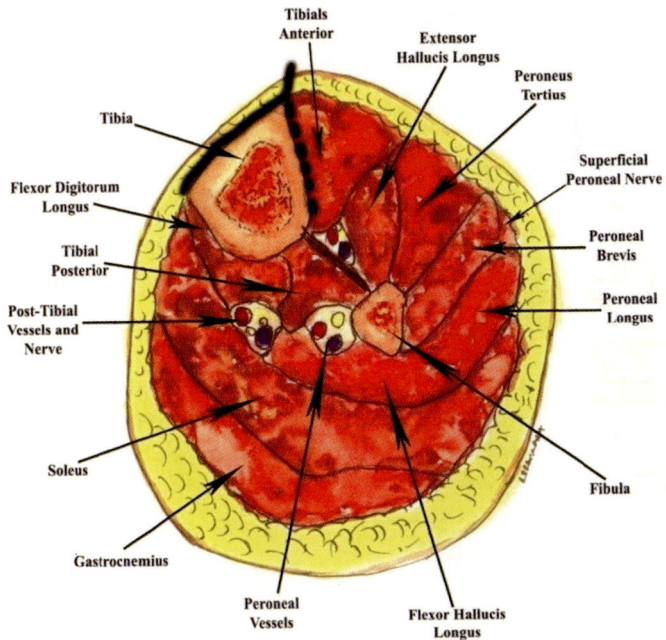

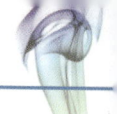

To expose the lateral border of the tibia, the fascia covering the anterior compartment muscle is detached from the crest of the tibia throughout the length of the incision.

Care should be taken to avoid injury to the anterior tibial artery and deep peroneal nerve. They are prone to injury where they enter the anterior compartment in the proximal limit of this approach.

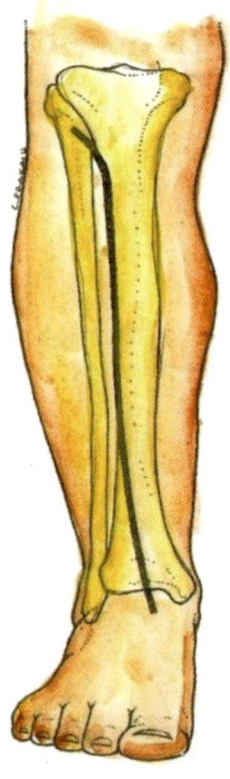

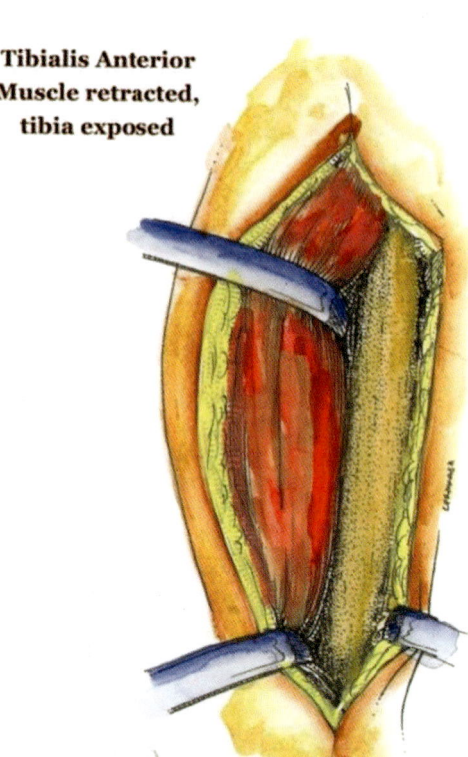

Tibialis Anterior Muscle retracted, tibia exposed

Indications: For the exposure and internal fixation of fractures of the tibia. The incision affords excellent exposure for open reduction and internal fixation of fractures of the proximal, middle or distal thirds.

Medial Approach

Access: Almost the whole length of posterior border of the tibia.

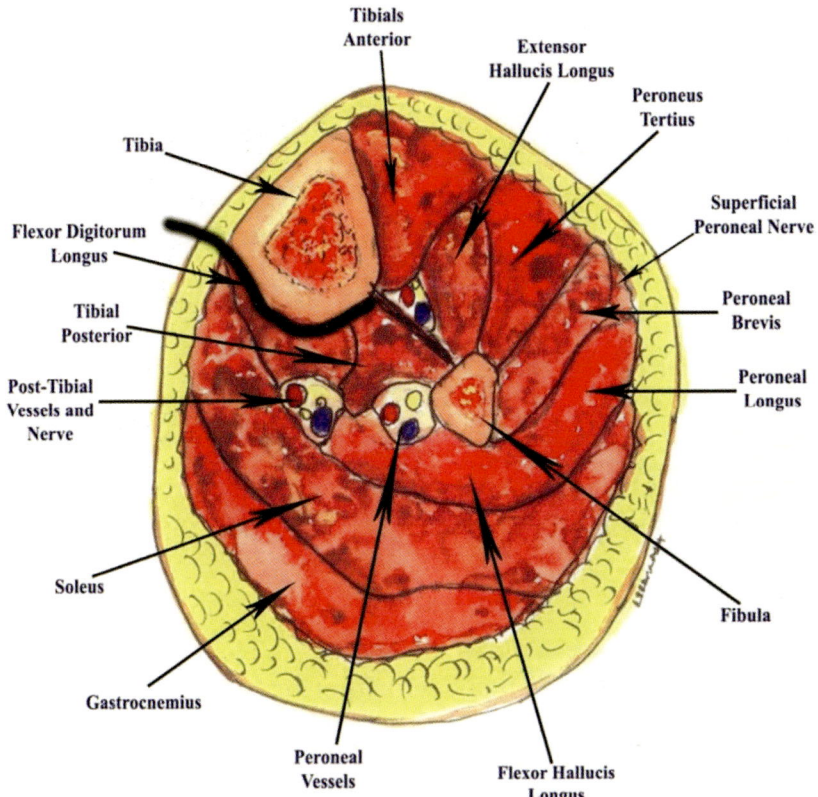

Incision: The skin incision is straight, parallel to the postero-medial border of the tibia 1 cm behind the posteromedial border.

Care should be taken to identify and protect the saphenous vein and nerve.

Approach: The periosteum overlying the posteromedial border of the tibia is now exposed and incised.

Subperiosteal dissection is carried out posteriorly to expose the entire posteromedial surface of the tibia.

In bone grafting procedures, it is preferable to expose the posterior surface of the tibia by using a sharp chisel to raise a corticoperiosteal flap.

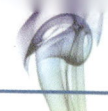

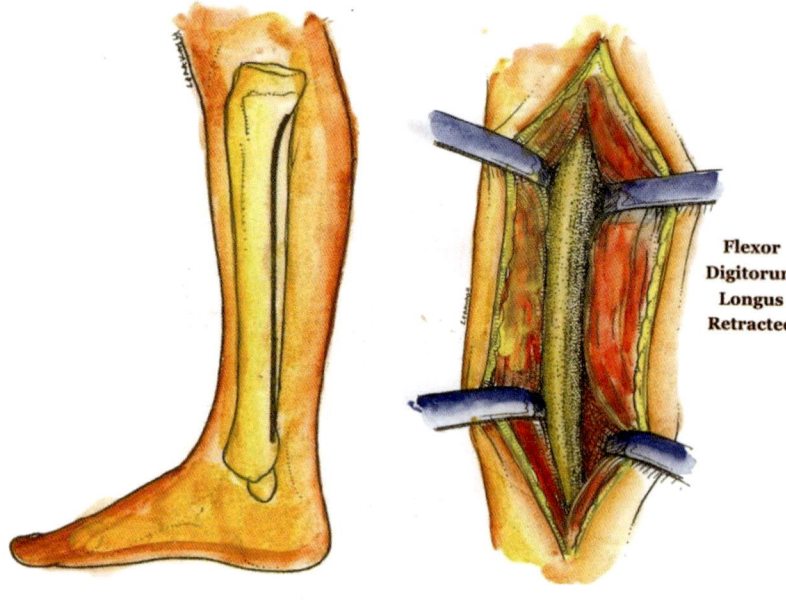

Flexor Digitorum Longus Retracted

Indications:
- Bone grafting procedures throughout the length of the tibia.
- It is not used for the management of acute fractures.

Posterolateral Approach (Harmon)

History: Paul H Harmon described this approach in 1945. He was a brilliant scientist and surgeon.

Paul H Harmon, MD (1906–1988): Born in Gallatin, Missouri, on July 6, 1906, Paul Harmon was the son of a school superintendent and an occupational therapist. He received a Bachelor of Science degree in Chemistry in 1925 and a Doctor of Philosophy in bacteriology in 1929, both from the University of Chicago. In 1930, he earned a Doctor of Medicine degree from Rush Medical College, University of Chicago.

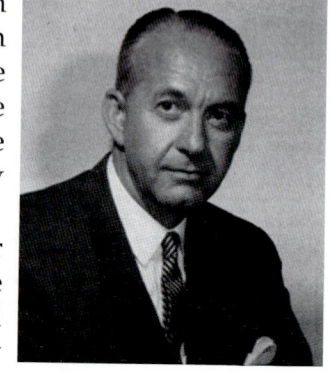

At Rush, he was awarded the Freer Prize for excellence in scholarship. He was president of the senior class and held memberships in Sigma XI honorary

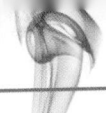

fraternity and Alpha Omega Alpha honorary medical scholastic fraternity.

At the University of Chicago, Dr Harmon and two other physicians isolated the preparalytic poliomyelitis virus in monkey.

Dr Harmon served his internship at the Johns Hopkins Hospital. Baltimore, Maryland from 1930 to 1931. He then returned to the University of Chicago to complete his residence in general and orthopaedic surgery, serving as instructor and assistant professor of orthopaedic surgery from 1935 to 1937.

From 1940 to 1945, Dr Harmon was chief of orthopaedic surgery at the Guthrie Clinic and the Robert Packer Hospital in Sayre, Pennsylvania. He was also an orthopaedic surgery consultant for the Crippled Children's Division of the State Department of Health in Pennsylvania and an associate surgeon for the Lehigh Valley Railway.

In 1947, he moved to Oakland, California to become chief of orthopaedic surgery at the Kaiser Foundation Hospital. In 1951, he accepted an appointment as orthopaedic surgeon for the Branch Medical Clinic in Hollywood. He was chief of staff at Hollywood Presbyterian Hospital and later was affiliated with the Moore White Clinic in Los Angeles. In 1957, he returned to northern California, where he served as chief orthopaedic surgeon for the Kaiser Foundation Hospital until 1965, when he entered private practice – first in West Covina, California and later in Covina. He continued to work until he had a heart attack in the fall of 1987.

Dr Harmon was responsible for a number of professional innovations. He pioneered high density polyethylene cups for arthritic joints; these cups were the forerunners of today's total joint replacements.

He also designed instruments for, and preferred the technique of, anterior (frontal) excision and vertebral body fusion for inner vertebral disc syndromes of the spine.

A frequent contributor to medical literature, he wrote books as well as articles.

Access: This approach allows access to the posterior border of the tibia and the interosseus membrane.

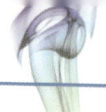

Position: The patient is positioned prone or in a lateral position with the affected leg prepared and draped free.

Incision: The incision is a straight line behind the shaft of the fibula extending in the interval between the peroneal tendons anteriorly and the gastrocnemius–soleus complex posteriorly.

Sural nerve is in the distal part of the incision and care must be taken to avoid damaging it.

Approach: The interval between the peroneous longus and brevis anteriorly and the gastrocnemius and soleus posteriorly is identified and opened down to the fibula.

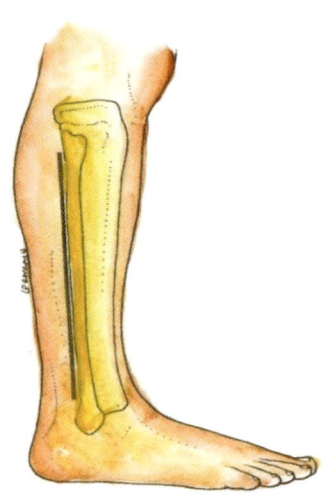

Widening this interval will expose the fibres of flexor hallucis longus, posterior to the fibula.

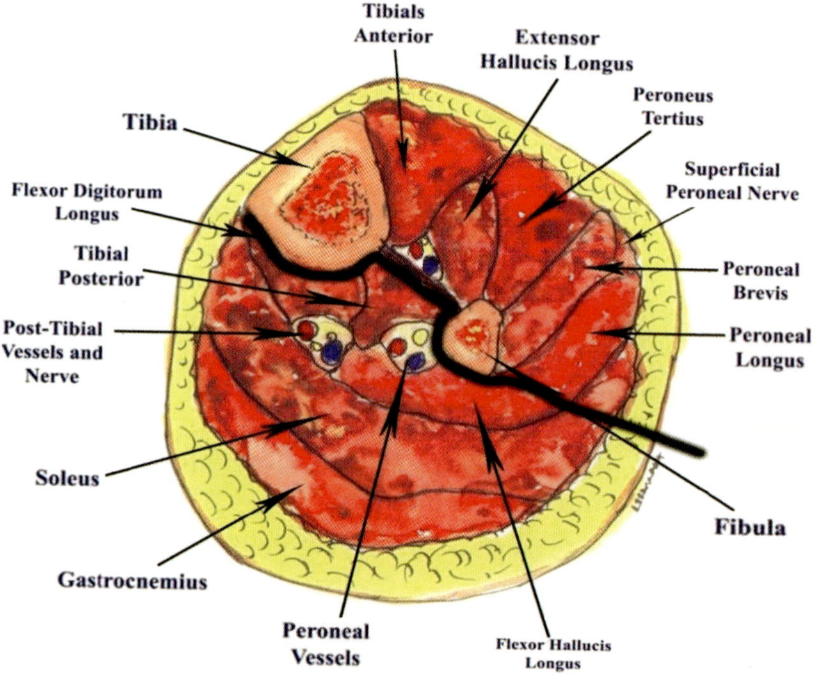

Tibials Anterior

Extensor Hallucis Longus

Peroneus Tertius

Tibia

Superficial Peroneal Nerve

Flexor Digitorum Longus

Tibial Posterior

Peroneal Brevis

Post-Tibial Vessels and Nerve

Peroneal Longus

Soleus

Fibula

Gastrocnemius

Peroneal Vessels

Flexor Hallucis Longus

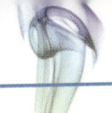

The fibres of of flexor hallucis longus are detached to expose the posterior border of the fibula.

Flexor hallucis longus is retracted posteriorly and medially with the gastrocnemius–soleus complex; peroneus longus and brevis are retracted anteriorly.

The posterior surface of the shaft of the fibula is now exposed.

By carefully remaining subperiosteal along the posteromedial border of the fibula, the fibres of tibialis posterior are detached from the interosseus membrane and retracted posteriorly to expose the posterior border of the tibia.

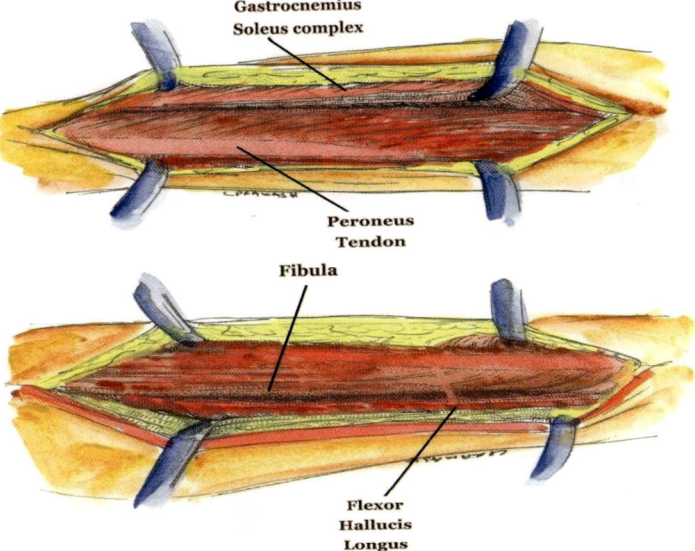

The posterior tibial artery and vein lie between the tibialis posterior and flexor hallucis longus; they are not seen in this dissection but are protected by retracting tibialis posterior and flexor hallucis longus medially.

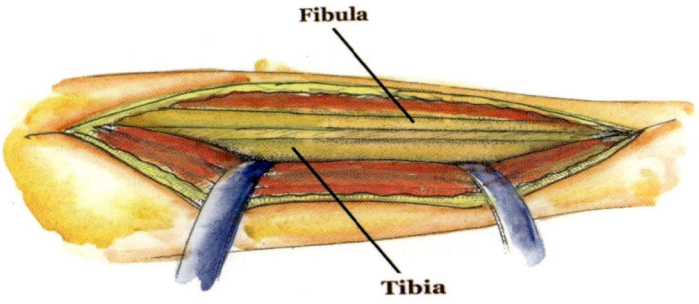

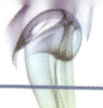

Muscular branches of the peroneal artery are frequently encountered along with the peroneal artery in this incision and must be secured, if divided.

Indications: Bone grafting of the distal thirds of the back of the tibia.

Posterior Approach to the Superior Medial Region of the Tibia (Banks and Laufman)

Access: Posterior surface of the proximal metaphyseal region of the tibia.

Position and draping: The patient is positioned prone and the leg is draped free to allow for knee movements.

Incision: The incision uses the distal popliteal crease as a landmark and the medial border of the gastrocnemius–soleus complex as the other landmark.

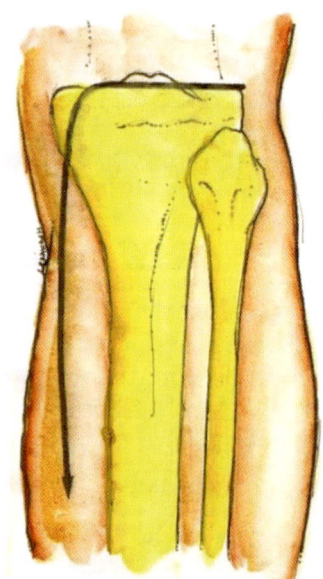

The incision follows the transverse popliteal crease and is then extended distally along the medial border of the calf.

Care must be taken to identify and protect terminal branches of the posterior cutaneous nerve of the thigh as well as terminal branches of the medial cutaneous nerve of the thigh.

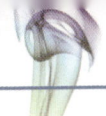

Approach: After the fascia is incised, the medial head of gastrocnemius is identified along with the lateral border of the semitendinosus muscle.

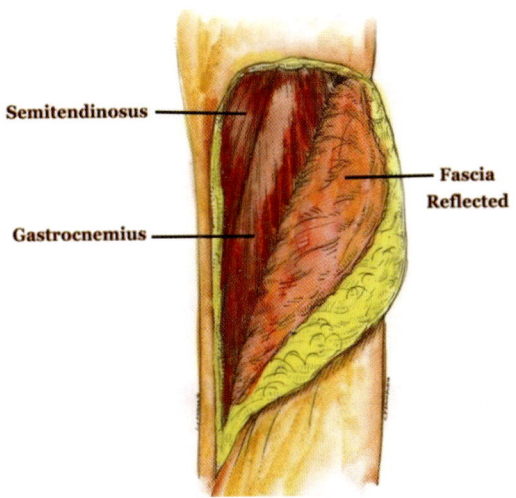

The semitendinosus is retracted medially and gastrocnemius is retracted laterally to expose the underlying popliteus muscle crossing the incision in its depth.

Flexor digitorum longus is seen in the floor of the incision, distal to the popliteus muscle.

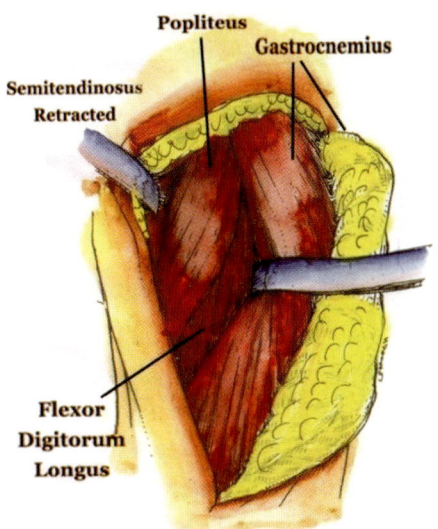

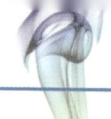

The clevage between flexor digitorum longus and popliteus is next explored.

Flexor digitorum longus is elevated subperiosteally from the posteromedial border of the back of the tibia and retracted distally, while popliteus is retracted proximally.

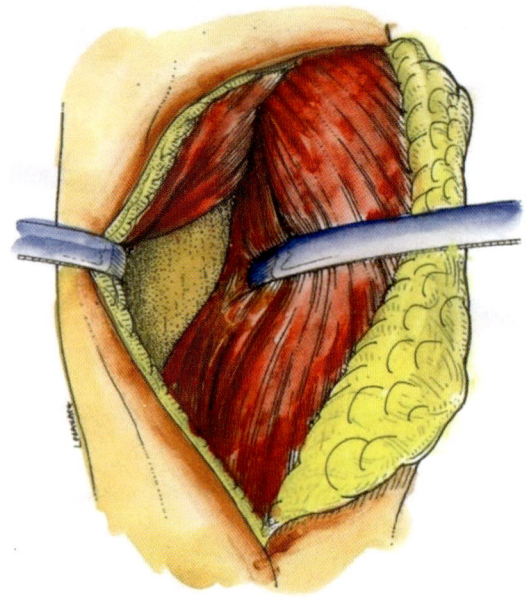

One should not look for the neurovascular bundle, as it runs adjacent to the deep surface of soleus.

Care must be taken in the lateral retraction of the gastrocnemius–soleus complex to avoid damage to these structures.

Indications:

- Neoplastic lesions of the superomedial corner of the back of the tibia.
- Posterior capsule and posterior cruciate region of the knee joint.

SURGICAL APPROACHES TO THE FIBULA

Posterolateral Approach

Access: The entire shaft of the fibula, except the proximal quarter, which can be difficult.

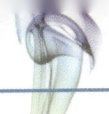

Position: The patient is positioned in the straight lateral or prone position.

Incision: The interval between the superficial posterior compartment and the lateral compartment is identified.

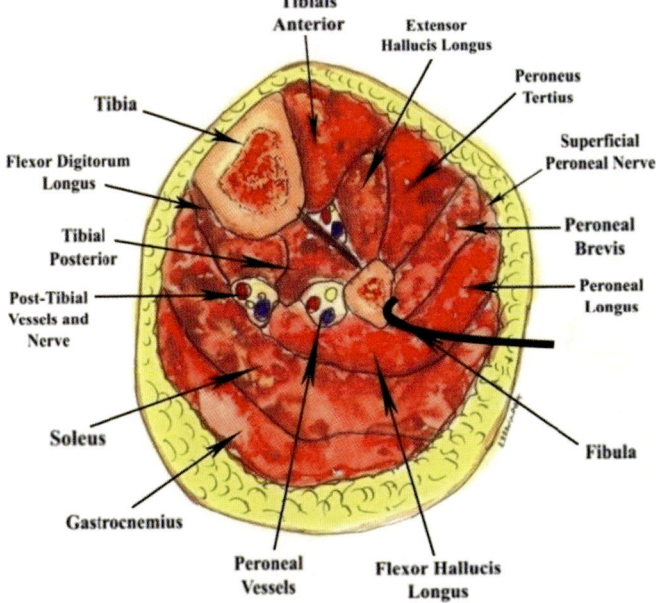

The fibula is subcutaneous in its distal quarter and a straight incision is used with this as a landmark.

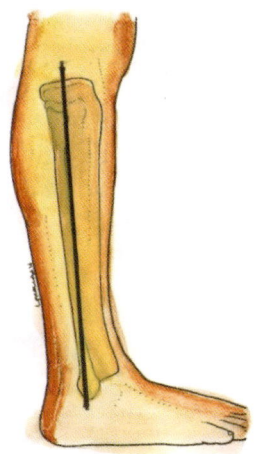

Approach: The gap is separated between the superficial posterior compartment posteriorly and the peroneal muscles anteriorly.

The incision is carried proximally and the peroneal nerve is isolated at the level of the posterior aspect of the biceps tendon.

The nerve crosses the proximal end of the wound and enters the substance of peroneus longus.

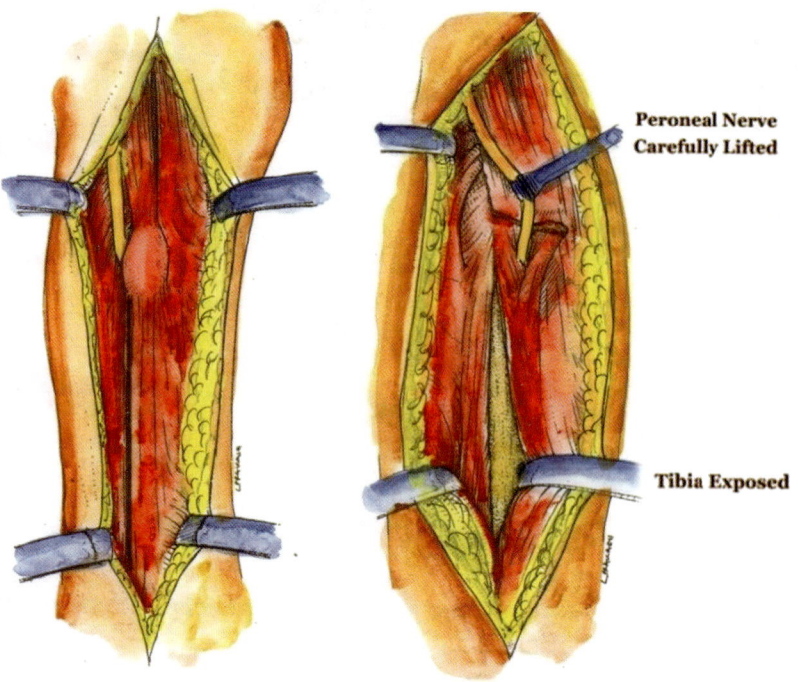

Peroneal Nerve Carefully Lifted

Tibia Exposed

By isolating the nerve and by using gentle retraction, it can be carried anteriorly to expose the head of the fibula.

The interval between the soleus posteriorly and the peroneal muscles anteriorly is now developed, with the nerve safely out of the way and the dissection is carried down to expose the shaft of the tibia.

Indications:
- Fibular osteotomy preliminary to tibial osteotomy.
- Harvesting of vascularized or free fibular bone grafts, and for the surgery of painful fibular non-union.

The Ankle

RELEVANT ANATOMY

Cutaneous Nerves

Avoid damage to the cutaneous nerves, wherever possible.

Formation of a neuroma can result in painful disability from footwear pressure.

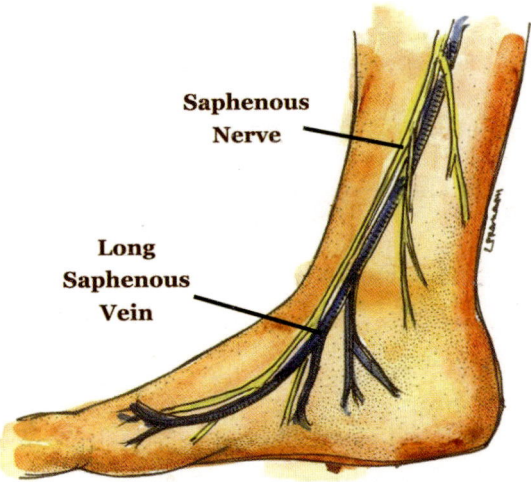

Superficial cutaneous nerves

Saphenous Nerve

This enters the ankle region, along with the long saphenous vein, along the line of the posteromedial border of the tibia.

Subsequently, this curves anteriorly to cross the ankle joint level just anterior to the medial malleolus.

It then divides into numerous small branches to supply an area on the dorsomedial aspect of the tarsus.

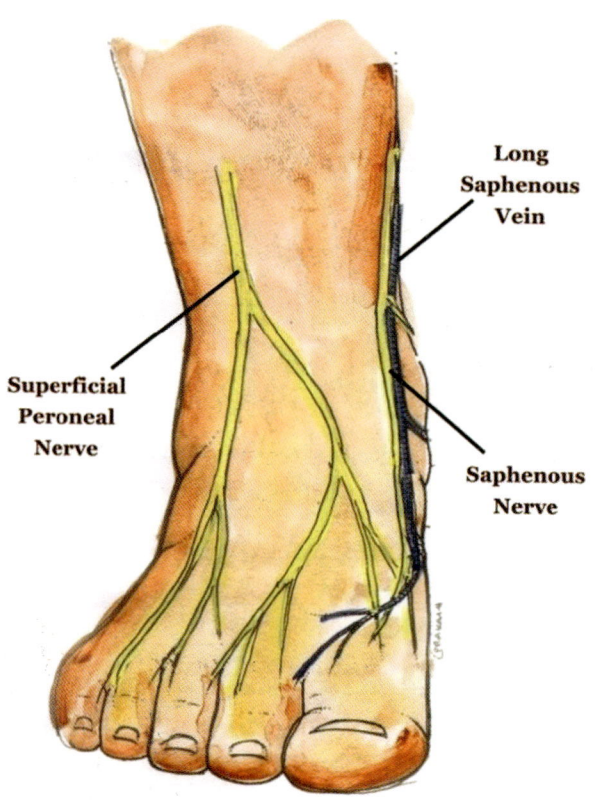

Long
Saphenous
Vein

Superficial
Peroneal
Nerve

Saphenous
Nerve

Superficial Peroneal Nerve

Arises at the bifurcation of the common peroneal nerve in the upper third of the leg.

It then gives branches to the peroneal muscles and then emerges through the deep fascia of the leg between the peronei and the extensor digitorum longus.

It next divides above the ankle into the medial and intermediate dorsal cutaneous nerves of the foot as shown in the drawing above.

The medial dorsal cutaneous nerve crosses the ankle joint just lateral to the midline and then divides into two branches which supply the medial aspect of the hallux and the adjacent sides of the second and third toes.

The intermediate branch crosses the ankle over the front of the inferior tibiofibular joint and supplies the adjacent sides of the third, fourth and fifth toes.

Sural Nerve

After originating from the tibial nerve and emerging from between the heads of gastrocnemius, the sural nerve pierces the deep fascia of the leg at the lateral edge of the Achilles tendon and descends to the interval between the lateral malleolus and the heel. From there, it curves below the malleolar tip to run along the lateral border of the foot as far as the fifth toe.

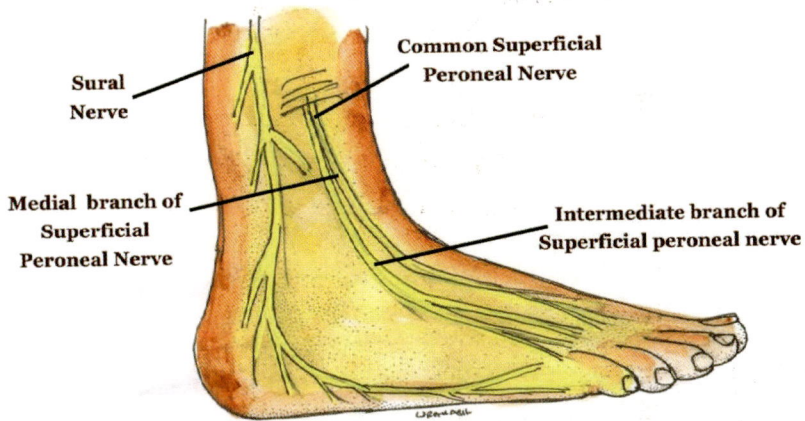

Deep Nerves and Vessels

Posterior Tibial Neurovascular Bundle

This large bundle passes down to the ankle region from the posterior compartment of the leg, running behind the medial malleolus to enter the medial plantar structures.

It lies on the posteromedial aspect of the distal tibial meta-physeal region between the tendons of flexor digitorum longus medially and of flexor hallucis longus laterally.

The nerve usually lies lateral to the vessels. The bundle, together with the tendons, is tethered by a thickening of the deep fascia which requires careful dissection, if they are to be explored and mobilized.

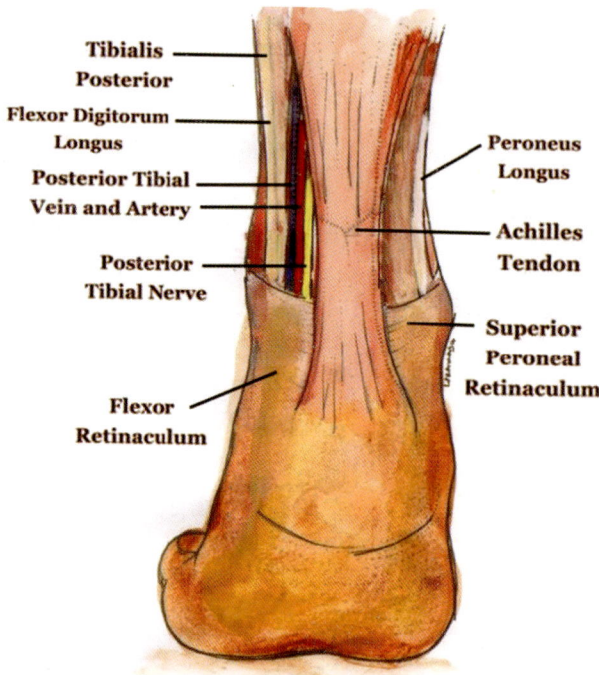

Just above the level of the ankle joint, the artery often gives a laterally running branch which joins with the peroneal artery.

PERONEAL ARTERY

This arises from the posterior tibial artery, in the middle third of the leg, and passes distally along the interosseous membrane, adjacent to the fibula, between the tibialis posterior and the flexor hallucis longus muscles.

It then crosses over the back of the inferior tibiofibular syndesmosis, deep to the flexor hallucis longus, and supplies branches to the lateral and posterior aspects of the heel.

Anterior Tibial Neurovascular Bundle

The anterior tibial vein, nerve and artery, VAN, (from lateral to medial) pass deep to the extensor retinaculum over the front of the ankle.

They lie between the tendons of tibialis anterior and extensor hallucis longus proximally, and then between the tendons of extensor hallucis longus and extensor digitorum longus distally.

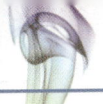

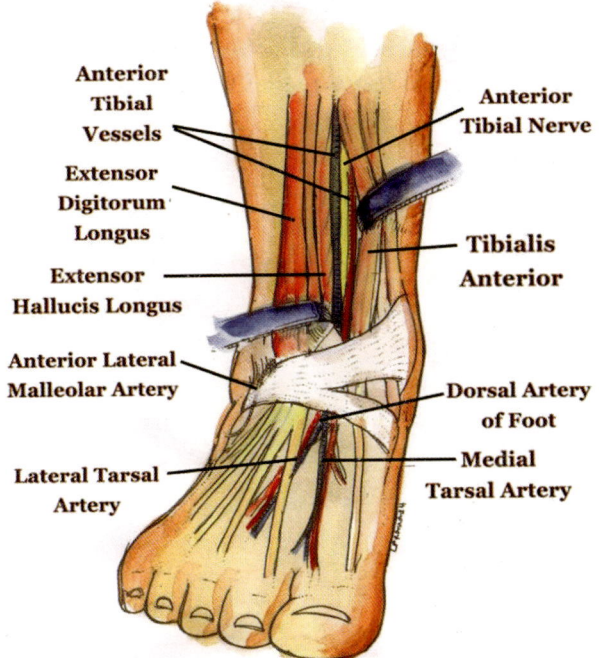

The tendon of the long extensor of the big toe crosses the bundle superficially from lateral to medial at about the ankle joint level.

The bundle then continues into the foot running towards the base of the second metatarsal, the artery becoming the dorsalis pedis vessel.

Ligaments

Lateral Ligament Complex

The lateral ligament complex of the ankle consists of two main units:

1. Anterior and posterior talofibular ligament.
2. Calcaneofibular ligament.

The anterior talofibular ligament arises from the anterior border of the lateral malleolus and is inserted into the lateral aspect of the talar neck between the articular surfaces of the ankle and the talonavicular joints.

It is always the first structure to be torn in inversion ankle injuries.

The calcaneofibular ligament is a strong band, originating from the tip of the lateral malleolus and inserted into the superolateral surface of the body of the calcaneum.

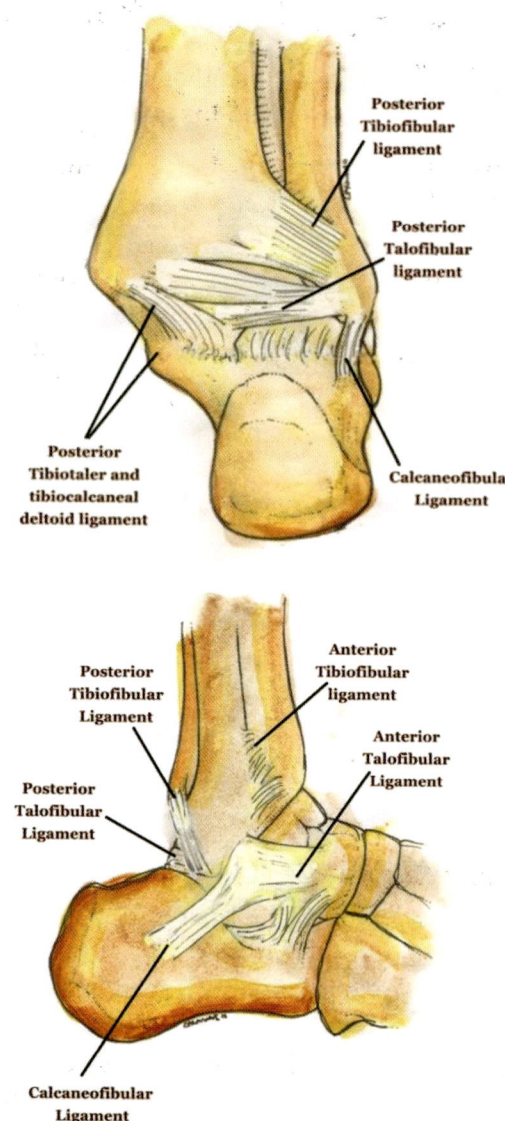

The posterior talofibular ligament arises from just behind the tip of the lateral malleolus and is inserted into the posterior tubercle of the talus.

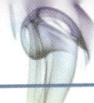

Deltoid Ligament

This is a strong triangular ligament arising from the tip of the medial malleolus and fanning out to a linear insertion along the medial aspect of the talus, above the medial articular facet.

A wider, superficial layer inserts more broadly into the navicular, the sustentaculum tali, the medial tubercle of the posterior process of the talus and into the intervening capsular fibres.

SURGICAL APPROACHES

- Anterolateral (Campbell, 1949)
- Anteromedial
- Posterolateral
- Posteromedial
- Posterior
- Transfibular (Gatellier and Chastang, 1924)
- Medial transmalleolar (Konig and Schafer, 1929)

Anterolateral Approach (Campbell)

History

Willis Cohoon Campbell (1880–1941): Willis Cohoon Campbell was born in Jackson, Mississippi, on December 18, 1880. His early education was received in his native state; his college and premedical training were at Hampden-Sydney College, Roanoke College; and his medical work at the University of Virginia, where he graduated in 1904.

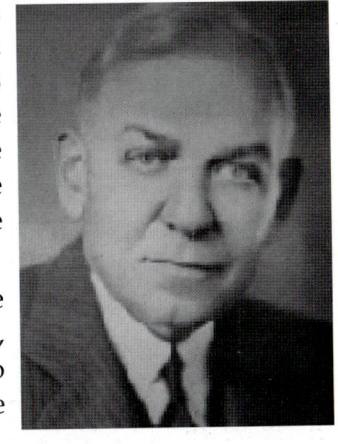

Early in his career, he became interested in orthopaedic surgery, and, surmounting many hardships, went to Europe to undertake the study of the specialty.

He studied in London and Vienna, and had further postgraduate study in New York and Boston with the celebrated orthopaedic surgeons of the country at that time.

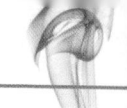

He returned to Memphis in 1909 and resumed his practice, specializing in orthopaedic surgery.

In 1910, he was asked to form a Department of Orthopaedic Surgery at the University of Tennessee Medical School and became the first professor of orthopaedic surgery in this institution, the office he held with distinction until his death.

His work in teaching was characterized by his desire to improve the teaching of orthopaedic surgery and postgraduate training.

Dr Campbell realized the need for properly organized surgical training and conducted institutions for the care of indigent cripples. He was one of the first to establish a crippled children's hospital school in that part of the South.

In 1920, he built the Willis C Campbell Clinic, an institution for the care of his private patients and for the postgraduate training of trainees desiring to specialize in orthopaedic surgery.

The fellowships in orthopaedic surgery, which he started in connection with the Willis C Campbell Clinic in 1924, provided essentially the same training required by the American Board for the Certification of Specialists.

Dr Campbell played an important role in the formation of the American Board of Orthopaedic Surgery. He served as a member of the examining board and was president from 1937 to 1940.

With a number of his colleagues, Dr Campbell founded the American Academy of Orthopaedic Surgeons. He was honoured by being made its first president in 1933.

His capacity for work was almost superhuman, and his interests were widely distributed. He contributed many articles to scientific programmes and to various medical journals, also chapters on orthopaedic surgery in many leading textbooks of surgery.

In addition to this, he published three volumes:
1. Orthopaedics of Childhood, 1927;
2. Textbook of Orthopaedic Surgery, 1930;
3. Operative Orthopaedics, 1939.

He described the anterolateral approach in 1949, and this is still one of the most extensively used approaches to the ankle.

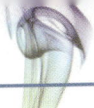
Positioning: Supine with a sandbag under the buttock to internally rotate the hip and bring forth the lateral surface.

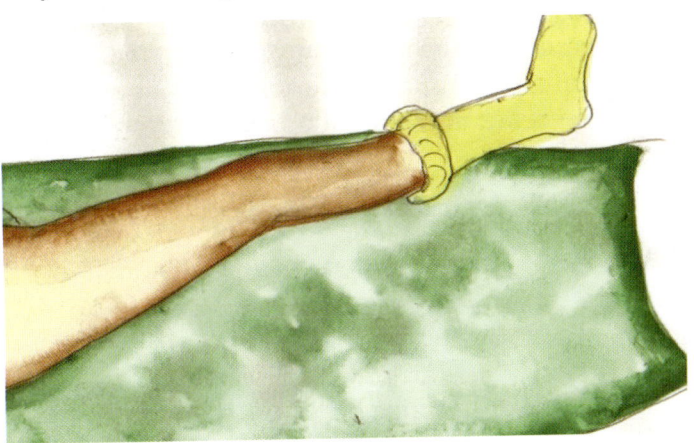

Access:
- Anterior surface of the distal tibia.
- The anterior talofibular ligament.

Incision: Starting approximately 8 cm above the ankle joint, 1 cm lateral to the anterior crest of the tibia and going down in a straight line towards the base of the fourth metatarsal.

The proximal part of the incision overlies the superficial peroneal nerve as it branches, and should be protected after identification.

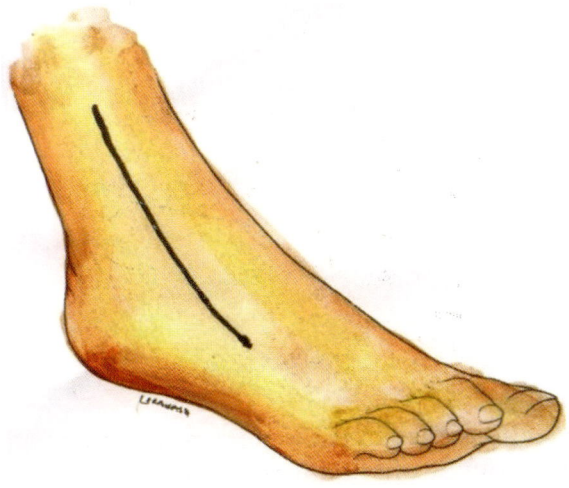

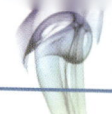

Approach: The extensor retinacular fibres are dissected in the line of the skin incision.

The tendons of the long toe extensors are retracted medially and that of peroneus tertius laterally.

The anterior capsule of the ankle joint and the anterior lateral malleolar vessels are now identified and protected.

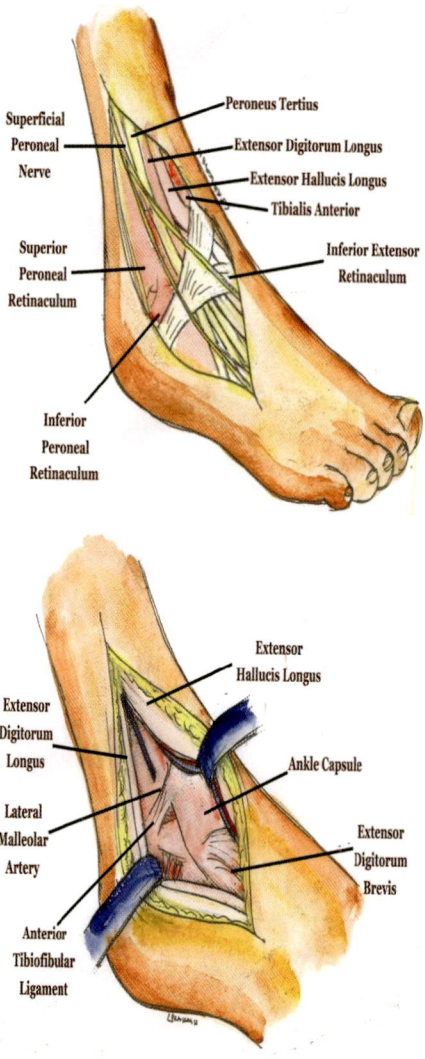

The ankle joint is entered by capsular incision, horizontal or vertical, according to the requirements.

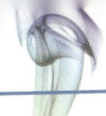

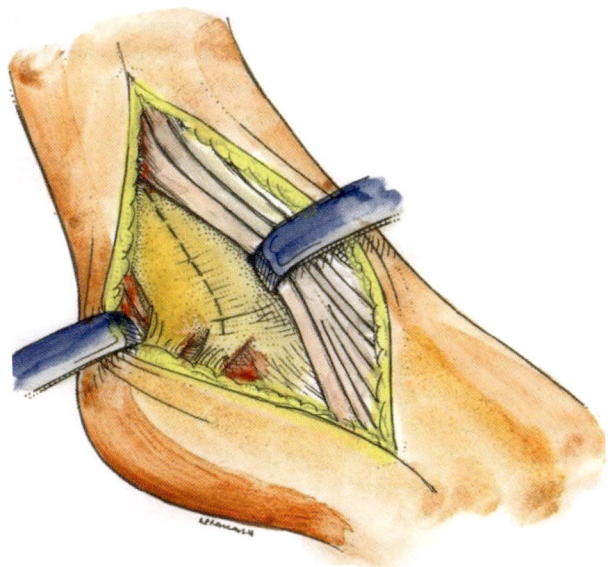

To reach the lateral aspect of the fibula, the tendon of peroneus tertius is mobilized medially, but the access here is limited.

Additional medial exposure is obtained by mobilization and medial retraction of the tendons of the extensor digitorum longus and the anterior neurovascular bundle. These can be relaxed by dorsiflexing the foot.

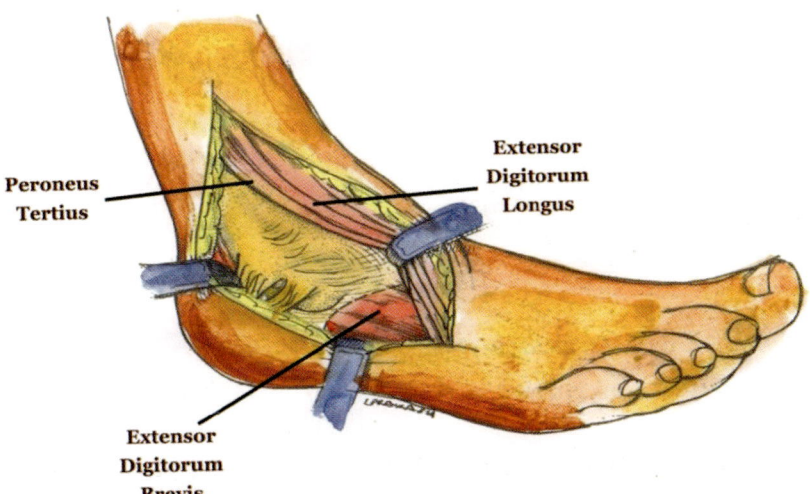

Peroneus Tertius

Extensor Digitorum Longus

Extensor Digitorum Brevis

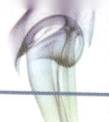

The exposure is distally developed by elevation and medial retraction of the belly of extensor digitorum brevis.

This permits exposure of the sinus tarsi and subtalar joint laterally, and of the talar neck and talonavicular joint medially.

During this exposure, the lateral tarsal vessels cross the field and may require identification and coagulation.

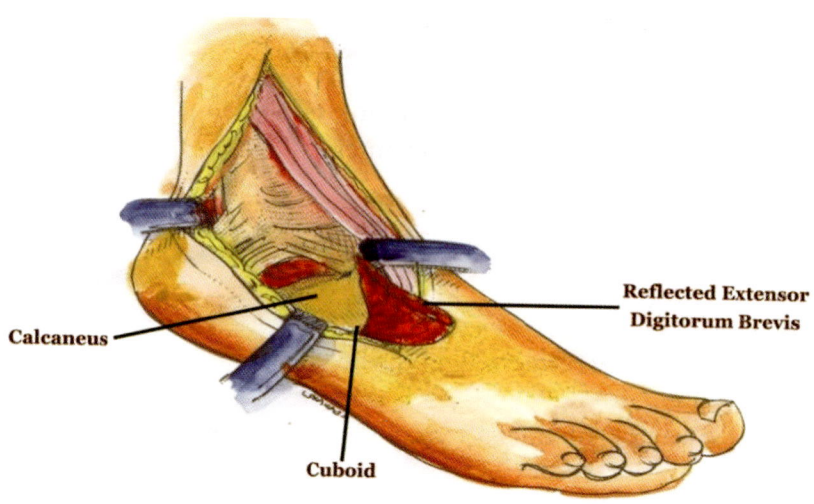

Calcaneus

Reflected Extensor Digitorum Brevis

Cuboid

Indications:

* Anterolateral marginal fractures of the tibia not involving the medial malleolus.
* Fractures of the lateral malleolus.
* Anterolateral dislocation of the talus.
* Surgery in the region of the sinus tarsi.
* Astragalectomy.

Anteromedial Approach

Positioning: The patient is positioned supine on the operating table.

A sandbag beneath the opposite buttock externally rotates the limb and brings the medial ankle into view.

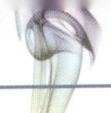

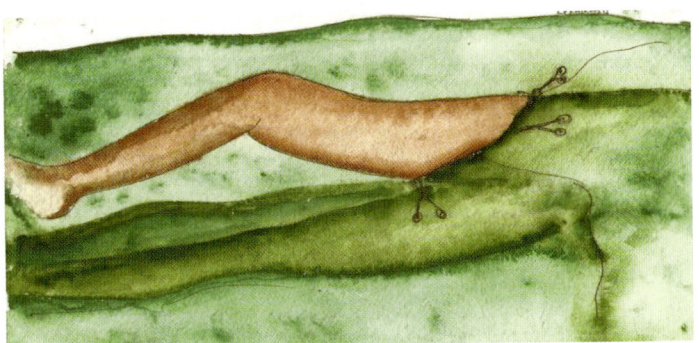

Access:
- The front of the distal tibia and ankle joint.
- The medial malleolus and the anterior tibial tubercle.

Incision: Beginning at the lower third of the leg, 1 cm lateral to the anterior crest of the tibia, running parallel to it.

This is then curved gently medially to midway between the tip of the medial malleolus and the navicular tubercle.

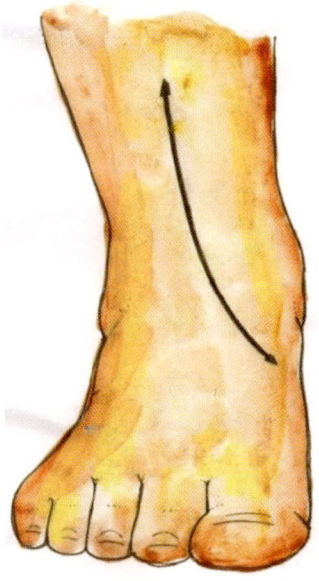

Approach: The long saphenous vein and saphenous nerve come in the path of the incision. The former is divided and ligated, while the latter is identified and preserved.

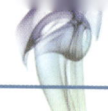

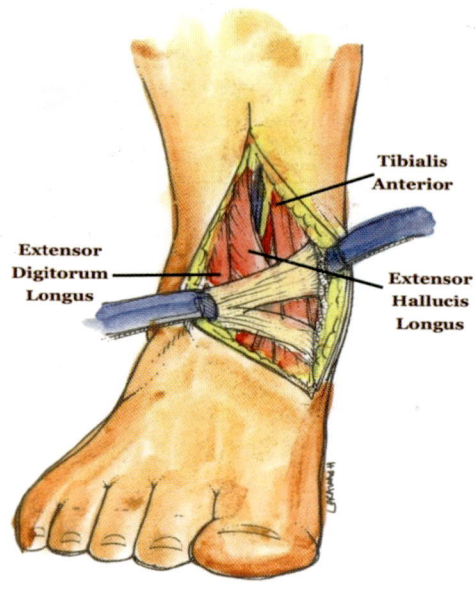

The medial border of the tibialis anterior tendon, along with the long extensor tendons and the neurovascular bundle are mobilized and retracted laterally with the foot dorsiflexed.

The dissection is deepened to periosteum along the same line.

It is now possible to reach as lateral as the anterior tibial tubercle.

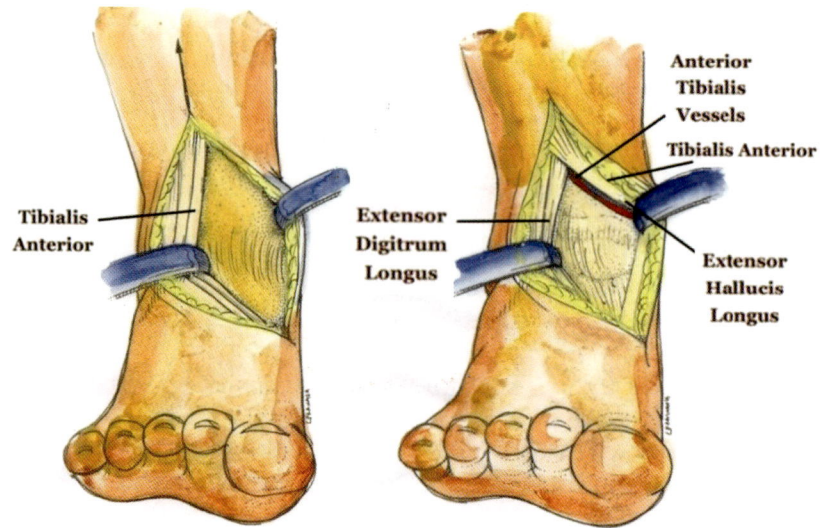

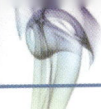

If additional exposure is desired, then a separate dissection is done between the extensor digitorum longus tendon and the neurovascular bundle medially and the extensor hallucis longus laterally.

Indications:

- Distal tibia ("pilon" fractures) and supramalleolar tibial fractures.
- Fractures of the tibial shaft extending down into the ankle.
- Tumours and other pathology of the anterior regions of the distal tibia and of the ankle joint.

Posterolateral Approach

Positioning: The patient is positioned supine with a sandbag under the buttock to shift the limb into internal rotation.

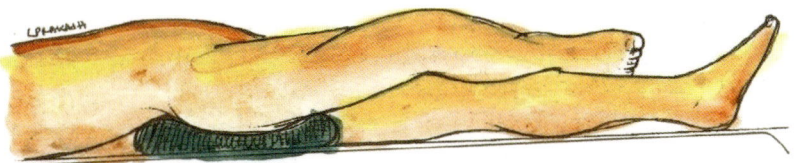

By flexing the knee and placing the heel on the opposite limb, additional posteromedial exposure can be achieved.

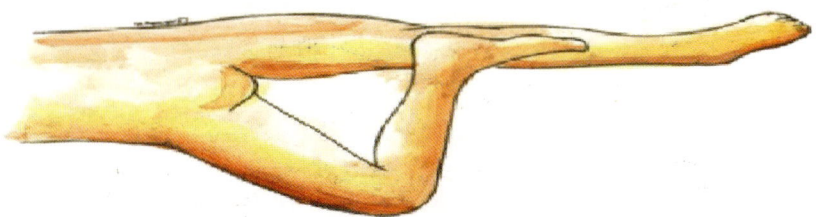

Access:

- Distal fibular shaft.
- Lateral malleolus.
- Anterior aspect of the inferior tibiofibular syndesmosis.
- Posterolateral quadrant of the distal tibia.

Incision: Along the posterior border of the lower third of the fibula, anterior to the surface marking of the sural nerve.

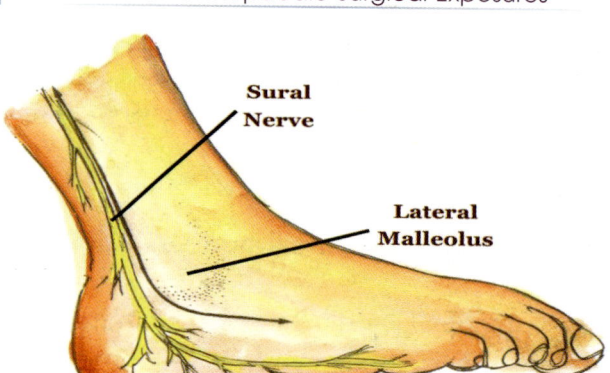

Below the tip of the lateral malleolus, the sural nerve curves in a lazy L fashion towards the peroneal tubercle.

In the lower curved portion, the sural nerve is close by and must be carefully located and protected.

Approach: Subcutaneous fascia over the lateral surface of fibula is dissected anteriorly, exposing the anterior inferior tibiofibular ligament and anterior tibial tubercle.

Dissection beneath the posterior edge of the incision exposes the sheath and retinaculum of the peroneus longus and brevis tendons.

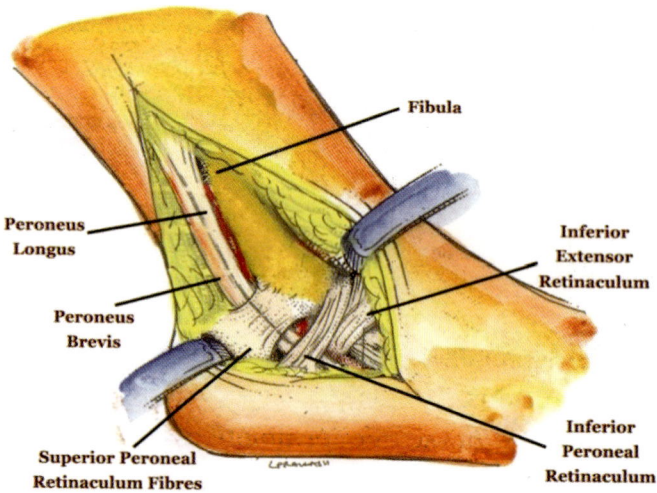

Incision of peroneal sheath allows mobilization of the tendons forwards, exposing the posterior border of the fibula.

At the level of the malleolus, the surface of the posterior talofibular ligament is separated by blunt dissection leading to the posterior aspect of the talus.

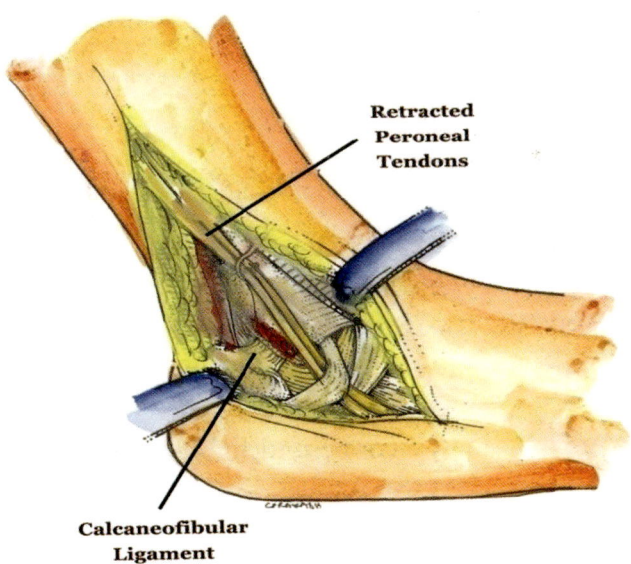

Retracted Peroneal Tendons

Calcaneofibular Ligament

Blunt dissection carried proximally reaches the posterior surface of the tibia.

Peroneal artery is ligated and secured, if it comes in the way and interferes with the procedure.

A long incision is preferable to avoid forceful soft tissue retraction and later wound healing problems.

Indications: Fixation of fractures of the distal fibula and of the lateral malleolus.

Associated posterior lip fracture of the tibia (Volkmann's fracture).

Procedures on the peroneal tendons, for reconstructive operations.

Posteromedial Approach

Positioning: Supine position with the knee flexed, the hip externally rotated, and the ankle placed on the shin of the other leg.

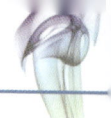

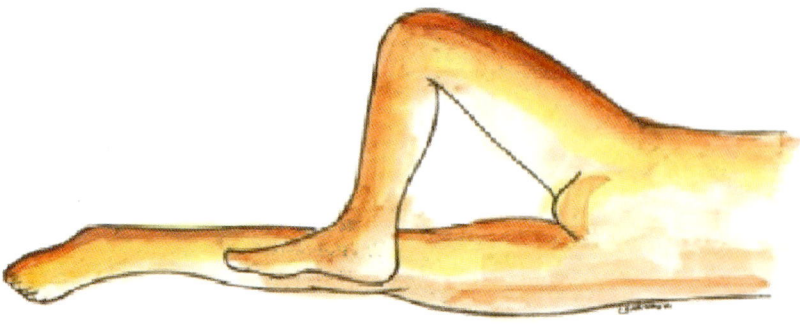

Access: Whole of the medial malleolus.

Medial and posteromedial aspects of the distal tibia.

Tendons and neurovascular bundle behind the lower medial tibia.

Incision: The incision begins in the lower third of tibia and runs distally, parallel to and 1 cm behind the posteromedial border of the tibia.

It then curves anteriorly, below the medial malleolus to the navicular tubercle.

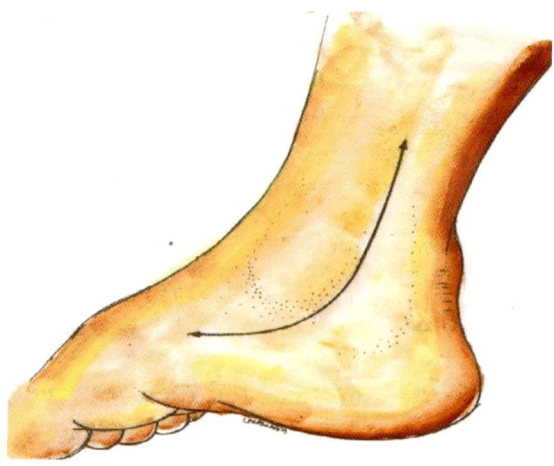

Approach: Dissection of subcutaneous fat and fascia reveals the deep fascia over the tendons of tibialis posterior and flexor digitorum longus, the posterior tibial neurovascular bundle and both tendon and belly of flexor hallucis longus.

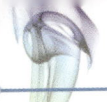

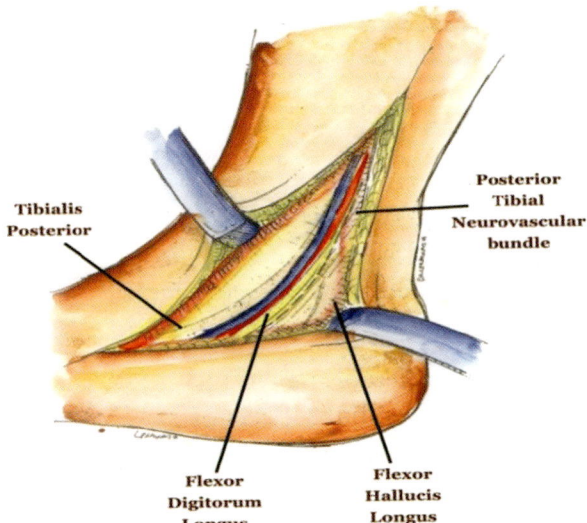

Tibialis
Posterior

Posterior
Tibial
Neurovascular
bundle

Flexor
Digitorum
Longus

Flexor
Hallucis
Longus

Further blunt dissection on the surface of this fascia leads to its anterior attachment to the posteromedial border of the tibia proximally and to the medial malleolus distally, where it thickens to form the flexor retinaculum.

For access to the posteromedial aspect, the deep fascia is carefully dissected from above, in the line of the incision, to expose the tendons and neurovascular bundle behind the tibia and medial malleolus.

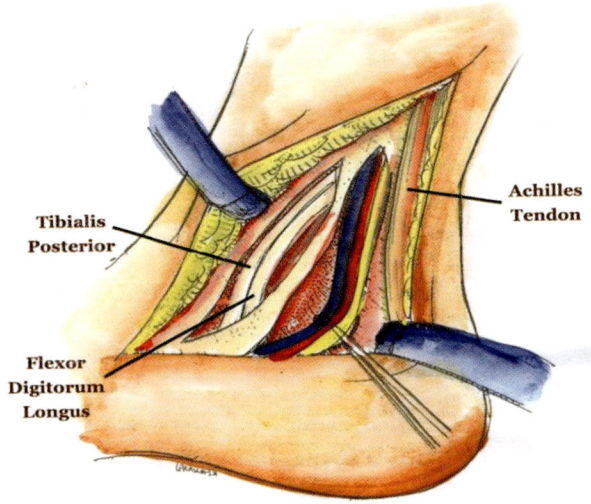

Achilles
Tendon

Tibialis
Posterior

Flexor
Digitorum
Longus

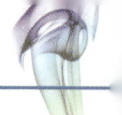

Plantar flexion of the foot slackens these posterior structures.

Just above the ankle, the posterior tibial artery usually gives off a lateral communicating branch to the peroneal artery, which is located and ligated.

Indications:

- Fixation of fractures of the medial malleolus.
- Posterior malleolar fractures of the tibia, where the fragment is more posteromedial than posterolateral.
- Exploration of the tendons and neurovascular bundle behind the medial malleolus.

Posterior Approach

Positioning: Prone with foam wedge support under chest and pelvis to keep abdomen free.

A pillow under the shin keeps the knee flexed at 30°.

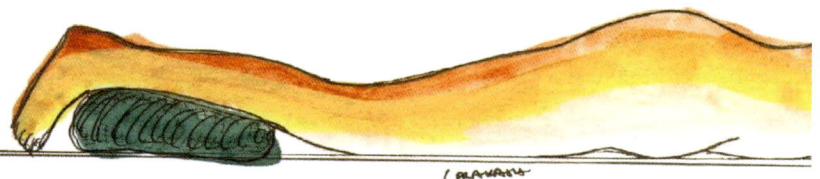

Access:

- Back of the distal tibia.
- Posterior aspect of the talus.
- Superior aspect of the body of the calcaneum.
- The exposure is limited between the inferior tibiofibular joint and the posterior lip of the medial malleolus.

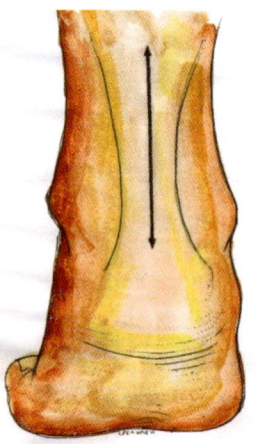

Incision: A straight midline skin incision over the length of the Achilles tendon, exposing its sheath and its insertion into the heel.

Approach: Z plasty of tendo-achillis. The separated ends are retracted north-south, and protected with repeatedly moistened swabs.

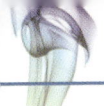

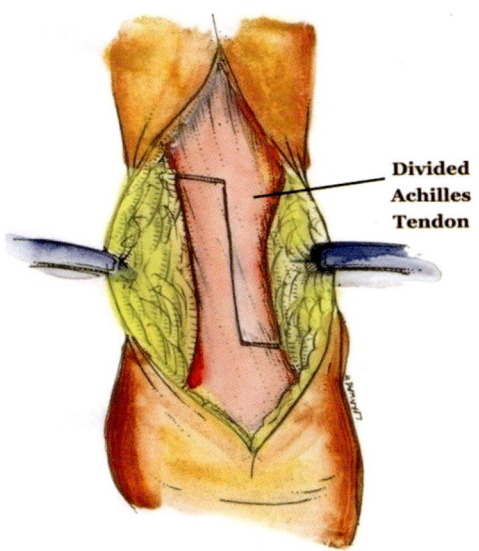

Divided
Achilles
Tendon

Deep fascia over the fat pad behind the ankle is incised and the fat pad removed.

The interval between the flexor hallucis longus medially and the peroneal muscles laterally is then developed to expose the back of the tibia and ankle, the posterior tubercle of the talus, and the upper surface of the calcaneum.

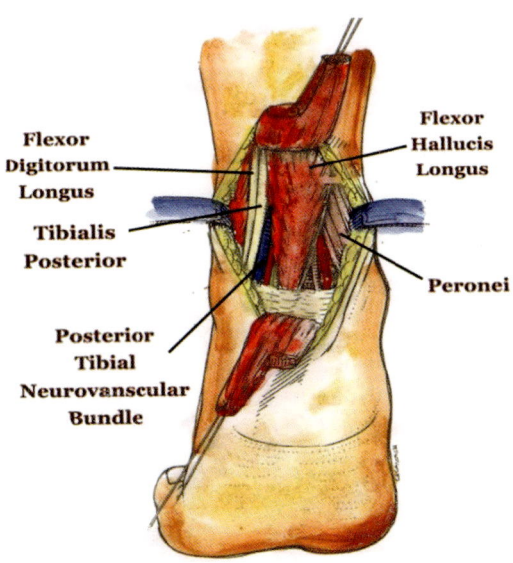

Flexor
Digitorum
Longus

Tibialis
Posterior

Posterior
Tibial
Neurovascular
Bundle

Flexor
Hallucis
Longus

Peronei

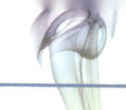

Care should be taken to locate the peroneal artery laterally and also any communicating vessels running horizontally across the back of the ankle capsule. They are later ligated.

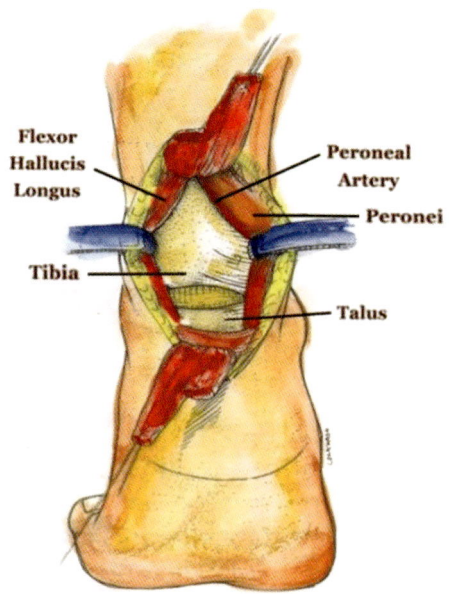

The Achilles tendon is repaired during closure of the wound.

Indications:
- Fractures of the posterior ankle.
- Posterior arthrodesis of the ankle.
- Lesions of bone or joint in the posterior aspect of ankle.

Transfibular Approach (Gatellier and Chastang)

Positioning: The patient is positioned supine on the operating table with a pad beneath the ankle.

A sandbag beneath the ipsilateral buttock improves lateral access.

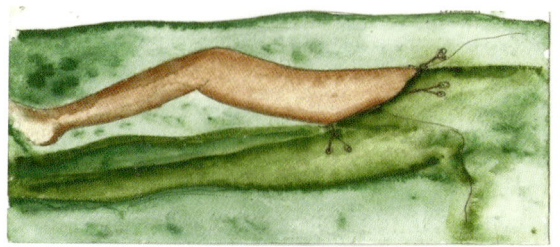

Access:
- The lateral portion of the ankle joint.
- Incisura fibularis.

Incision: Along the posterior border of the lower third of the fibula, anterior to the surface marking of the sural nerve.

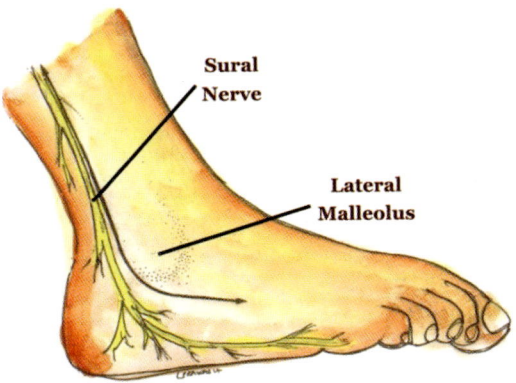

Sural Nerve

Lateral Malleolus

Approach: Osteotomy of the fibular shaft and turning down the distal portion, hinging on the lateral ligament complex.

At about 7.5 cm above the ankle, an oblique hole is drilled upwards and medially through the fibula.

An oblique fibular osteotomy is made in a plane perpendicular to the drill hole axis in the sagittal plane, so that the hole passes through the centre of the cut bony surface.

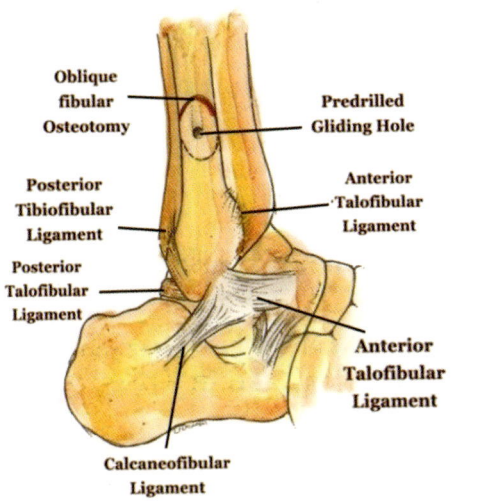

Oblique fibular Osteotomy

Predrilled Gliding Hole

Posterior Tibiofibular Ligament

Anterior Talofibular Ligament

Posterior Talofibular Ligament

Anterior Talofibular Ligament

Calcaneofibular Ligament

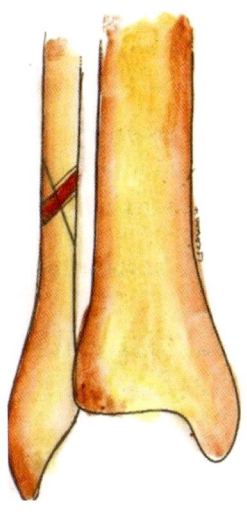

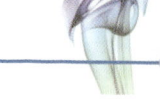

The lateral half of this hole is then over-drilled (lagged) to allow subsequent fixation with a screw through a fibular plate.

The distal fibular fragment is mobilized from the peronei and the ligaments of the inferior tibiofibular syndesmosis are carefully divided.

The fibula can now be turned down on lateral ligament, exposing the lateral aspect of talus and the lateral surface of the distal tibia.

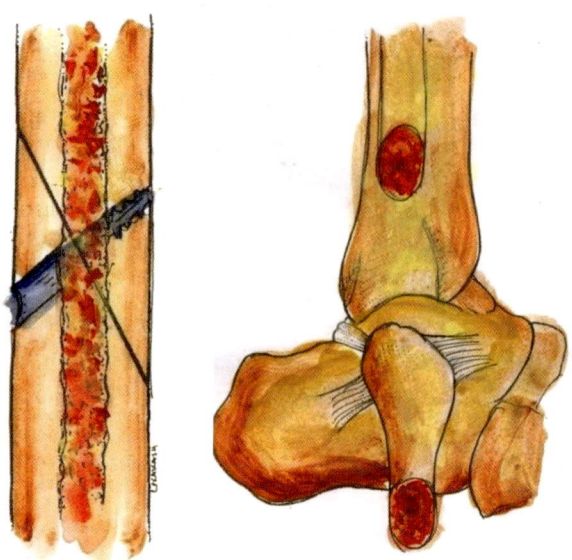

Repair is by suture of the ligaments of the syndesmosis after fixation of the fibular osteotomy as above.

Indications:
- Medial ankle fusion
- Ankle arthroplasty

Medial Transmalleolar Approach (König and Schafer)

History

Franz König (1832–1910): Franz König was a German surgeon born in Rotenburg an der Fulda and died in Grunewald near Berlin.

In 1855, he received his doctorate from the University of Marburg, and was later district wound surgeon in Hanau. Later he was a professor of surgery at the Universities of Rostock and Göttingen, and eventually the Charité, Berlin.

König is largely remembered for his work in bone and joint surgery. He was the first physician to identify the relationship between haemophilia and haemophilic arthropathy, as well as the first surgeon to perform a successful internal fixation of proximal femur fractures. In 1887, Franz König published a paper on the cause of loose bodies in the joint. In his paper, König concluded that: Lesser degrees of trauma might contuse the bone to cause an area of necrosis which might then separate.

Or in some cases, the absence of trauma made it likely that there existed some spontaneous cause of separation.

König named the disease "osteochondritis dissecans", describing it as a subchondral inflammatory process of the knee, resulting in a loose fragment of cartilage from the femoral condyle.

König's syndrome refers to abdominal symptoms caused by an incomplete obstruction of the small intestine. He described this exposure in 1929.

Positioning: The patient lies supine with a pad beneath the ankle. A sandbag is placed under the opposite buttock.

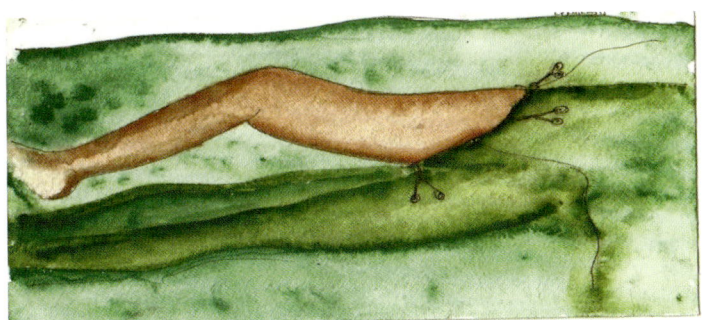

Access:
- Medial part of the ankle joint cavity
- Superomedial part of the dome of the talus.

Incision: Lower half of either the anteromedial or posteromedial incision.

Konig and Schafer originally described a horizontal curved incision, convex proximally, at the level of the ankle joint medially.

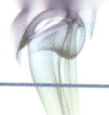

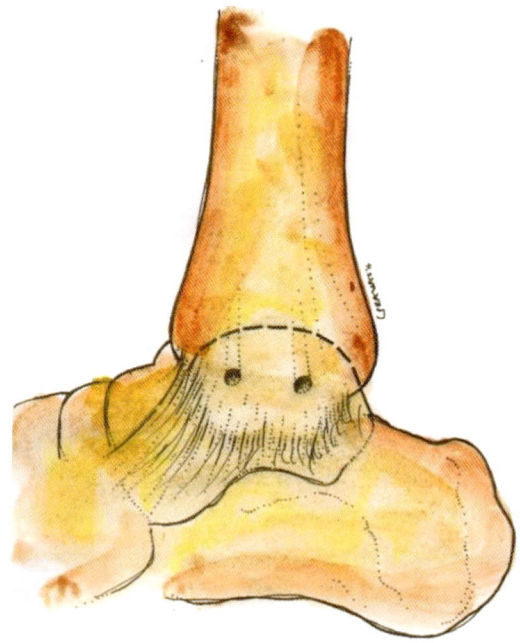

Approach: The medial malleolus is osteotomized and turned downwards, hinging on the deltoid ligament.

The base of the medial malleolus is exposed and a Hohmann retractor is passed posteriorly between the bone and the soft tissue structures behind the malleolus to protect them from injury during the osteotomy.

A near-vertical osteotomy is made to enter the ankle at the junction of the horizontal and vertical planes of the distal tibial articulation at the base of the medial malleolus.

Two drill holes are made through the middle of the proposed osteotomy site, to facilitate later reattachment with two cancellous lag screws.

The bone is then carefully divided with an oscillating saw in a near-vertical osteotomy. This step requires great care and precision.

The terminal thickness of the subchondral bone adjacent to the site of entry of the osteotomy is left uncut; the mobilization of the medial malleolar fragment is completed by osteoclasis to give an irregular, intra-articular fracture capable of being perfectly restored with the later fixation.

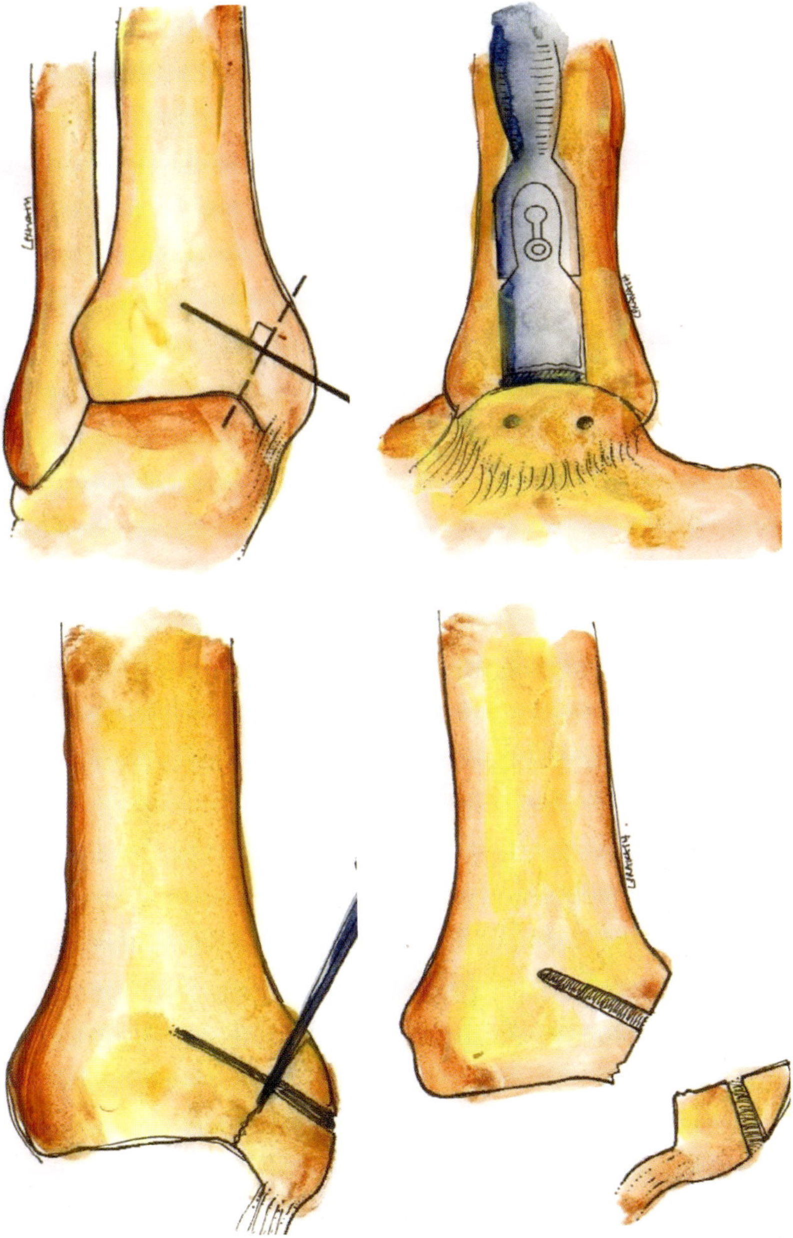

Soft tissue mobilization along the edges of the deltoid ligament will then permit downward tilting of the bony fragment and entry into the ankle joint.

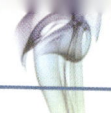

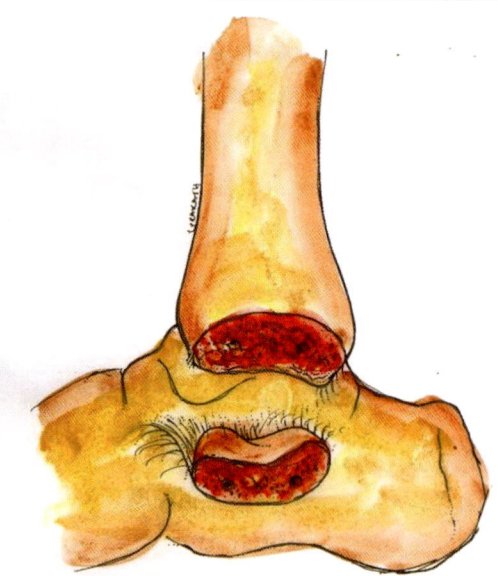

Indications: Intra-articular access to the medial side of the ankle for lesions of the superomedial dome of the talus, such as osteochondritis or osteochondral fractures.

The Foot

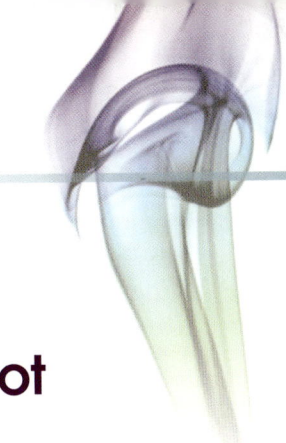

ANATOMY

Incisions on the foot should follow cleavage lines to allow formation of much finer scars.

On the plantar aspect and over the dorsum of the first ray, the cleavage lines are disposed longitudinally.

On the lateral aspect of the dorsum, they run obliquely from the medial side proximally to the lateral side distally.

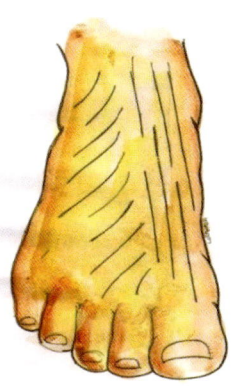

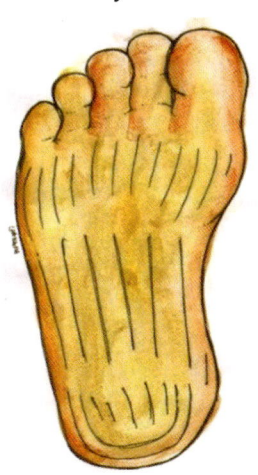

Peripheral Nerves

These should be spared and protected to avoid troublesome neuromas.

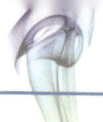

The main nerve trunks which supply the foot are as follows:

Sural Nerve

This passes into the foot just over 1 cm from the tip of the lateral malleolus and below the peroneal tendons at the base of the fifth metatarsal.

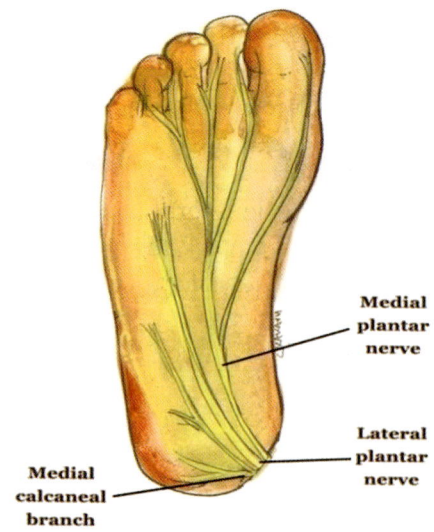

Medial plantar nerve

Lateral plantar nerve

Medial calcaneal branch

It divides into a lateral branch supplying the dorsolateral surface of the little toe, and a medial branch passing obliquely across the dorsolateral surface of the foot, to the fourth inter-osseous space, subdividing to supply the dorsomedial aspect of the little toe and the dorsolateral aspect of the fourth toe.

The sural nerve also gives off two lateral calcaneal branches above the lateral malleolus. The incisions on the lateral aspect should pass between this and the superficial peroneal nerve.

Superficial Peroneal Nerve

The first branch intermediate dorsal cutaneous nerve crosses the extensors to the fourth and fifth toes and divides distally in the third cleft to supply the dorsomedial side of the fourth toe and dorsolateral side of the third toe.

Its other division is the medial dorsal cutaneous nerve, which crosses the extensor retinaculum and runs lateral and parallel to the extensor hallucis longus tendon.

It gives off three branches. The medial branch crosses the tendon of extensor hallucis and runs distally on its medial side, anastomosing with the terminal part of the saphenous nerve, to supply the dorsomedial aspect of the great toe.

The lateral branch divides distally in the second cleft to supply the dorsomedial aspect of the third toe and the dorsolateral aspect of the second toe.

The middle branch divides distally in the first interspace to supply the dorsomedial aspect of the second toe and dorsolateral side of the great toe.

Plantar Aspect of the Foot

The sural nerve supply to the lateral side of the plantar aspect of the heel is thus:

The medial calcaneal branch of the posterior tibial exits just above the ankle and divides into a posterior branch to supply the medial and posterior aspects of the heel, and an anterior branch which supplies the medial side of the plantar aspect.

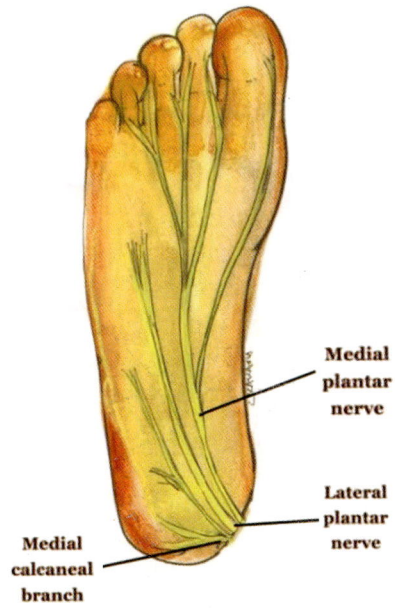

Medial plantar nerve

Lateral plantar nerve

Medial calcaneal branch

Part of the insole is supplied by the saphenous nerve. The base of the sole and plantar aspects of the medial three and a half toes are supplied by the medial plantar nerve; the other one

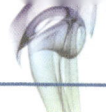

and a half by the lateral plantar nerve and a small area of the lateral border by the sural nerve.

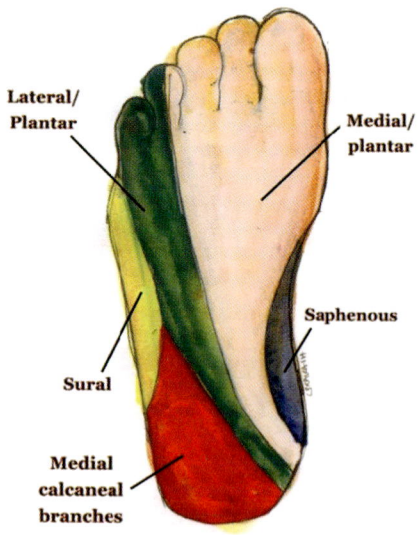

Neurovascular bundle on the dorsum of the foot includes the anterior tibial vessels and nerve.

They start in the centre of the ankle and run downward, between the extensor hallucis longus and the extensor digitorum, to the proximal end of the first intertarsal space.

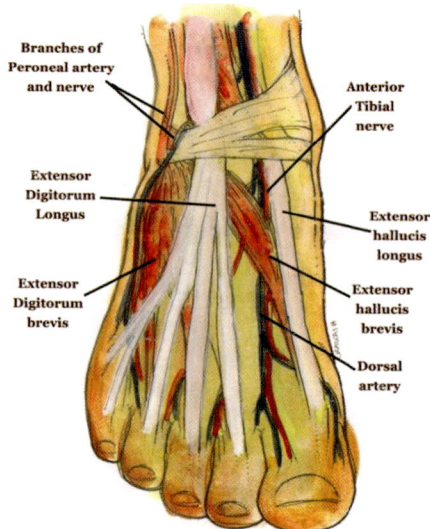

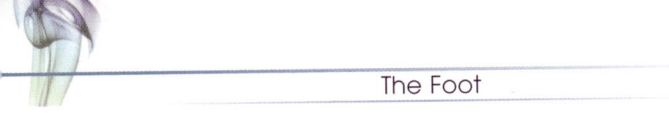

The main neurovascular bundles in the sole of the foot run deep to the first layer of muscles: The abductor hallucis longus and brevis, and flexor digitorum brevis.

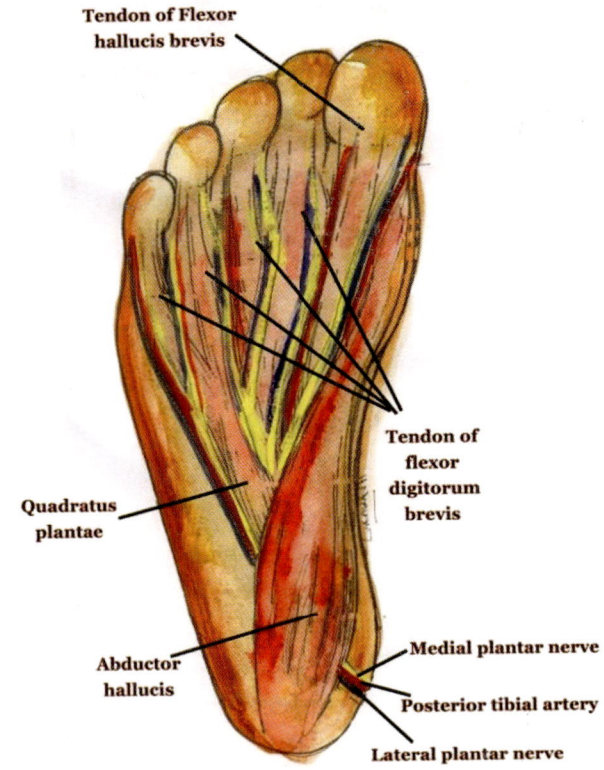

Tendon of Flexor hallucis brevis

Tendon of flexor digitorum brevis

Quadratus plantae

Medial plantar nerve

Abductor hallucis

Posterior tibial artery

Lateral plantar nerve

SURGICAL APPROACHES

- Anterolateral (Campbell)
- Lateral
- Medial (Henry)
- Plantar incisions
- Heel
- Medial calcaneum
- Plantar sagittal
- Dorsal sagittal
- Dorsal transverse
- Plantar transverse

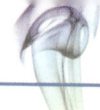

Anterolateral Approach (Campbell)

Position: The patient is placed supine, with a sandbag beneath the ipsilateral buttock.

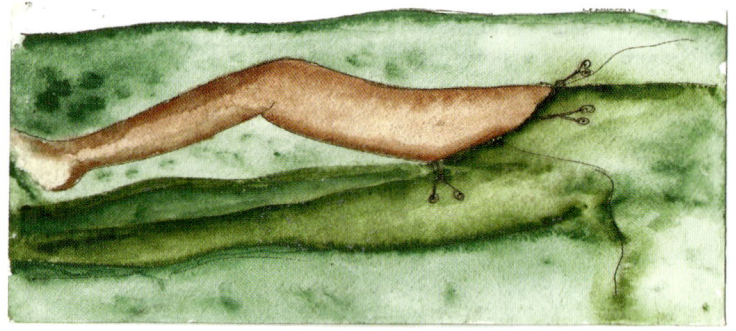

Access:
- Anterior aspect of the ankle
- Superolateral part of calcaneum
- Lateral aspect of the subtalar joint
- Sinus tarsi
- Calcaneocuboid and talonavicular joints.

Incision: The skin incision begins 3 to 4 cm above the lateral malleolus.

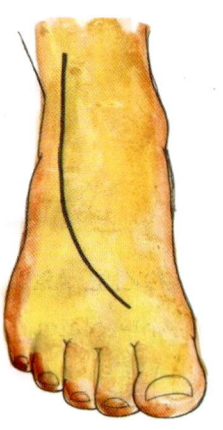

It passes downwards, following the anterior border of the fibula, to a point 1 cm below the malleolus.

It then curves gently medially across the dorsum of the foot in a line towards the base of the great toe.

Passing dorsal to the peroneal tendons, the cleavage is between the lateral and medial dorsal cutaneous nerves.

Approach: The deep fascia and the extensor retinaculum are divided, lateral to peroneus tertius and extensor digitorum brevis, which are partially reflected from their origin.

The medial flap thus created is freed from the underlying bones and joint capsules. This interval is developed inferiorly under the extensor tendons, which are elevated and retracted medially.

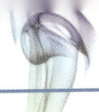

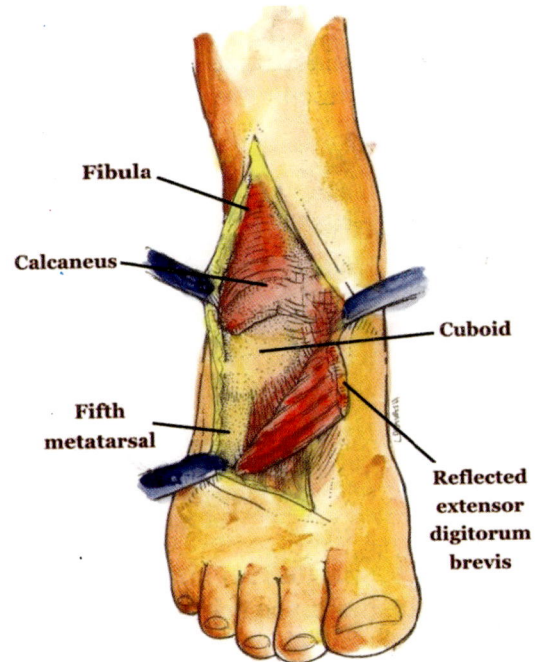

Fibula

Calcaneus

Cuboid

Fifth
metatarsal

Reflected
extensor
digitorum
brevis

The peronei are separated from the underlying fascia and retracted posteriorly.

The cleavage thus created exposes the anterior aspect of the ankle, the superolateral part of the calcaneum, the lateral aspect of the subtalar joint, the sinus tarsi, the calcaneocuboid joint and the talonavicular joint.

Advantages:
- The most versatile of dorsal approaches.
- Gives the greatest access to the tarsal joints.
- Wound closes easily.
- Being in the line of a vascular anastomosis, it heals well.

Indications:
- Ankle joint replacement
- Ankle arthrodesis
- Anterior tibiofibular ligament repair
- Tarsal fusions
- The full extent of the incision is not always needed, and can be tailored according to circumstances.

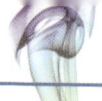

Lateral Approach

Position: The patient is placed supine, with a large sandbag beneath the ipsilateral buttock.

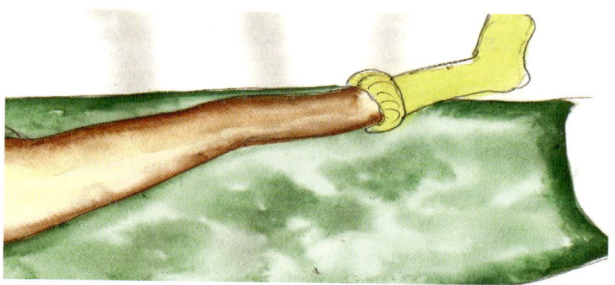

Access:
- Calcaneum
- Peronei
- Lateral ligaments of the ankle
- Subtalar joint
- Base of the fifth metatarsal

Incision: The incision begins just anterior to the lateral border of the Achilles tendon.

It passes obliquely forwards and downwards, skirting the apex of the lateral malleolus.

It then passes across the peroneal tubercle to reach the lower border of the calcaneum and the base of the fifth metatarsal.

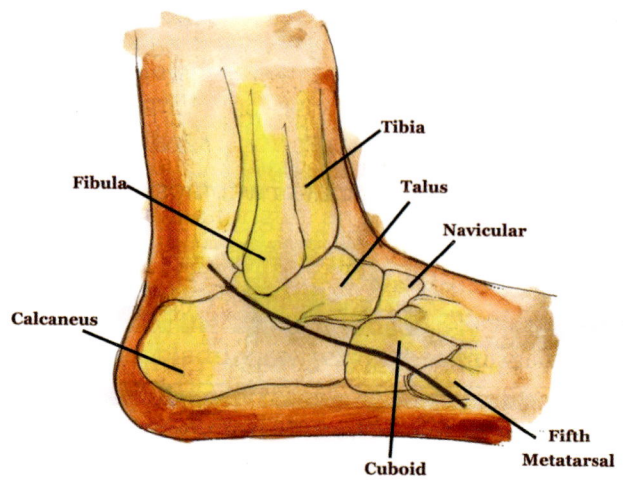

Approach: The incision is deepened, the peroneal sheath opened, and the peronei retracted out of the way.

The deep incision lies parallel to the peronei, beneath and behind them.

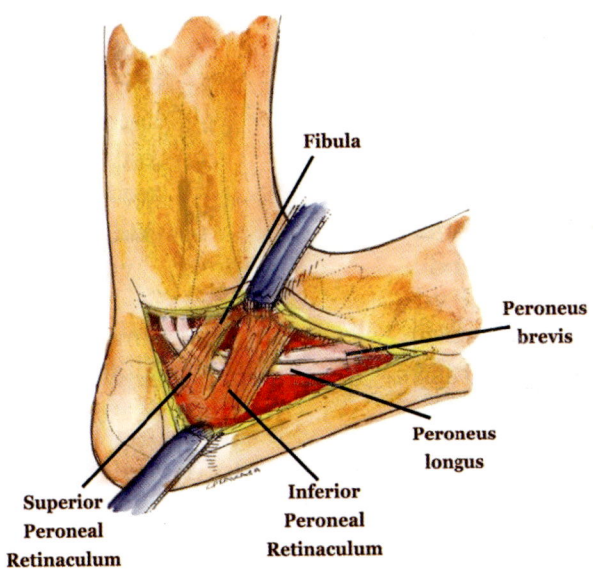

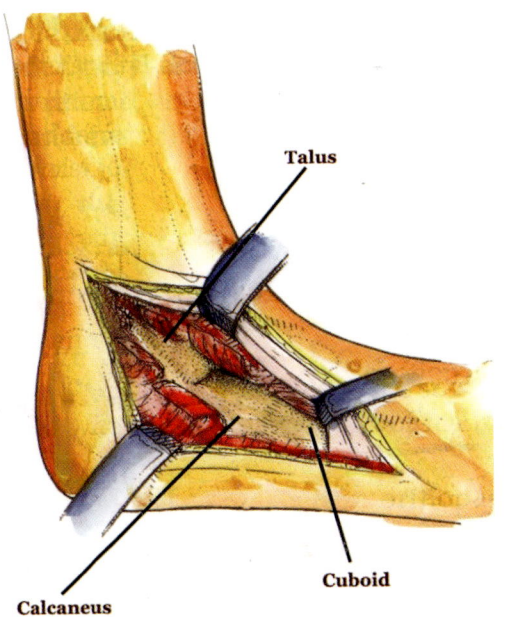

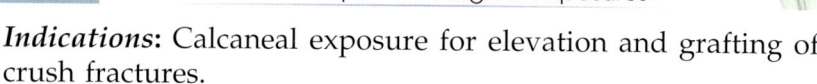

Indications: Calcaneal exposure for elevation and grafting of crush fractures.

Osteotomies of the calcaneum.

Problems of peronei and the lateral ligaments of the ankle.

Medial Approach (Henry)

Position: Supine with a sandbag beneath the contralateral buttock. With the knee flexed and the hip externally rotated, excellent access is provided.

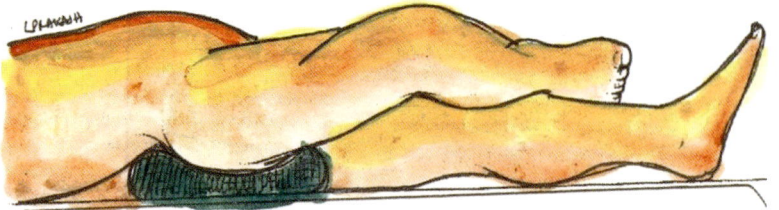

Access: Posterior tibial compartment.

Medial aspects of both the tarsus and the plantar aponeurosis.

Incision: Starts 3 cm above the medial malleolus, midway between the tendo-Achilles and the posteromedial border of the tibia.

It passes down behind the medial malleolus to just beyond its tip and then curves towards the base of the first metatarsal.

Medial calcaneal nerve branches are vulnerable to damage here.

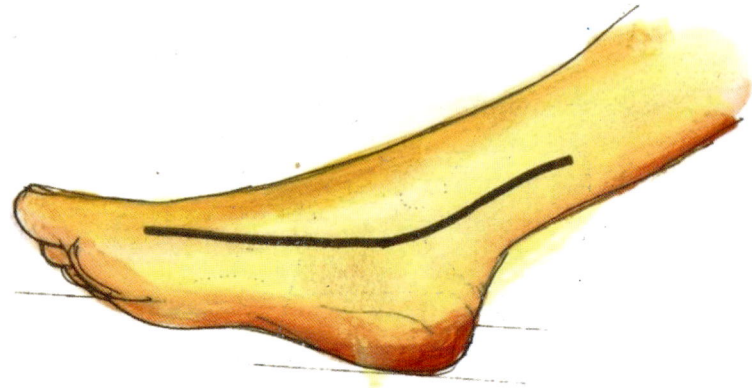

Approach: The deep fascia and the retinaculum of the posterior tibial compartment are cut to expose the tarsal tunnel containing flexor digitorum and hallucis longus, the tibialis posterior tendon, and the posterior tibial neurovascular bundle.

Inferior to the medial malleolus lies the abductor hallucis muscle, whose tendon passes on the belly of the flexor hallucis brevis, below the first metatarsal base.

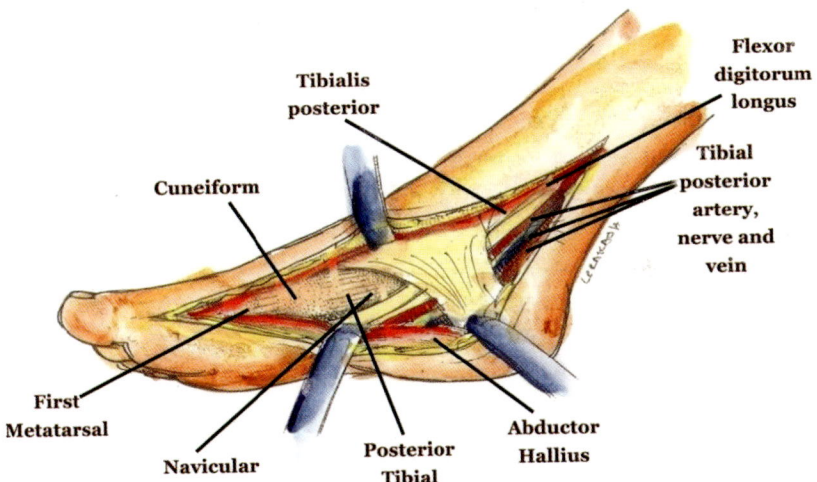

The abductor hallucis is swung plantar-wards by partially detaching its origin.

The medial plantar nerve and artery are seen on its deep surface.

At this point, 2 cm proximal to the navicular tuberosity, the flexor digitorum crosses medial to the flexor hallucis longus tendon.

The posterior tibial nerve divides 2 cm below the medial malleolus into lateral and medial plantar nerves.

The lateral plantar nerve passes along the lateral border of flexor digitorum brevis.

All these nerves should be identified and protected.

The posterior portion of the insertion of tibialis posterior tendon into the navicular tuberosity may be partially lifted anteriorly, to improve the access.

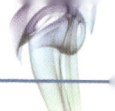

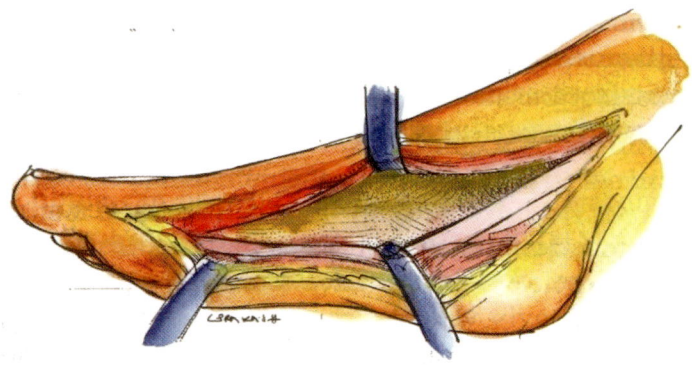

***Indications*:** Access to:

- Plantar aspect and medial side of the inner column of the calcaneum, navicular, medial cuneiform and first metatarsal, and the joints between them.
- Medial release in club foot.
- Tarsal tunnel decompression.

Plantar Incisions

Plantar Approach to the Heel

A midline incision to the long axis of the foot is made in the heel pad down to the plantar ligament.

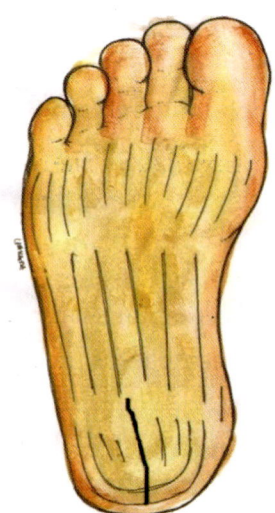

Indications: Lesions of calcaneum in this area.

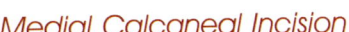

Medial Calcaneal Incision

The skin is incised parallel with the inferior bony border of the calcaneum.

Indications:

- Plantar fasciotomy
- Steindler fasciotomy

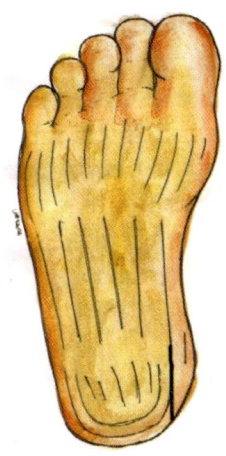

Plantar Sagittal Incisions

These can be used anywhere on the plantar surface.

2 cm incisions over the appropriate cleft are used for excision of digital neuromas.

The fat is incised and retracted. The deep fascia is then divided, to expose the bifurcations of the vessels and nerves to the cleft.

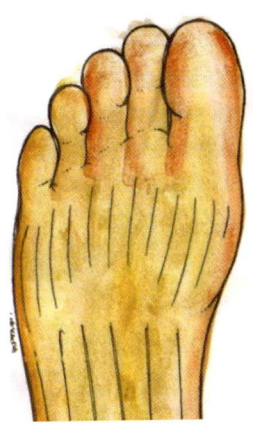

A 2 cm incision beneath any metatarsal head provides access to either sesamoid or to the flexor sheath and the flexor tendon.

The flexor sheath is incised and the tendon retracted away from the sesamoid to be excised.

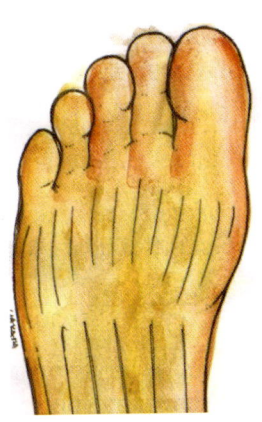

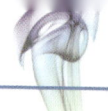

Dorsal Sagittal Incisions

Access: Metatarsal heads and necks from the dorsum.

Incisions: 2 cm skin incisions over the first and fifth metatarsals and a single 3 cm incision over the middle metatarsal provide adequate access to the distal thirds or the metatarsals mentioned.

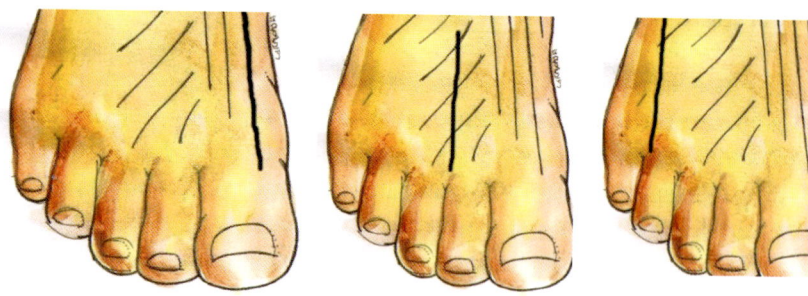

Approach: Dissection proceeds down to the bone, avoiding section of cutaneous nerves, veins and extensor tendons.

Small Hohmann levers are placed round the bone, the soft tissues separated, and the bone further exposed proximally and distally by gentle blunt dissection.

A sharp periosteal elevator is used to strip the periosteum and interossei from the bone to be exposed.

Indications:
- Osteotomies of the metatarsals.
- Metatarsophalangeal arthroplasties.

Dorsal Transverse Approach

Access: Dorsal aspect of metatarsal heads and necks and the metatarsophalangeal joints.

Incision: The skin is incised transversely across the line of the metatarsal heads.

Approach: The skin is retracted and the incisions deepened in the sagittal plane on the medial sides of the extensors, down to the dorsal capsules of the joints. These are incised transversely (if access to the joint alone is required) or longitudinally (if the necks and shafts of the metatarsals also need to be exposed).

Indications: Synovectomy of the metatarsophalangeal joints.

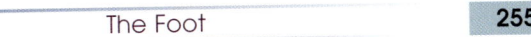

Plantar Transverse Approach

Access: Metatarsal heads from the plantar aspect.

Incision: A transverse incision is made over the metatarsal necks.

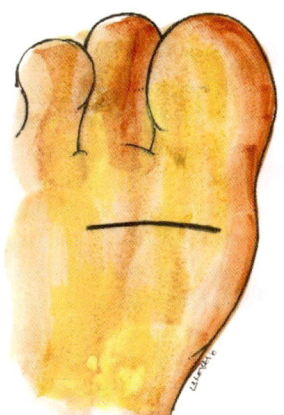

Approach: There is usually little subcutaneous fat and the deep fascia and joint capsules are exposed through longitudinal incisions.

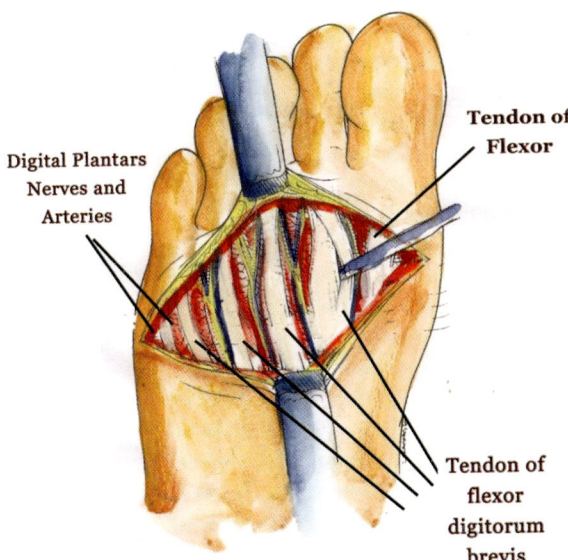

Indications:
- Excision of metatarsal heads.
- Repositioning of a distally migrated metatarsal fat pad, usually in rheumatoid arthritis.

The Shoulder

ANATOMY OF THE SHOULDER

The shoulder has two *true* joints; the glenohumeral and the acromioclavicular and one *false* subacromial joint, which allows the supraspinatus tendon to glide under the coracoacromial arch.

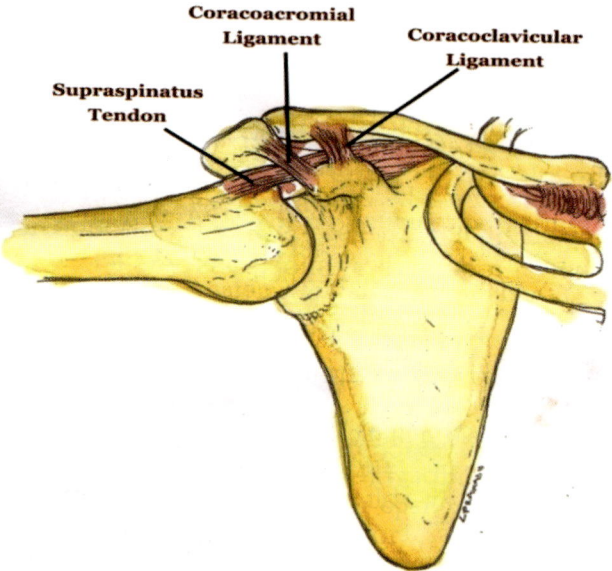

The function of the glenohumeral joint depends on the muscles around the shoulder, of which the deltoid is the most important.

The deltoid cloaks the shoulder region and must be either retracted, split longitudinally or detached and reattached to give access to the glenohumeral and subacromial joints.

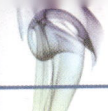

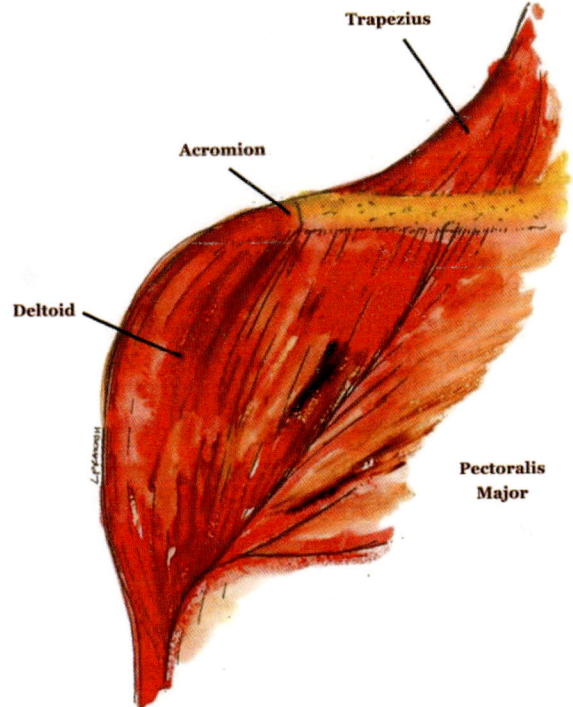

The deltoid should not be detached from its origins (the acromion, the lateral spine of the scapula and the lateral third of the clavicle) unless absolutely necessary for exposure, as repair is difficult and will delay the start of the postoperative physiotherapy.

Nerves at Risk

Anteriorly

The musculocutaneous nerve leaves the brachial plexus opposite the lower border of the pectoralis minor muscle.

It passes laterally, giving one or two small twigs to the coracobrachialis.

It then pierces the coracobrachialis about 7.5 cm below the tip of the acromion and runs down laterally in the groove between the biceps and the brachialis.

On reaching the lateral side of the arm, it ends as the lateral cutaneous nerve of the forearm.

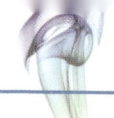

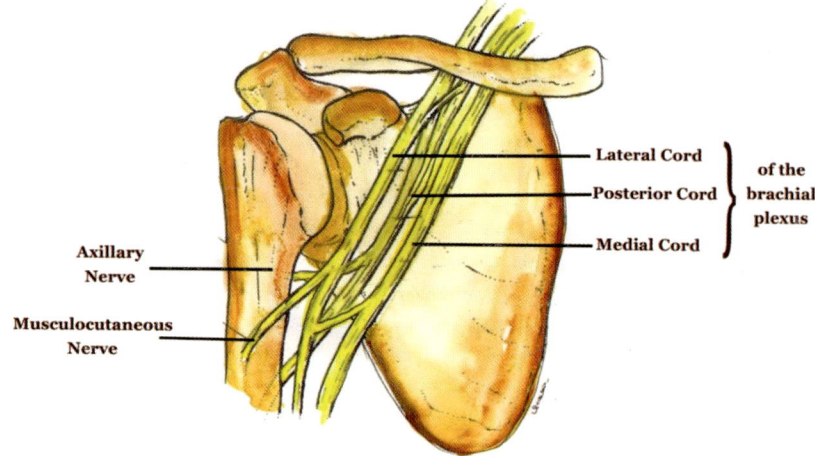

It may be injured due to traction as it passes through coraco-brachialis or it can be caught in sutures inserted inferior to the glenoid.

Inferiorly

The axillary nerve is at risk, as it passes around the back of the neck of the humerus. It is located 5 cm distal to the tip of the acromion, where it passes through the quadrilateral space and then into the deltoid muscle. Finally, as the lateral cutaneous nerve of the arm, it provides the sensory supply over the lateral aspect of the upper arm.

Posteriorly

The suprascapular nerve travels around the scapular notch at the lateral end of the spine of the scapula when passing from the supraspinatus to the infraspinatus muscles and ends in terminal branches a little short of medial scapular border.

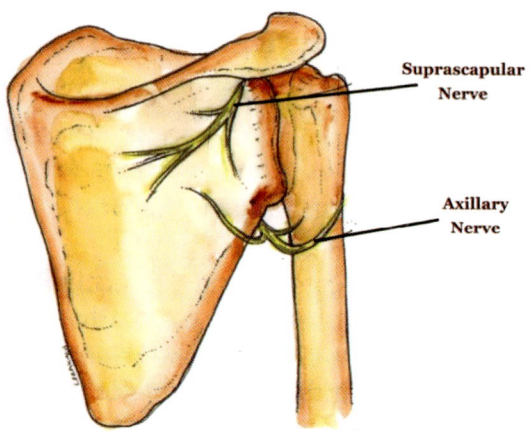

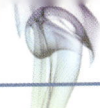

Positioning

Two standard positions are used for shoulder surgery.

The dental chair position for all anterior and superior surgery and the lateral position for posterior surgery.

Dental Chair Position

The shoulder is elevated by adjusting the trunk to a 45° tilt, reducing venous pressure and the risk of bleeding.

The shoulder is stabilized by placing a small sandbag under the medial border of the scapula. This is the ideal position for most shoulder operations and is the most commonly used.

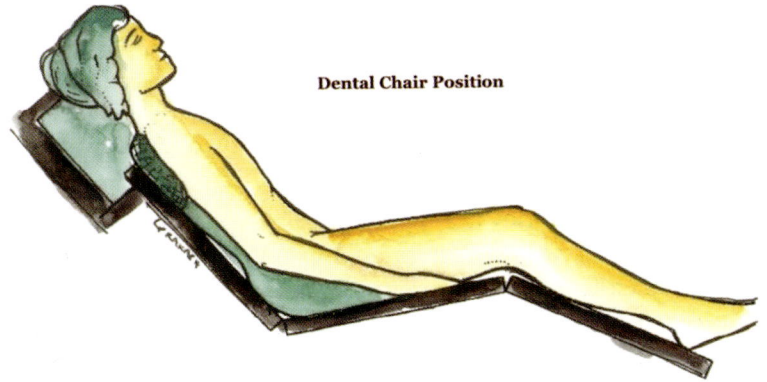

Dental Chair Position

Lateral Position

This again ensures elevation of the shoulder region and allows access to both the back and the front of the shoulder. The trunk must be stabilized with supports anteriorly against the lower chest cage and posteriorly with a firm pad applied to the middle of the thoracic spine. This position is used both for posterior shoulder surgery and for arthroscopy of the shoulder.

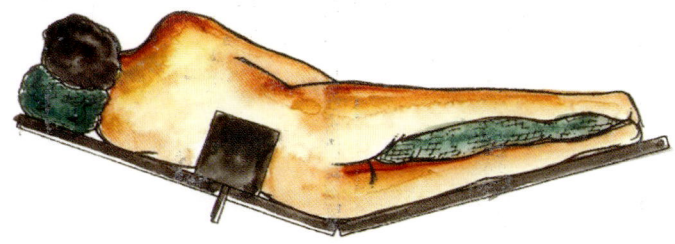

Lateral Position

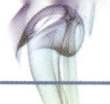

SURGICAL APPROACHES

- Anterior deltopectoral (Neer)
- Long anterior deltopectoral (Watson and Stanton, 1932)
- Anterior extensile (Redfem, Wallace and Beddows, 1989)
- Axillary
- Deltoid-splitting transacromioclavicular joint (AC joint) (Ha'Eri and Wiley, 1981)
- Transacromial (Kessel, 1982)
- Posterior
- Coronal for acromioclavicular joint
- Parasagittal for acromioclavicular joint

Anterior Deltopectoral Approach

History: Dr Charles Neer II, was born in Vinita, Oklahoma in 1917, the son and grandson of physicians. He graduated from Dartmouth College and obtained his MD from the University of Pennsylvania.

He began a residency at Presbyterian Hospital, New York City, and his training was interrupted by WWII. After the war, he returned to Columbia University to complete his residency, and join the faculty, where he remained throughout his career. He retired as an Emeritus Professor in 1990.

Dr Neer, a prolific writer, published his first paper on hip fractures in 1948, and his last paper in 1992. Though he wrote on many topics, the majority were related to the shoulder.

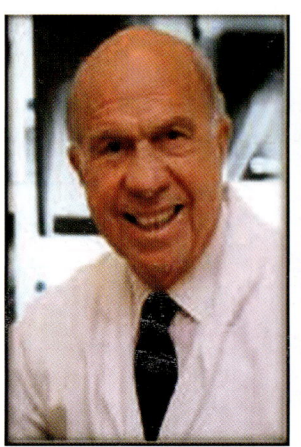 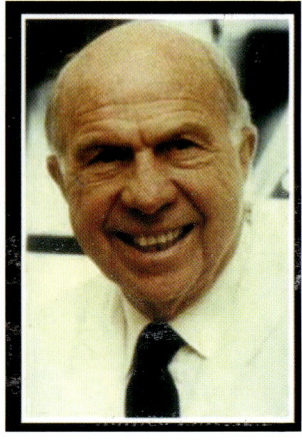

In 1968, Dr Neer organized a symposium titled "The Clavicle", in which the papers reviewed the development and anatomy of the clavicle, and the treatment of various injuries. He was a founding member and the first president of the American Shoulder and Elbow Surgeons in 1982, served on the American Board of Orthopedic Surgery, the Board of Trustees of The Journal of Shoulder and Elbow Surgery, and the International Board of Shoulder and Elbow Surgery.

Among his most popular works is a classification of shoulder fractures reported in 1970 and still widely used today. He has also made many other contributions, including an understanding of the impingement syndrome and a procedure to alleviate the impingement.

Neer was a pioneer in shoulder arthroplasty, and developed the first practical and widely-used prosthesis for the shoulder.

In his view, all comminuted fractures of the proximal humerus treated by internal fixation, resection arthroplasty, or arthrodesis had "unsatisfactory" outcomes. He reasoned that replacement of the humeral articular surface provided better pain relief and function, and designed a device and surgical technique for implantation. Neer reported 12 patients in his initial series, all of whom had acute or long standing "extra-articular extrusion and detachment of the humeral head or a long-standing painful incongruity of the humeral articulation." 11 of the 12 patients had pain relief, the exception being a patient with "improper seating of the prosthesis."

He described the anterior deltopectoral approach, the most popular for all anterior affections of the shoulder.

Access:
- Front of the shoulder.
- Exploration of the glenohumeral joint.
- The anterior glenoid rim can be exposed.
- However, access to the rest of the glenohumeral joint and the humeral neck is limited.

Incision: A vertical incision about 7.5 cm long is made from the tip of the coracoid down to the axillary fold. This is deepened through fat to the fascia overlying the deltoid and pectoralis major.

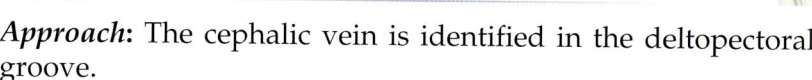

Approach: The cephalic vein is identified in the deltopectoral groove.

The deltoid and pectoralis major are separated with the cephalic vein retracted medially, and side branches are ligated.

Some surgeons routinely ligate this at the proximal and distal ends.

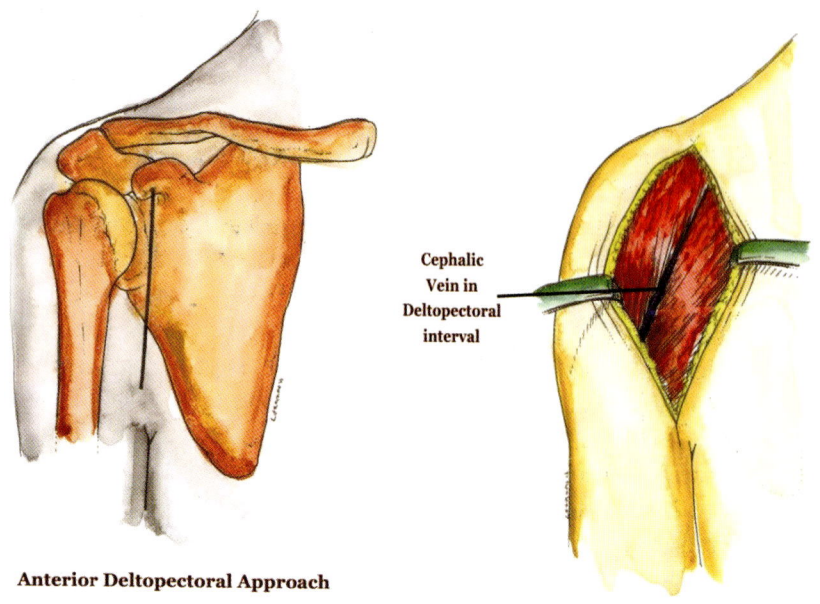

Cephalic
Vein in
Deltopectoral
interval

Anterior Deltopectoral Approach

Retractors are inserted into the cleavage between deltoid and pectoralis major. The coracoid is now exposed proximally and a small, plus-shaped incision is made over the tip of the coracoid which is predrilled with a 2.5 mm diameter drill along the length of the distal part.

The direction of drilling is determined by palpation of the coracoid. The depth of the hole is then measured, tapped with a 3.5 mm tap and thus prepared for reattachment later with a 4.0 mm small cancellous screw. The soft tissues are divided across the coracoid 1.5 cm from its tip and haemostasis achieved before cutting the coracoid with a power saw or osteotome. The divided tip of the coracoid is gently retracted downwards and soft tissue dissected away from the tendon, while preserving the musculocutaneous nerve at its medial edge.

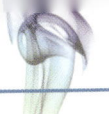
Coracoid
Process

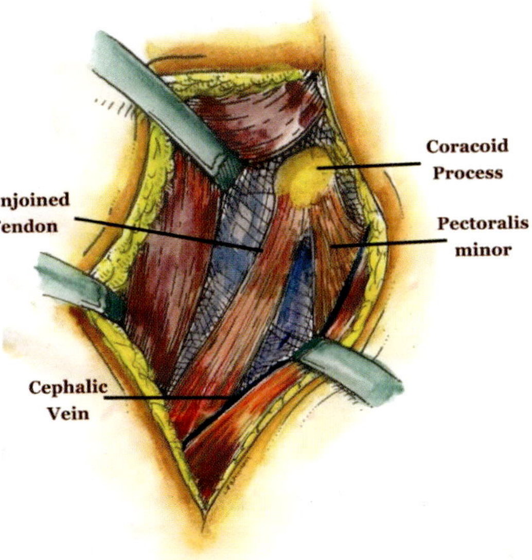

Conjoined
Tendon

Pectoralis
minor

Cephalic
Vein

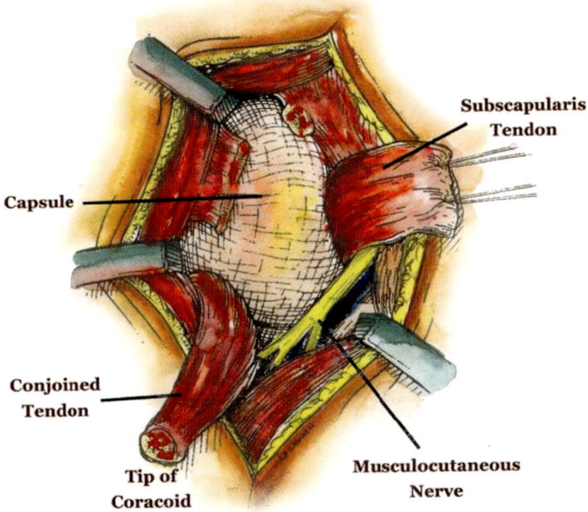

Subscapularis
Tendon

Capsule

Conjoined
Tendon

Tip of
Coracoid

Musculocutaneous
Nerve

The coracoid and conjoined tendon should now be gently placed in a subcutaneous pocket just inferior to the distal end of the incision. Unnecessary traction may result in injury to the musculocutaneous nerve.

The subscapularis tendon overlies the front of the humeral head. Its upper border is identified by palpation just inferior to the base of the coracoid and its lower border by a bunch of veins coursing along this border.

These veins are cauterized and the anterior capsule separated from the subscapularis by gentle dissection. Two stay sutures should now be inserted into the subscapularis to control retraction and its tendon divided 2.5 cm from its lateral attachment. By external rotation of the arm, the anterior capsule is exposed and can be divided vertically to expose the glenohumeral joint and the anterior rim of the glenoid.

Indications:

- Repair of recurrent anterior dislocation of the shoulder.
- Removal of loose bodies.
- Drainage of a septic arthritis.
- Limited synovectomy.

Long Anterior Deltopectoral Approach (Neer, Watson and Stanton)

Access:

- Front of the glenohumeral joint
- Upper humeral shaft
- Humeral head

Incision: The incision extends from the clavicle, across the tip of the coracoid to the anterior border of the deltoid.

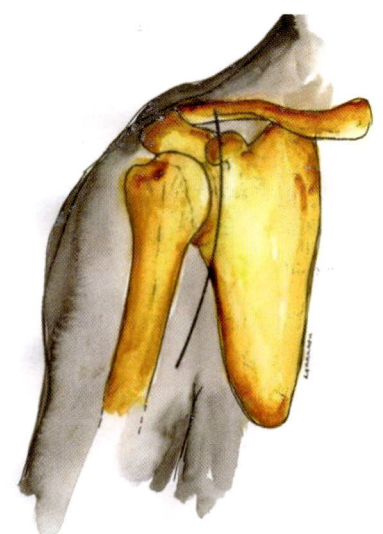

Long Anterior Deltopectoral Approach

Approach: The cephalic vein is ligated distally and proximally.
   The deltoid is retracted laterally.
   The arm is abducted 50°.
   The clavipectoral fascia is then incised.
   A broad elevator is placed under the acromion as a retractor. Improved exposure is obtained by dividing the proximal 1.25 cm of the insertion of pectoralis major.
   The anterior insertion of deltoid can be released as described by Neer.

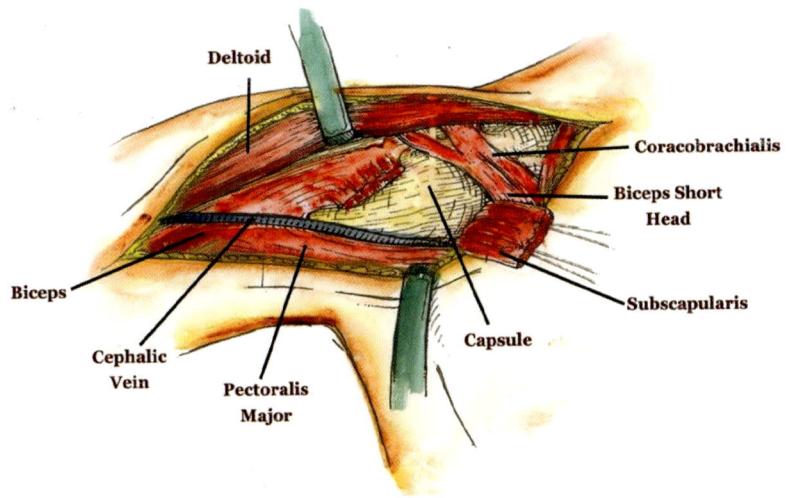

Flexion and external rotation facilitate coagulation of the anterior circumflex vessels.
   Stay sutures are inserted into the subscapularis and its tendon is divided 2.5 cm medial to the bicipital groove.
   Tight subscapulares should be divided in an oblique or 'Z' manner.
   The joint capsule is released anteriorly and inferiorly.
   Care is taken to protect the axillary nerve.
   The glenohumeral joint is dislocated anteriorly by abduction and external rotation to expose the head and neck.

Indications: Humeral hemiarthroplasty or total shoulder replacement.
   The currently recommended approach by Neer for total shoulder replacement.

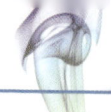

Anterior Extensile Approach (Henry, Redfern, Wallace and Beddows)

History

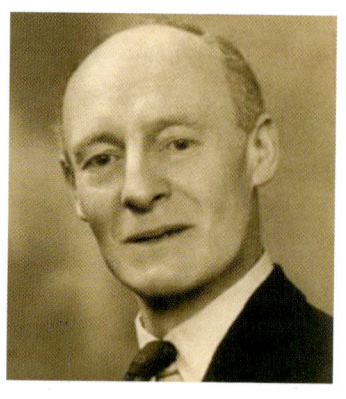

Professor AK Henry (1886–1962): Professor Arnold K Henry graduated from Trinity College in 1911 and obtained his fellowship of the Royal College of Surgeons in Ireland (RCSI) in 1914. In the First World War, he served as a surgeon in both the Serbian and French armies and was decorated by both. He was accompanied by his wife, Dr Dorothy Milne Henry, a close collaborator and assistant.

Subsequent to this, he worked as a surgeon in Dublin, then as Professor of Surgery at the University of Cairo and at the Postgraduate Medical School at Hammersmith. In 1947, he returned to Dublin as Professor of Anatomy at the RCSI. Professor Henry was a trendsetter in many respects. At the time of his appointment to RCSI, he was a retired surgeon and not a "pure" anatomist. Consequently, he was never at ease with the classroom, and swiftly abandoned this for teaching on the cadaver. His lectures were always very practical, demonstrating for example that the strap muscles of the neck were a barrier to surgical "damage". He also demonstrated in the cadaver that pulmonary emboli could be removed surgically, a technique that was long before its time.

His classic "Extensile Exposure Applied to Limb Surgery" is an absolutely amazing book and even today one cannot put it down, if he or she begins to read it.

I am copying below the first paragraph of his wonderful book and the word play speaks of his genius:

If, as one keeps on hearing, the sort of anatomy untastefully called 'gross' were really finished, this re-edition would count only as a further impertinence. But while its predecessor was received with unexpected kindliness, the not-intolerant climate held just the echo of a salutary feline note: "It's all very interesting," said the Miller's Cat to the Mill-race, "but if you could manage to do your work-whose value I don't in the least dispute-a little more soberly, I for one should be grateful."

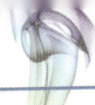

Meanwhile, however, Time, which finds ways of settling sobriety's worse disorders, has not been idle. The present progress in surgery is so rapid that one year now is like a former hundred, and ten can leave us not outstripped but at the post. Even simple straight incisions have been altered, and I am most grateful for the chance of taking my impressions of their modern trends from a variety of patients, with scars long-healed and admirable, put at my disposal by the courtesy of Mr JC Sugars of the Adelaide Hospital, Dublin.

He gets the undoubted credit for describing all exposures of femur together in one place and has detailed the anterior, antero-lateral, and lateral approaches in detail.

This approach is essentially modified from Henry's classic extensile approach to the shoulder (Henry, 1973).

Access
- Wide exposure of the whole of the front of the shoulder.
- Glenohumeral joint.
- Whole of the humeral head.
- Subacromial region.
- Humeral neck up to the insertion of deltoid.

Incision: An five incision starting 2.5 cm above the clavicle, passing vertically down, across the tip of the coracoid, and ending lateral to the anterior axillary fold.

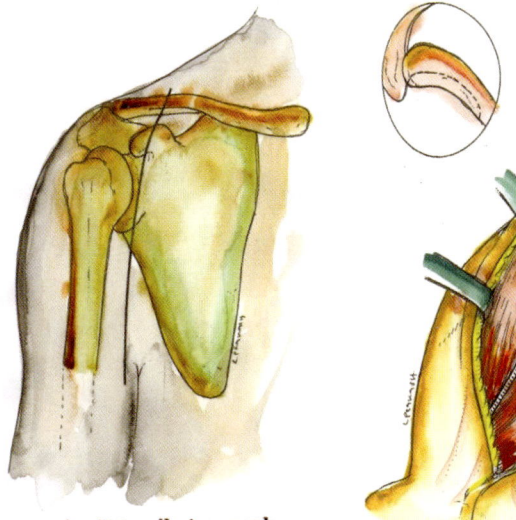

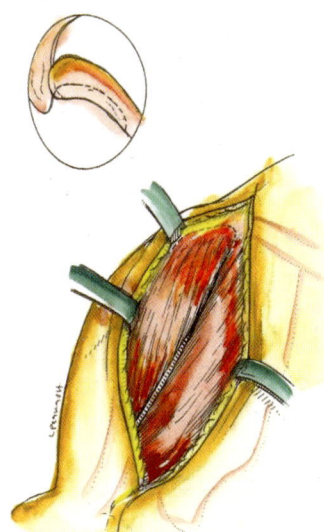

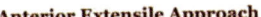

Anterior Extensile Approach

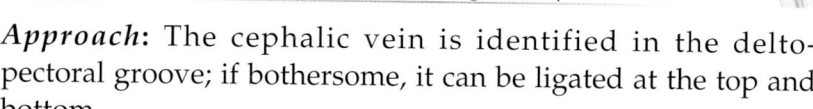

Approach: The cephalic vein is identified in the delto-pectoral groove; if bothersome, it can be ligated at the top and bottom.

The lateral third of the clavicle is exposed and the acromio-clavicular joint identified. The periosteum over the lateral third of the clavicle is now divided longitudinally retaining the muscular attachments of the deltoid below and the trapezius above.

The anterior one-third of the clavicle is osteotomized with an oscillating saw, leaving the clavicular attachment of the deltoid attached to the separated bony piece.

The split clavicle is gently levered apart using a periosteal elevator and the clavicular head of deltoid is gently reflected downwards and laterally.

The rotator cuff is now be exposed by excising the coraco-acromial ligament and access to the glenohumeral joint is be gained by dividing the subscapularis 2.5 cm from its insertion, or by osteotomizing the lesser tuberosity from the humeral head.

The subscapularis tendon is separated from the supraspinatus tendon along the line of the rotator interval. Exposure of the proximal humeral shaft is decent, providing adequate exposure of the proximal humerus for plating. Closure is carried out by repair of the subscapularis (or lesser tuberosity) with strong non-absorbable sutures, and reattachment of the clavicular osteotomy with absorbable cerclage sutures.

Indications: Proximal humerus for fractures or fracture-dislocations.

Total shoulder replacement, when the glenohumeral joint is stiff, preventing abduction required for the long anterior deltopectoral approach.

Axillary Approach

Access: Exposure of the front of the shoulder from below.

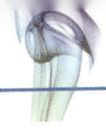

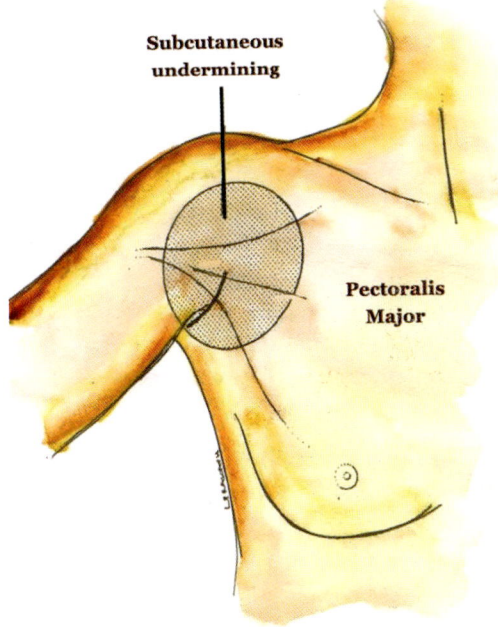

Incision: From the middle of the anterior axillary fold to the middle of the axilla.

Approach: The lowest segment of pectoralis major tendon is divided vertically.

Abduction of the arm and retraction of the pectoralis major tendon exposes the subscapularis tendon, the coracobrachialis and short head of biceps.

Indications: Only indicated in females who insist on no visible scar after surgery.

Access is poorer than in other approaches.

Scarring in the axilla can be uncomfortable.

Deltoid-splitting Transacromioclavicular Joint Approach (Ha'Eri and Wiley)

Access: Whole of the supraspinatus tendon.

The entire extent of infraspinatus and subscapularis tendons.

The entire supraspinatus muscle can be exposed by proximal extension of the incision.

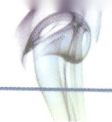

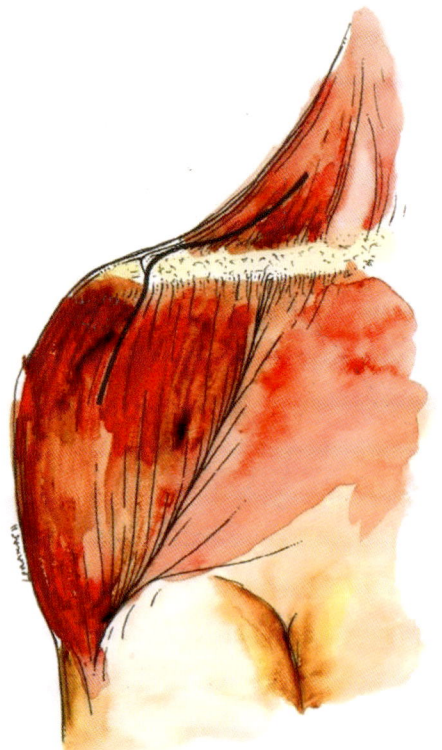

**Deltoid-splitting transacromioclavicular
Joint Approach**

Incision: A 10 cm straight incision, over the acromioclavicular joint.

From the middle of the trapezius proximally, then over the acromioclavicular joint, passing down in the direction of the fibres of deltoid.

The incision can be extended proximally or distally, if any additional exposure is needed.

Approach: The fibres of the trapezius are split longitudinally in line with the acromioclavicular joint.

Distally, the deltoid is split for just 5 cm. Going further distally endangers the anterior branch of the axillary nerve.

The superior acromioclavicular ligament over the AC joint is now divided in line with the joint.

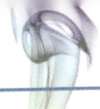

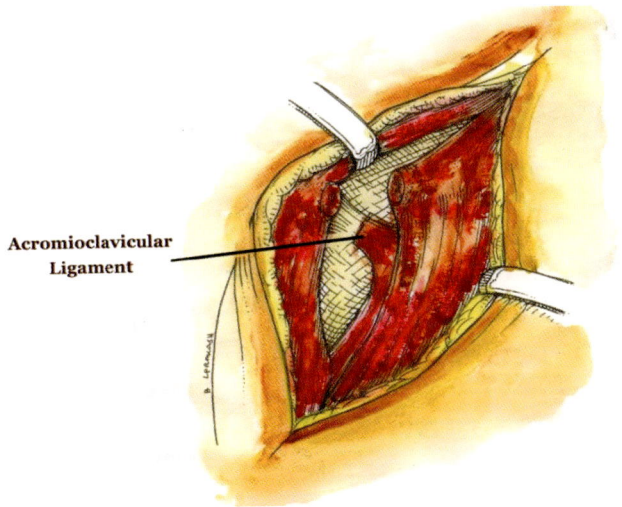

**Acromioclavicular
Ligament**

Subperiosteal dissection of the periosteum on the lateral side of clavicle is done, followed by an osteotomy of the lateral 1.25 cm of the clavicle with an oscillating saw in the plane of the AC joint.

The periosteum over the acromion is now carefully dissected to expose the whole of the anterior acromion.

A lamina spreader separates the clavicle medially and the articular surface of the acromial side of the AC joint laterally.

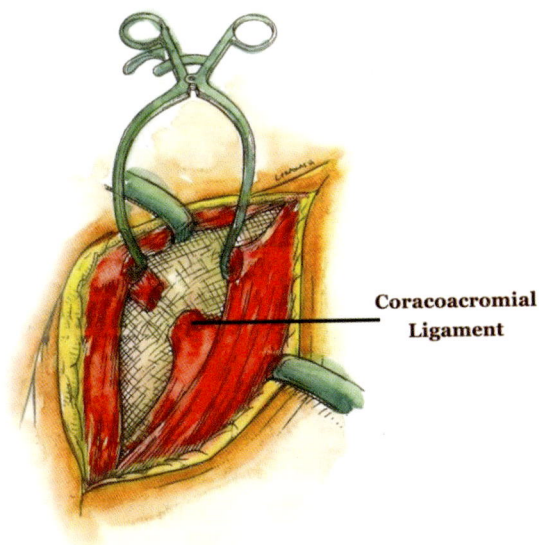

**Coracoacromial
Ligament**

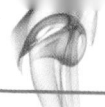

Next, the supraspinatus tendon is exposed by excision of the coracoacromial ligament.

In rotator cuff surgery, the undersurface of the anterior part of the acromion is excised.

The muscles and tendons can now be visualized by manipulating the arm. The subscapularis is brought into view by flexion of the shoulder and external rotation, while the infraspinatus is visualized by internal rotation and extension.

The trapezius muscle is split proximally to expose the supraspinatus, which can be dissected from the supraspinous fossa.

Indications

- Rotator cuff lesions.
- Impingement lesions.
- Gives limited exposure to infraspinatus, especially postero-inferiorly.

Transacromial Approach (Kessel)

History

Lipmann Kessel (1914–1986): Professor Lipmann Kessel was born in South Africa, educated at the University of Witwatersrand, and went to England to attend St Mary's Hospital Medical School, from where he graduated in 1937.

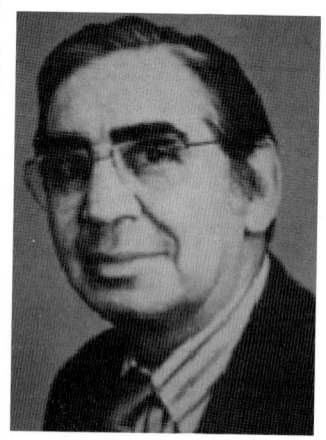

After holding various junior resident posts, he joined the Royal Army Medical Corps, volunteered for parachute duties and, as surgeon in command of a parachute team, took part in the battle of Arnhem, where with exceptional skill and courage he was directly responsible for saving many lives. He managed to escape his German captors and, with the help of the Dutch Resistance, eventually made his way back. He has narrated these experiences in his book *Surgeon at Arms*. He was appointed MBE (Military) and awarded the Military Cross.

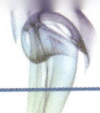

He then became clinical assistant at the Institute of Orthopaedics under Sir Herbert Seddon and was appointed consultant at Fulham and St. Mary Abbot Hospitals in 1952. He took a keen interest in the casualty services of UK, and established accident and emergency departments, with adequate training programmes for the staff. At the end of his time at Fulham and St. Mary Abbot Hospitals, he was 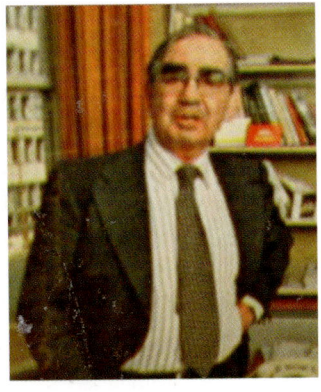 involved in the planning and smooth integration of these hospitals with the Charing Cross Hospitals to form the existing New Charing Cross Hospital.

In 1974, he became professor of orthopaedics of London University and established specialist departments at the Royal National Orthopaedic Hospital that would help to maintain its identity and reputation. He was instrumental in the setting up of the spinal injuries unit and a specialist shoulder unit, his own particular lifelong interest.

His list of publications is long and ranges from articles about his early experiences with the parachute surgical team, to many publications about the shoulder joint, which remained his ardent interest. He published several authoritative books on this subject and formed an international society for the study of the shoulder joint and related diseases. He was executive member of the Council of the British Orthopaedic Association and served on the editorial board of The Journal of Bone and Joint Surgery (JBJS). He had an international reputation and lectured all over the world.

Lipmann Kessel died in London on June 5, 1986, aged 72.

He described this approach in his book on shoulder surgery published four years before his death.

Access: Superior part of the rotator cuff.

Infraspinatus muscle and tendon posteriorly.

The access to the inferior part of the subscapularis tendon anteriorly is a little difficult with this approach.

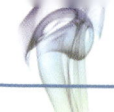

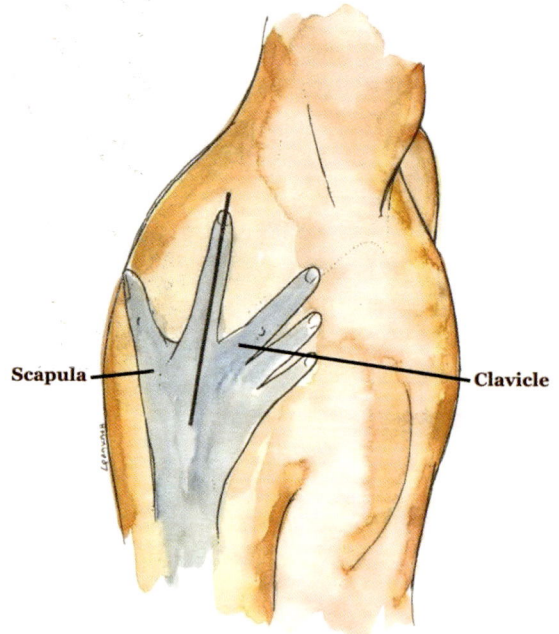

Scapula —   — Clavicle

Transacromial Approach

Incision: The line formed in the centre of the imaginary angle between the scapula and clavicle.

The surgeon places his middle finger in the line of the clavicle, and his thumb along the line of scapular spine.

His index finger now lies along the line of the incision which is about 10 cm on either side of the acromion.

Approach: The trapezius and deltoid are split in the line of their fibres above and below the acromion.

An osteoperiosteal flap is raised from the acromion, maintaining the continuity of the two muscles.

The distal incision in deltoid is restricted to the level of the axillary nerve, present 5 cm below the tip of the acromion, as it curves posteriorly around the humeral neck.

The acromion is divided in the coronal plane using a power saw, and a self-retaining retractor is used to spread the osteotomy and complete the exposure.

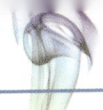

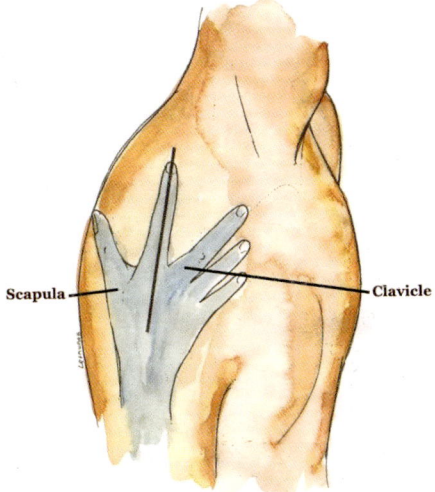

Scapula — — Clavicle

Transacromial Approach

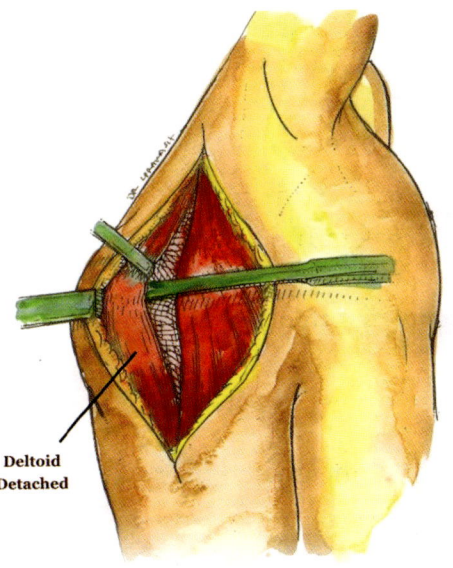

Deltoid
Detached

The superior part of the rotator cuff now comes into view; rotating the humerus and moving it into flexion and extension will allow a full inspection of the rotator cuff.

The acromion osteotomy is reattached by Vicryl or stainless steel wires. If the tip is excised for decompression, anterior deltoid needs to be reconstructed.

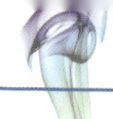

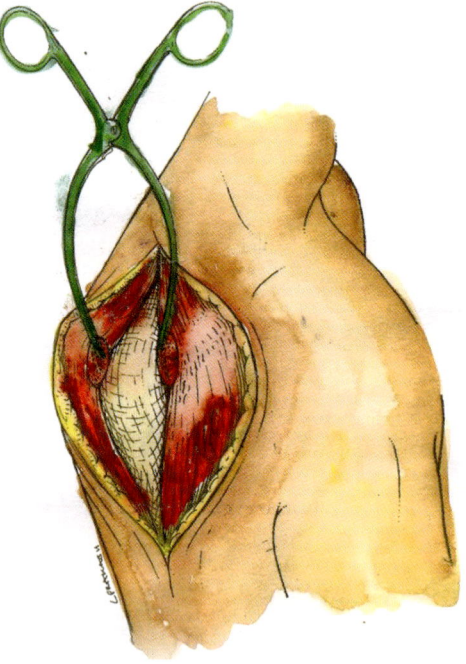

Indications

- Repair of large tears of the rotator cuff.
- Extensive rotator cuff tears affecting the infraspinatus tendon.
- This is unsuitable for internal fixations of proximal humerus.

Posterior Approach

Access

- Posterior aspect of the glenohumeral joint
- Posterior glenoid rim
- Tendon of infraspinatus

Incision: Straight midline back strap incision about 10 cm long, ending at the lower border of scapula.

Approach: Deltoid is detached with periosteum from its origin along the lateral one-third of the scapular spine and the posterior belly of deltoid is reflected downwards and laterally.

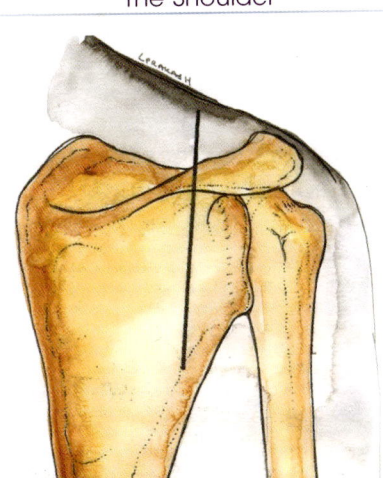

Posterior 'bra-strap' Incision

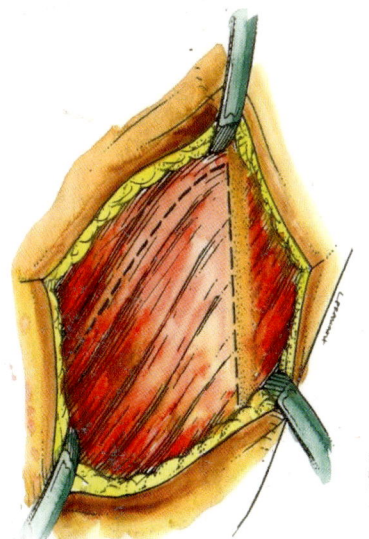

The axillary nerve is seen as it emerges from the quadrilateral space giving a number of muscular branches here. Gentle retraction should be used to avoid traction injury to the nerve.

The infraspinatus and teres minor muscles lying deep to the deltoid are separated.

Division of the infraspinatus tendon 1.25 cm medial to its insertion allows access to the posterior aspect of the glenoid.

Care must be taken to avoid stretch or damage to the supra-scapular nerve along the lateral ridge of the scapular spine. Internal rotation of the glenohumeral joint exposes the capsule which is divided vertically to gain access to the posterior glenoid rim.

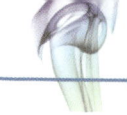

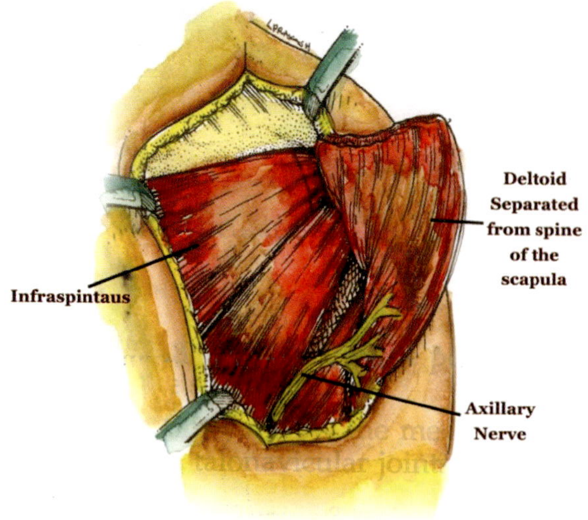

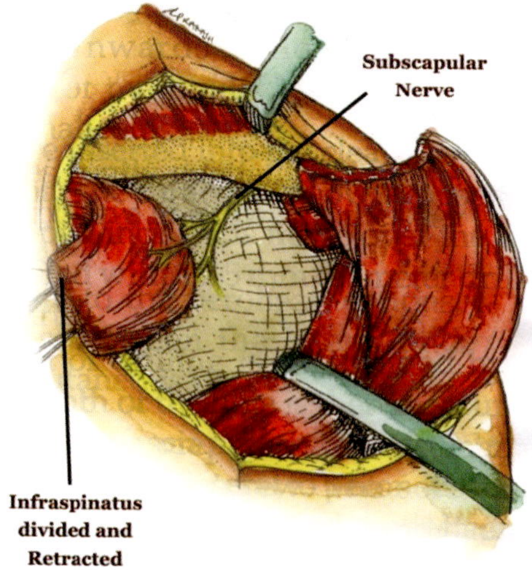

The posterior third of the deltoid is reattached to the scapular spine with absorbable sutures passed through drill holes in the scapular spine.

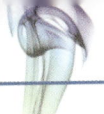

Indications: Recurrent posterior subluxation or dislocation of the shoulder (Reverse Bankart).

Approach to Acromioclavicular Joint in Coronal Plane

Access: Limited approach to the acromioclavicular joint by a concealed cosmetic incision.

Incision: Parallel to the lateral one-third of clavicle.

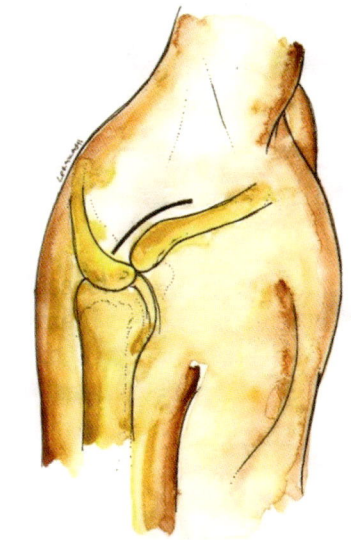

Coronal Approach

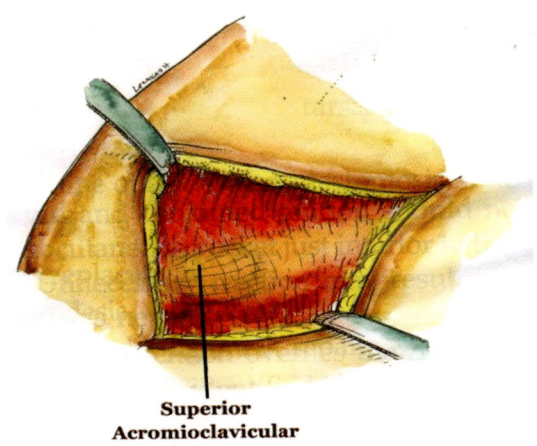

**Superior
Acromioclavicular
Ligament**

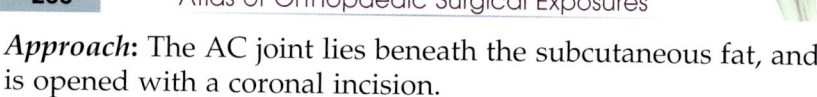

Approach: The AC joint lies beneath the subcutaneous fat, and is opened with a coronal incision.

Indications
- Clearance of the acromioclavicular joint.
- Excision at the lateral tip of the clavicle for osteoarthritis.
- Open reduction and fixation of AC joint dislocation.

Parasagittal Approach to the Acromioclavicular Joint

Access
- Excellent exposure to the AC joint.
- Scars are unpredictable.

Incision: Vertical from above the clavicle and passing down over the tip of the coracoid. (Bra strap)

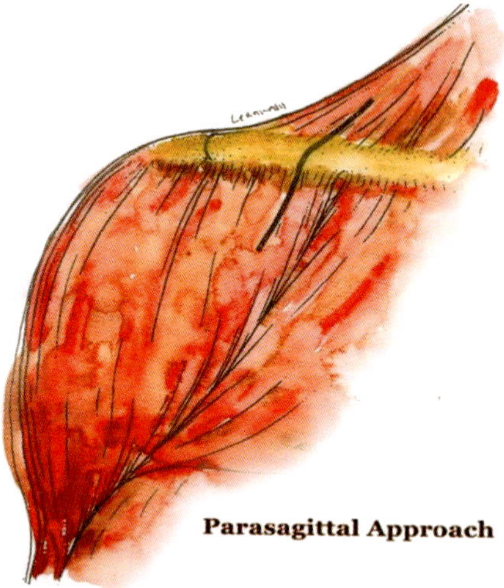

Parasagittal Approach

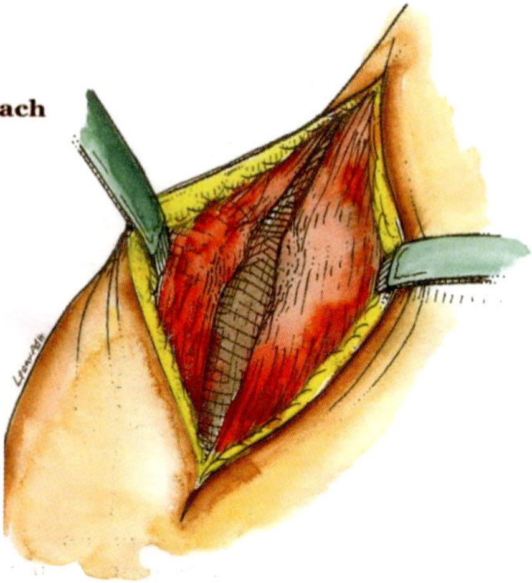

1 cm of Clavicle excised

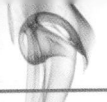

Approach: The joint lies below the subcutaneous fat.

Indications

- Trauma to the AC joint.
- Subacromial rotator cuff decompression.
- Excision of the coracoacromial ligament and anterior acromioplasty. (Neer's procedure)

The Humerus

ANATOMY

Superficial Cutaneous Nerves

Knowledge of their anatomy prevents accidental damage.

Intercostobrachial Nerve

This enters the axilla through the intercostal and serratus anterior muscles. Occasionally, there is a second contributing branch from the third intercostal nerve. There are communicating branches between the intercostobrachial and the medial brachial cutaneous nerves.

Medial Brachial Cutaneous Nerve

The medial brachial cutaneous nerve is the smallest branch of the brachial plexus arising from the medial cord. It crosses the axilla to lie medial to the brachial artery and vein, and often communicates with the intercostobrachial nerve.

Medial Antebrachial Cutaneous Nerve

The medial antebrachial cutaneous nerve arises from the medial cord of the brachial plexus just distal to the origin of the medial brachial cutaneous nerve. It courses on the medial side of the brachial artery anterior to the ulnar nerve giving off its superior branch, which penetrates the deep fascia, supplying the anterior skin of the upper arm over the biceps. The main body of the nerve pierces the deep fascia, with the basilic vein, at the middle of the arm and then divides just proximal to the elbow into anterior and posterior branches.

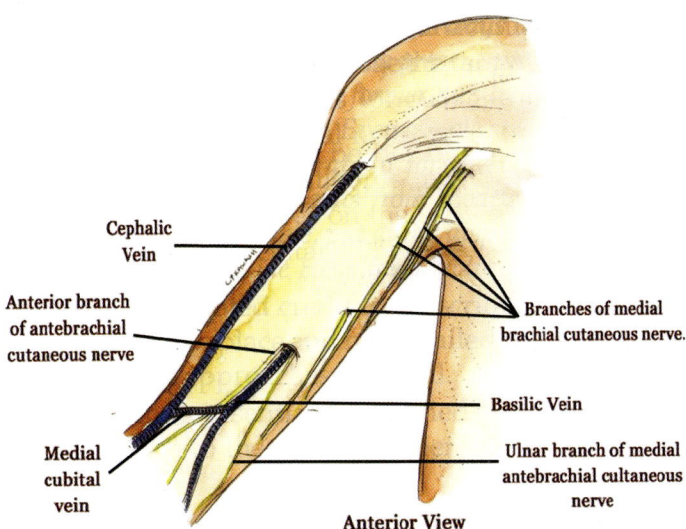

Anterior View

Superior Lateral Brachial Cutaneous Nerve

This is a continuation of the posterior axillary nerve containing only sensory fibres, and penetrates the deep fascia at the posterior edge of the deltoid as the superior lateral cutaneous nerve. It then branches to supply the skin over the inferior deltoid and superior aspect of the long head at the triceps.

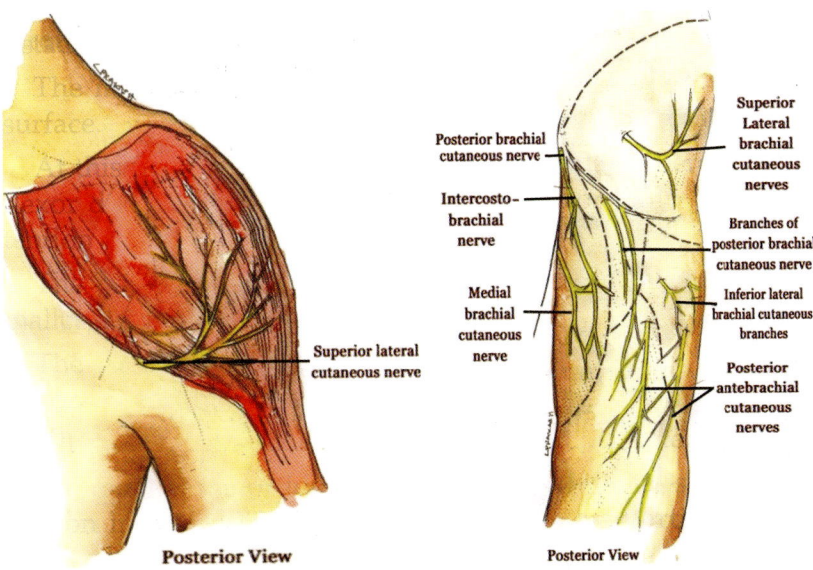

Posterior View **Posterior View**

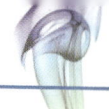

Posterior Brachial Cutaneous Nerve

This arises from the radial nerve in the axilla, pierces the deep fascia and supplies skin over the posteromedial aspect of the upper arm.

Inferior Lateral Brachial Cutaneous Nerve

This arises from the radial nerve at the level of the lateral head of the triceps, penetrates this and the deep fascia over it to travel beside the cephalic vein and supplies the posterior and anterolateral portions of the distal arm.

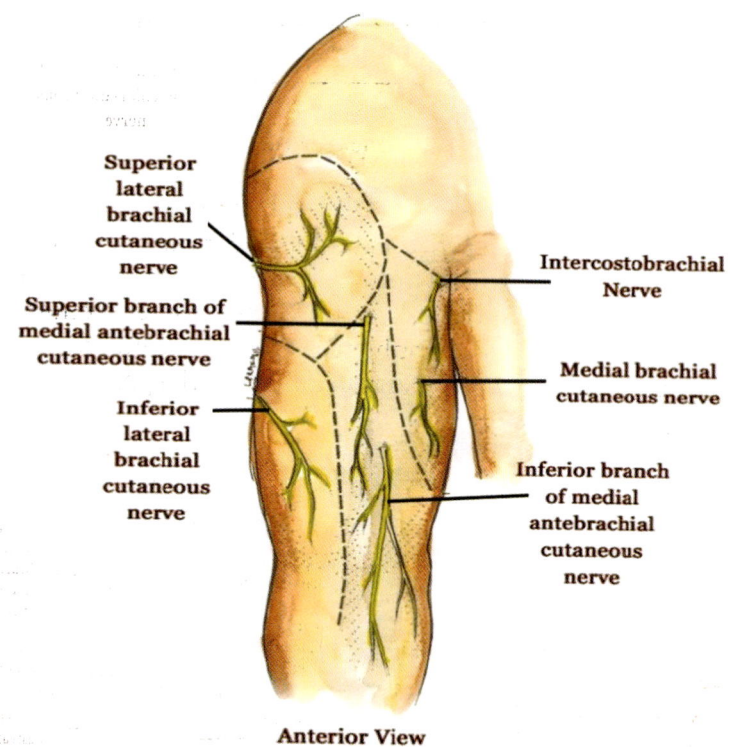

Anterior View

Posterior Antebrachial Cutaneous Nerve

The posterior antebrachial cutaneous nerve, a branch of the radial nerve, penetrates the lateral head of the triceps just before the radial nerve penetrates the lateral intermuscular septum. It then goes posterior to the lateral humeral epicondyle, enervating the lower arm and upper part of the back of the forearm.

Deep Nerves and Vessels

Muscles of the upper arm are innervated by the radial and musculocutaneous nerves.

The median and ulnar nerves cross the upper arm to innervate the muscles of the forearm and hand.

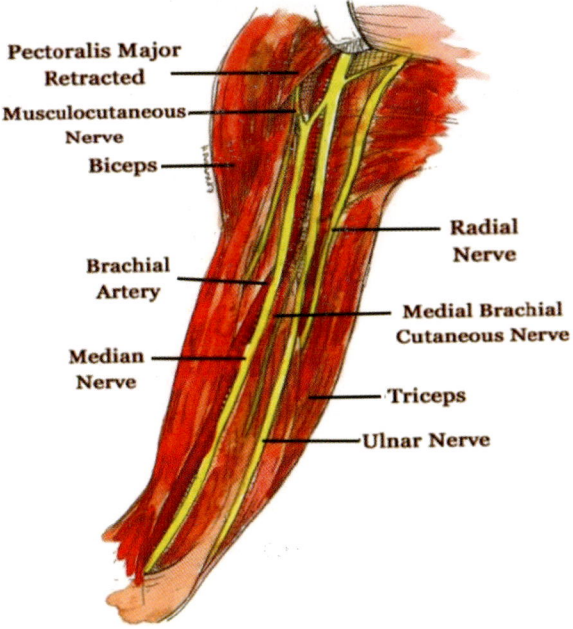

Median nerve enters the arm lateral to the brachial artery, crossing it and then descends medial to the artery to enter the antecubital fossa.

Ulnar nerve enters the arm medial to the brachial artery and at the midarm level, diverges posteriorly, piercing the medial intermuscular septum to the posterior aspect of the medial epicondyle.

Musculocutaneous nerve enters the arm just below the inferior border of the pectoralis minor and lies between the biceps and the brachialis. It then branches at the midarm to supply the brachialis, after which it continues as a purely sensory nerve in the lower arm, renamed as the lateral antebrachial cutaneous nerve.

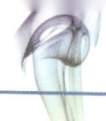

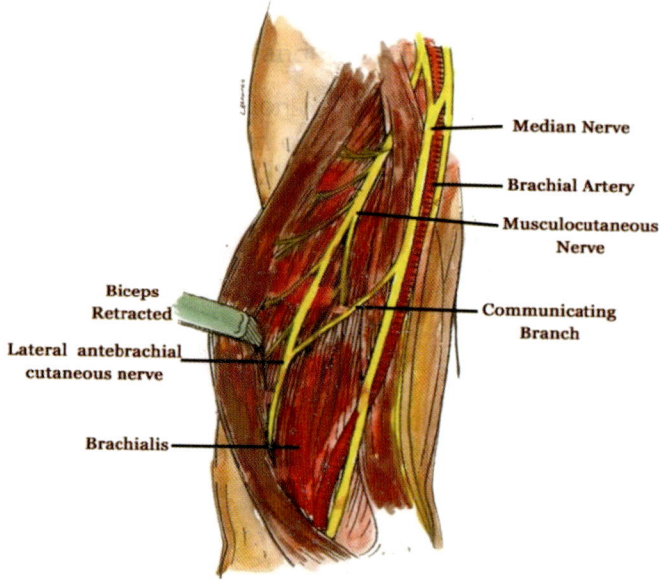

Radial nerve is the largest branch of the brachial plexus and a continuation of the posterior cord.

Entering the arm behind the brachial artery, it descends obliquely and laterally, arriving in the posterior arm with the profunda brachii artery and takes a spiral course down the arm close to the humerus.

It then pierces the lateral intermuscular septum with the radial collateral branch of the profunda brachii artery.

The medial branches of this nerve originate in the axilla, the posterior branches supply the triceps, and the distal branches supply the brachioradialis and the extensor carpi radialis longus muscles. It also gives a few sensory branches.

Brachial artery is the continuation of the axillary artery from the inferior border of the teres major. Passing from medial side of the humerus, it turns anteriorly at the elbow. The biceps lie anterolaterally, while medially it is covered by skin, subcutaneous fat and deep fascia. It is accompanied by two brachial veins, and gives off several branches: the profunda brachii artery, the nutrient artery of the humerus, the superior and inferior ulnar collateral arteries and muscular branches in the arm.

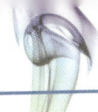

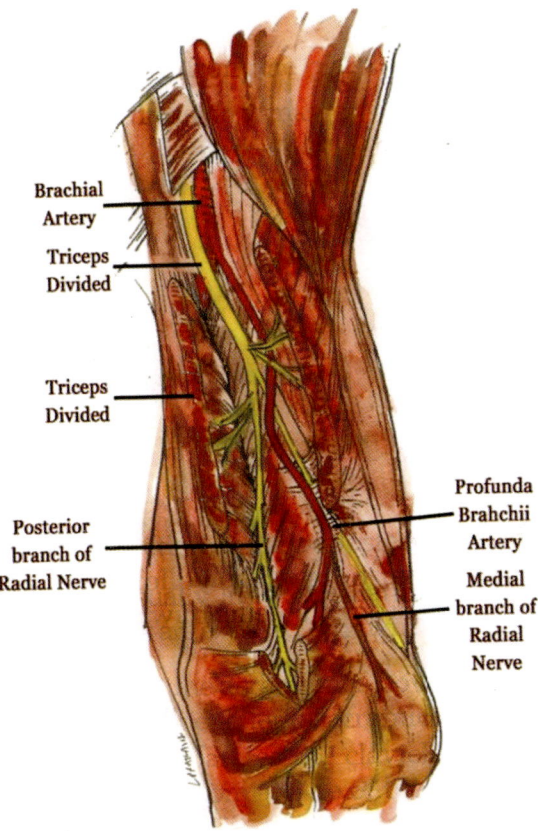

Brachial
Artery

Triceps
Divided

Triceps
Divided

Posterior
branch of
Radial Nerve

Profunda
Brahchii
Artery

Medial
branch of
Radial
Nerve

The profunda brachii artery is the largest branch of the brachial artery. Arising from the posteromedial side of the brachial artery in the upper arm, it passes downwards behind the brachial artery, running parallel with the radial nerve. As it approaches the lateral intermuscular septum, it branches into the middle collateral artery (which supplies the medial head of the triceps) and the radial collateral artery, which continues with the radial nerve through the remaining course in the arm supplying adjacent muscles.

Cephalic vein ascends subcutaneously in the arm, superficial to the groove between the brachioradialis and the lateral edge of the biceps, until it courses medially in the upper arm to lie in the deltopectoral interval.

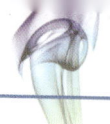

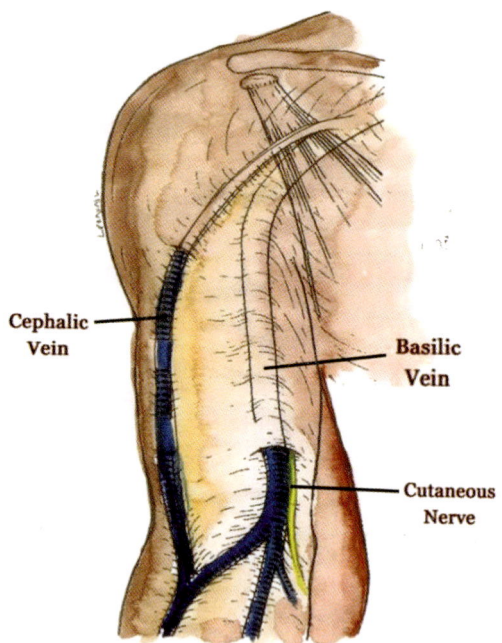

Cephalic Vein

Basilic Vein

Cutaneous Nerve

Basilic vein runs subcutaneously, medial to the biceps and perforates the deep fascia a little below the middle of the upper arm, accompanied by the medial antebrachial cutaneous nerve. It enters the anterior compartment to lie medial to both the brachial artery and medial brachial vein, until it reaches the inferior border of the teres major, where it joins with the medial brachial vein to become the axillary vein.

SURGICAL APPROACHES

- Posterior triceps splitting (Henry, 1924)
- Proximal anterolateral (Thompson, 1973 and Henry, 1918)
- Distal anterolateral

Posterior Triceps Splitting Approach (Henry)

About Henry and his masterly wonderful book *Extensile.*

Approaches , description has been given earlier. This is the most commonly deployed incision for fractures of the humerus, and passes through safe corridors.

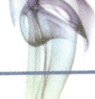
Access
- Central two-thirds of the posterior humeral shaft.
- Radial nerve in middle arm.

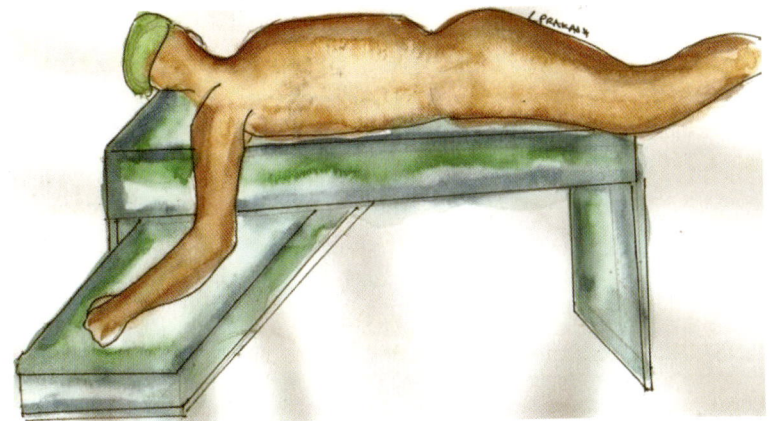

Position: Prone with the arm abducted, resting on a side-table.

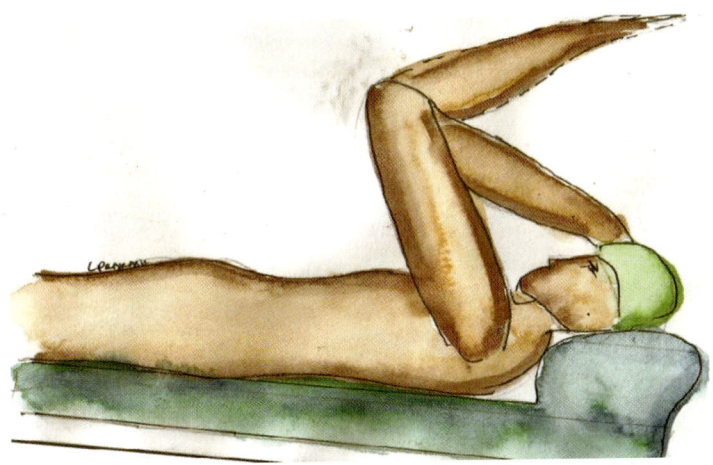

Alternatively, supine with the arm flexed, adducted and internally rotated.

In both cases, the elbow is draped free to provide a lever arm to rotate the shoulder.

Incision: The midline posterior incision is parallel to the long axis of the humerus, from the posterior border of the deltoid, to the olecranon fossa.

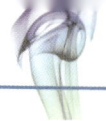

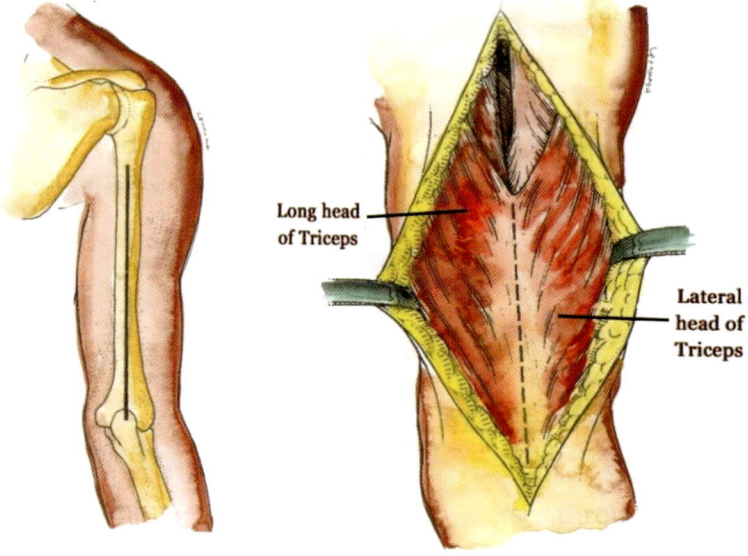

Long head of Triceps

Lateral head of Triceps

Approach: Superficial and deep fasciae are incised in line with the incision.

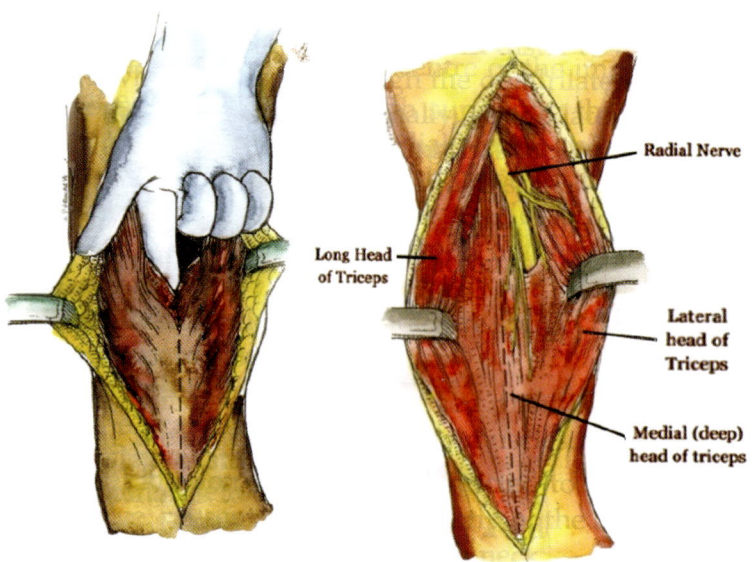

Radial Nerve

Long Head of Triceps

Lateral head of Triceps

Medial (deep) head of triceps

The interval between the long and lateral heads of the triceps is identified; the fascia is lifted with a finger and split distally.

The neurovascular bundle, containing the radial nerve and profunda brachii artery, travels obliquely laterally and distally along deep medial head of the triceps; this is protected.

The muscle belly of triceps is split in the midline in the direction of its fibres, and the humerus is exposed subperiosteally.

As the outer part of the deep medial head of the triceps is raised from the back of the humerus, the lateral intermuscular septum is visualized, and so are the origins of the brachioradialis and extensor carpi radialis longus.

Division of these exposes the radial nerve.

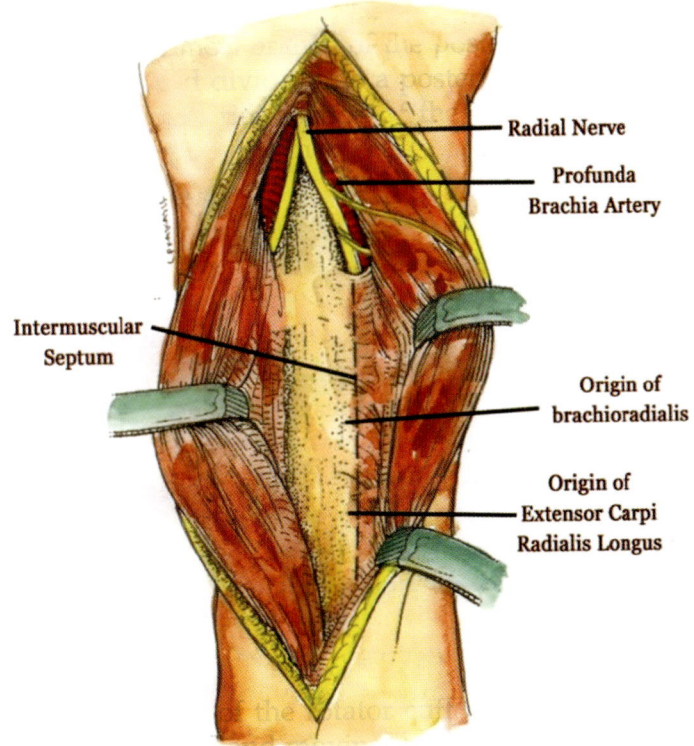

Indications
- Fractures and lesions of the middle two-thirds of the humerus.
- Radial nerve exposure.

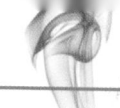

Proximal Anterolateral Approach (Thompson and Henry)

History

Frederick Roeck Thompson (1907–1983): Frederick Thompson was former director of the Department of Orthopaedic Surgery at St. Luke's Hospital Centre in New York City.

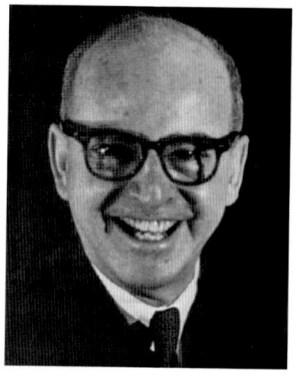

Born in Galveston, Texas, in 1907, he received a Bachelor of Arts degree from the University of Texas in 1927 and a Doctorate of Medicine from the University of Texas Medical School in 1931.

He pursued postgraduate training in surgery at the Roosevelt Hospital in New York City and became a Fellow at the New York Orthopaedic Dispensary and Hospital in 1934, finishing his orthopaedic training in 1939.

Following a tour of the orthopaedic clinics in Europe, Dr Thompson joined the staff at St. Luke's Hospital in 1935. His interests in orthopaedic surgery were widespread. He wrote 41 medical manuscripts and was the author of 9 medical motion pictures. Although his primary interests involved hip and spine surgery, his publications included articles on trauma and adult and paediatric reconstructive surgery.

Dr Thompson's most outstanding contribution was the development of the hip prosthesis that bears his name. This design became a prototype for many later prostheses, including the femoral component for the total hip replacement in use today.

He was the president of the Association of Bone and Joint Surgeons in 1961, a founding member of the Hip Society, and vice-president of the American Academy of Orthopaedic Surgeons from

Dr Thompson was a devoted sportsman with great interest in hunting and fishing. An active member of several fish and game clubs, he spent long hours studying the art of fly-fishing and participating in outdoor events.

Access: Proximal and middle thirds of the humeral shaft.

This can be combined superiorly with deltopectoral exposure of shoulder.

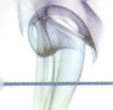

Position: The patient is positioned supine. The arm is placed on an arm board perpendicular to the long axis of the operating table. The arm is then rested on this support so that the shoulder may be abducted, adducted or rotated internally or externally.

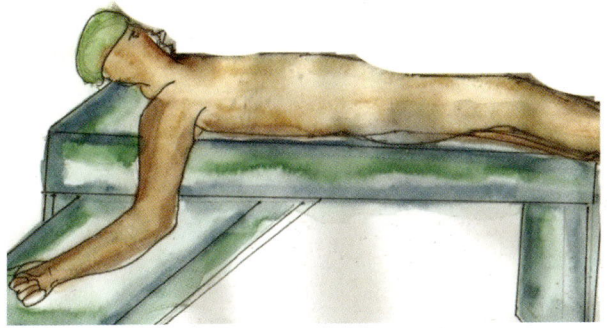

Incision: The incision starts proximally along the anterior margin of the deltoid, a little below the acromion.

At the I insertion of the deltoid, it is curved distally, parallel to the lateral border of the biceps ending 5 cm above the elbow, proximal to the origin of the brachioradialis.

Approach: The cephalic vein, lying under the superficial and deep fascia, is protected and retracted medially.

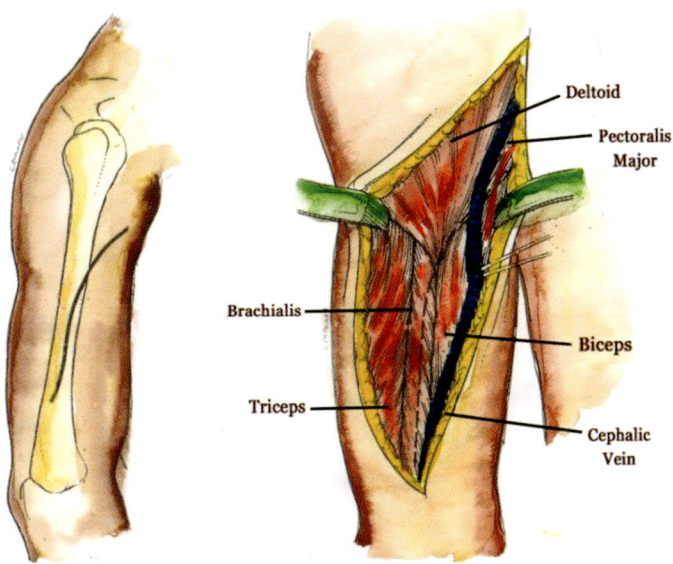

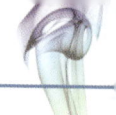

The interval between the deltoid and the pectoralis major muscles is developed.

Below the insertion of the deltoid, the brachialis is split longitudinally along its lateral third and medial two-thirds.

The humerus is exposed by subperiosteal dissection. All structures are relaxed when the elbow is flexed to loosen the brachialis muscle.

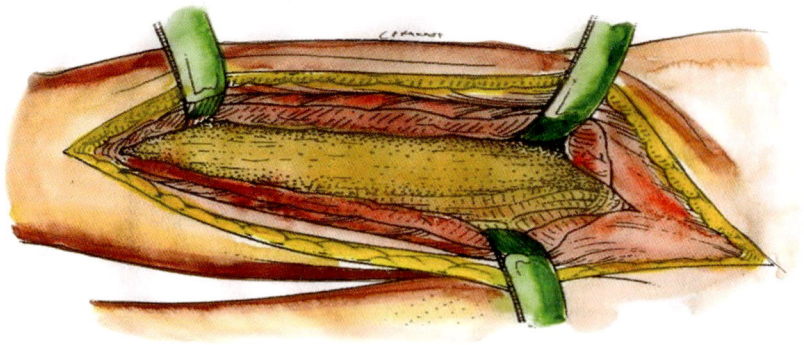

The lateral third of the brachialis protects the radial nerve, though some surgeons look for it, isolate it, and protect it.

Indications

- Trauma
- Tumours
- Sepsis

Distal Anterolateral Approach

Access

- Middle and distal thirds of the humeral shaft.
- Radial nerve at this level.
- The incision can be extended up and down for proximal and distal exposure, right up to the anterolateral border of lower forearm.

Incision: The incision lies in the groove between the biceps and the brachioradialis, its length depending on the needs.

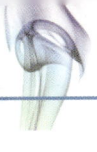

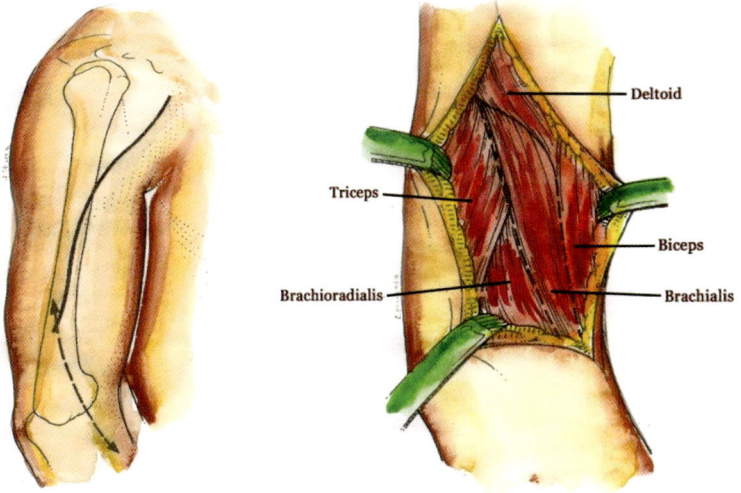

Approach: The subcutaneous and deep fasciae are cut in line with the incision. The interval between the brachioradialis and brachialis and biceps is developed.

The radial nerve is identified deep in the incision along the anterolateral aspect of the humerus and can either be left alone or mobilized and retracted laterally.

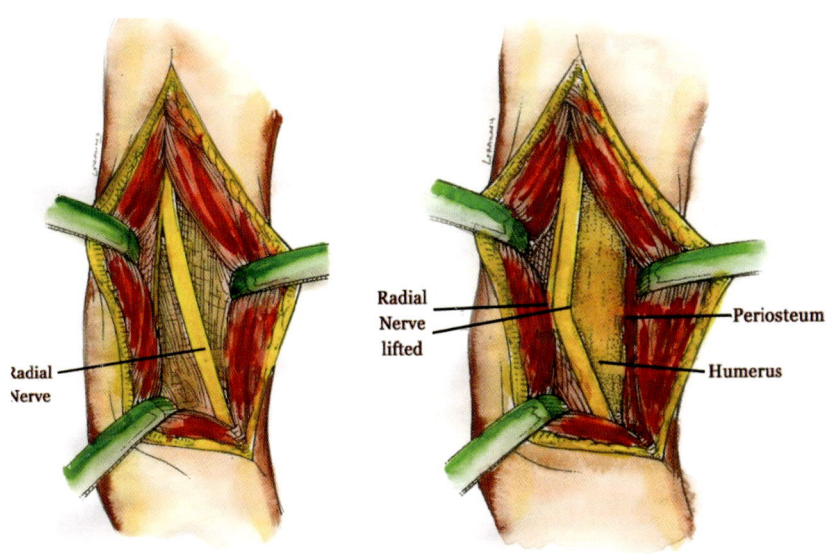

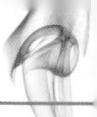

The periosteum is incised in line with the lateral margin of the brachialis and the junction of the middle and distal thirds of the humerus exposed.

Indications
- Trauma
- Tumours
- Sepsis
- Exposure of radial nerve in this area

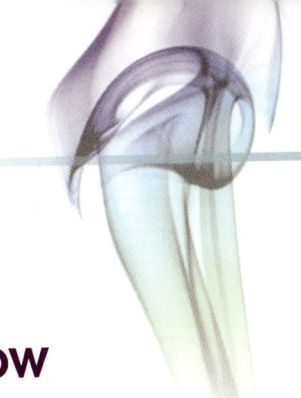

The Elbow

ANATOMY OF THE ELBOW

Lateral antebrachial cutaneous nerve is an extension of the musculocutaneous nerve, which penetrates the deep fascia near the lateral border of the biceps tendon and supplies the lower anterolateral portion of the elbow region.

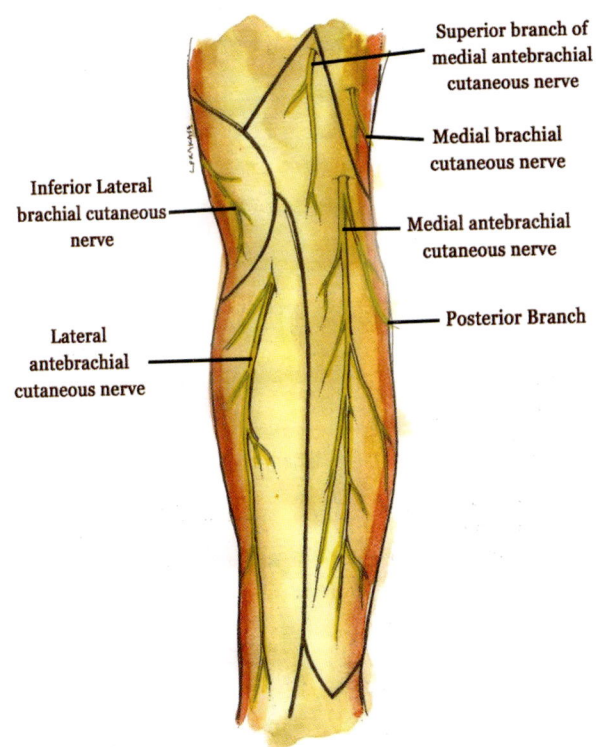

Superior branch of medial antebrachial cutaneous nerve

Medial brachial cutaneous nerve

Inferior Lateral brachial cutaneous nerve

Medial antebrachial cutaneous nerve

Lateral antebrachial cutaneous nerve

Posterior Branch

Posterior antebrachial cutaneous nerve is a part of the posterior group of radial nerve branches. Descending along the posterolateral aspect, it supplies skin over the posterior elbow.

Cubital fossa is the triangular area lying in front of the elbow. its base formed by an imaginary line drawn between the two humeral epicondyles. The sides are formed by brachioradialis and pronator teres, converging distally to meet at the apex. The floor is the brachialis and the supinator.

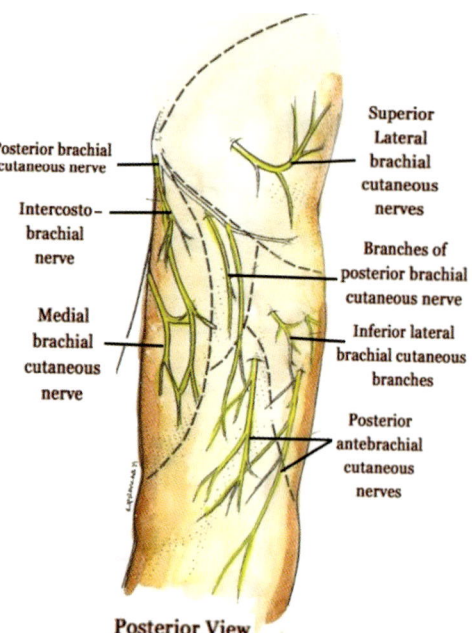

Posterior brachial cutaneous nerve

Intercosto-brachial nerve

Medial brachial cutaneous nerve

Superior Lateral brachial cutaneous nerves

Branches of posterior brachial cutaneous nerve

Inferior lateral brachial cutaneous branches

Posterior antebrachial cutaneous nerves

Posterior View

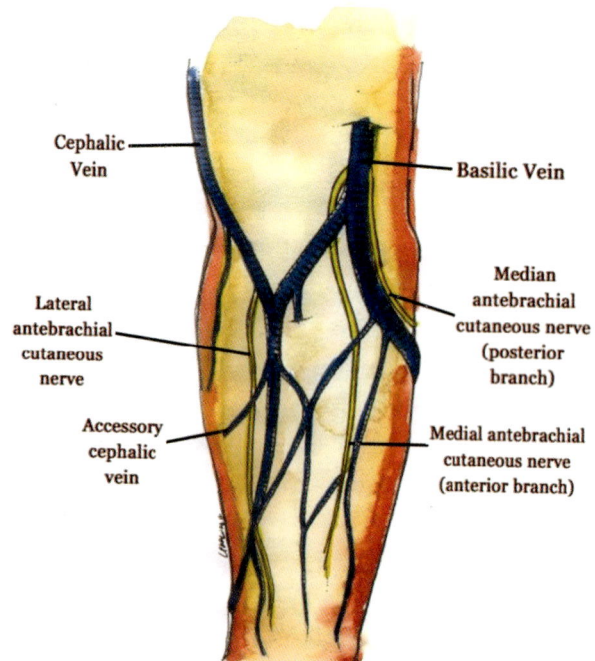

Cephalic Vein

Basilic Vein

Lateral antebrachial cutaneous nerve

Median antebrachial cutaneous nerve (posterior branch)

Accessory cephalic vein

Medial antebrachial cutaneous nerve (anterior branch)

It contains the median nerve, branchial artery and biceps tendon. Near the apex, brachial artery divides into its radial and ulnar branches.

Ligament of Struthers extends from the tip of the supracondylar process to the junction of the medial epicondyle and the humeral metaphysis; it lies anterior to the medial intermuscular septum.

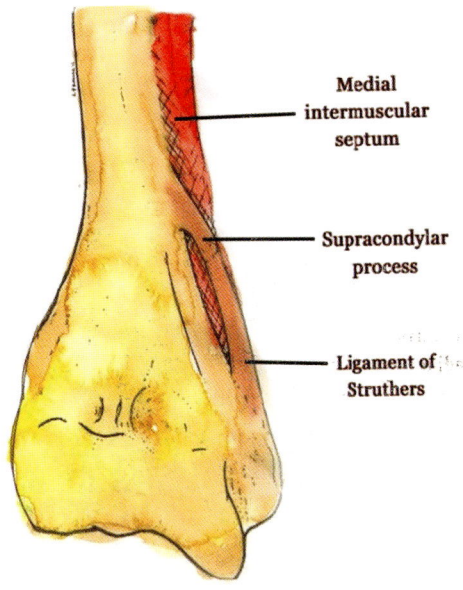

Medial intermuscular septum

Supracondylar process

Ligament of Struthers

The supracondylar process is a bony spur found in a small percentage of population.

The median nerve and brachial artery pass deep to these structures and occasionally cause an entrapment syndrome.

Deep nerves and vessels: All three major nerves of the upper extremity leave the elbow between two muscular heads: the median nerve (between the two heads of pronator teres), the ulnar nerve (between those of the flexor carpi ulnaris) and the posterior interosseous branch of the radial nerve (between the two heads of the supinator).

Median nerve enters the cubital fossa medial to the brachial artery and courses obliquely from medial to lateral over the brachialis muscle. It then crosses over the ulnar artery from

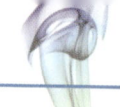

medial to lateral entering between the superficial and deep heads of the pronator teres, the deep head separating it from the ulnar artery.

Radial nerve crosses the lateral intermuscular septum, passes anterior to the lateral humeral epicondyle behind the brachialis muscle and between it and the brachioradialis. It then divides into its superficial (sensory) and posterior interosseous (motor) branches around the epicondylar level of the elbow.

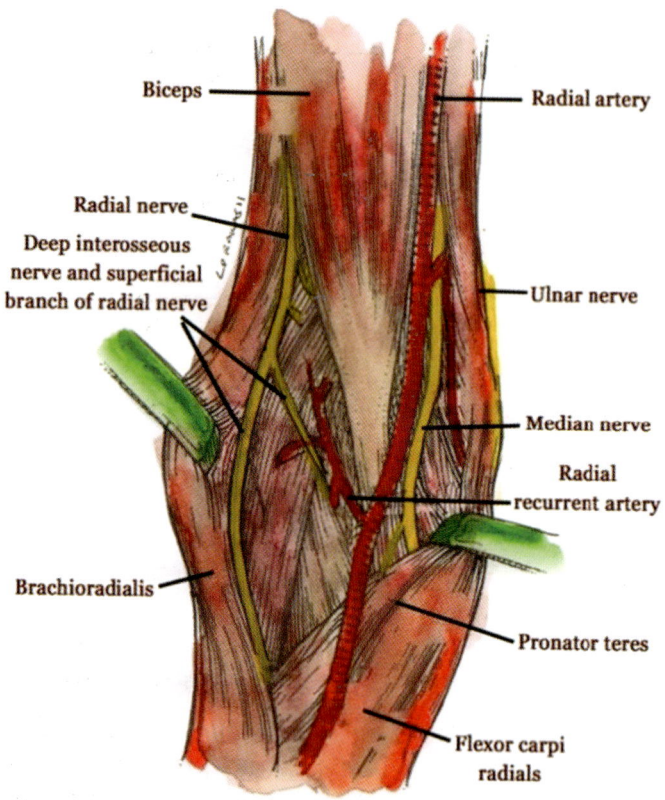

Ulnar nerve pierces the medial intermuscular septum, courses medially joined by the superior ulnar collateral artery on the medial head of the triceps to reach ulnar groove on the dorsum of the medial humeral epicondyle.

Here it branches and gives off motor supplies to the joint, flexor carpi ulnaris and flexor digitorum profundus.

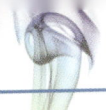

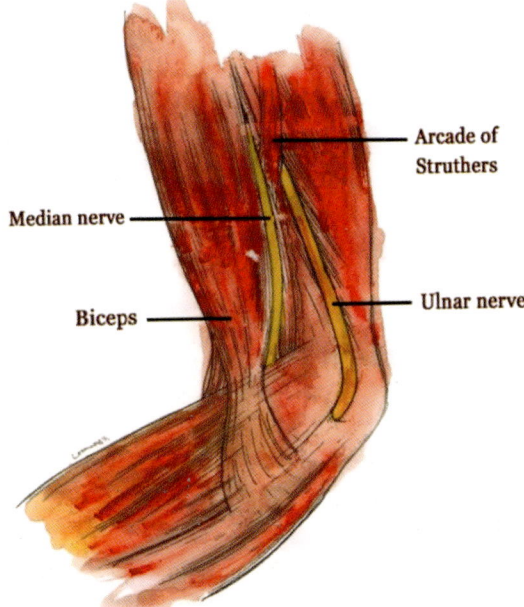

Brachial artery lies medial to the biceps and anterior to the brachialis, as it enters the cubital fossa, and terminates about 1.25 cm below the elbow by dividing into the radial and ulnar arteries.

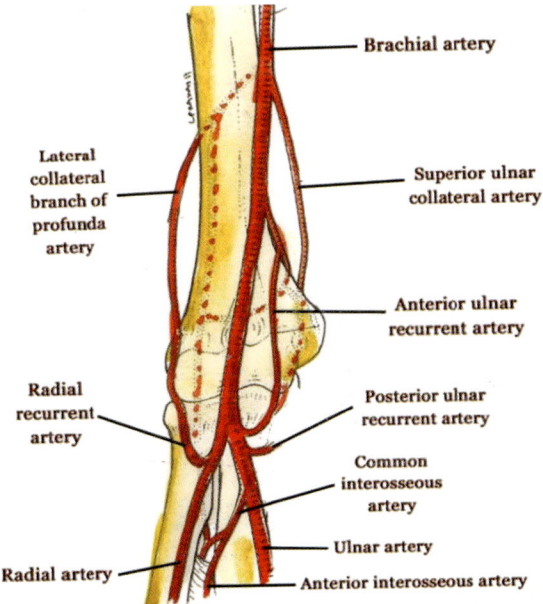

Cross branches between these form the collateral circulation around the elbow.

Ulnar collateral ligament is thick, triangular, and attached between medial humeral epicondyle and medial side of olecranon.

Radial collateral ligament originates at the inferior lateral humeral epicondyle and fans distally to insert into the annular ligament and the proximal supinator crest of the ulna.

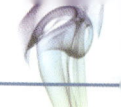

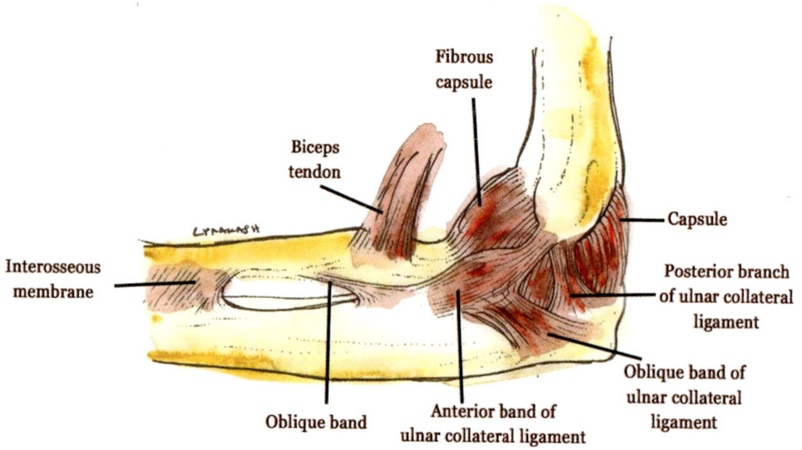

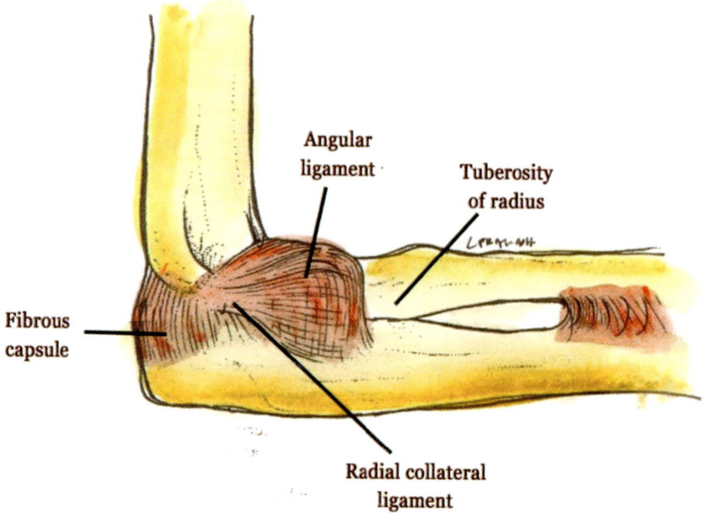

The **annular** and **quadrate** are the other ligaments of the elbow.

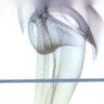

SURGICAL APPROACHES

- Posterior (Campbell, Van Gorder).
- Posterior with osteotomy of olecranon.
- Posterior transolecranon 'U' (MacAusiand).
- Lateral.
- Posterolateral (Kocher).
- Anterior (Pheasant).
- Medial (Molesworth, Campbell, Learmouth).
- Posterior approaches to olecranon and proximal ulna.

Posterior Approach

History: This approach was independently described by RE Campbell and Van Gorder in 1932.

Access: Distal humerus including its articular surface.

Position: A wide arm board is affixed perpendicular to the table and the patient is positioned prone to expose the posterior aspect of elbow.

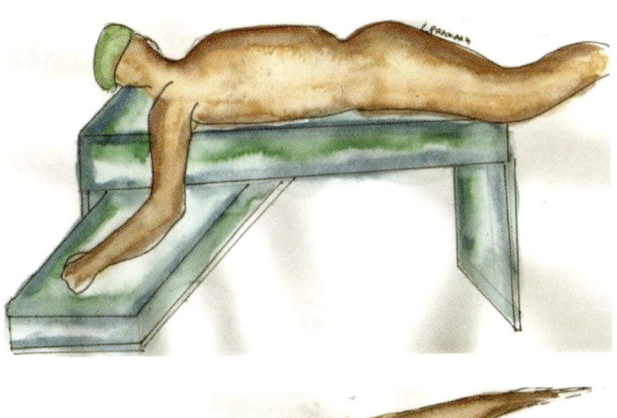

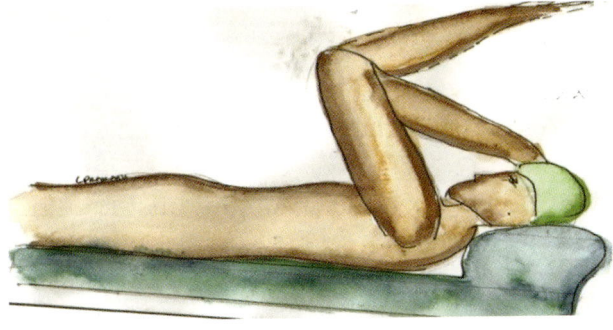

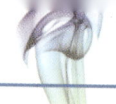

Alternatively the patient is supine with this shoulder adducted and the elbow flexed across, with an assistant holding the wrist and forearm.

Incision: Curved posterior midline incision over the olecranon, skirting laterally to avoid the olecranon bony prominence.

Approach: The lower part of the triceps and its tendon is located, exposed, and the ulnar nerve is protected using a thin moist tape gauze.

The triceps tendon is cut in the shape of a tongue with the apex about 7.5 to 10 cm above the olecranon.

The base extends to the level of the humeral condyles at the joint line.

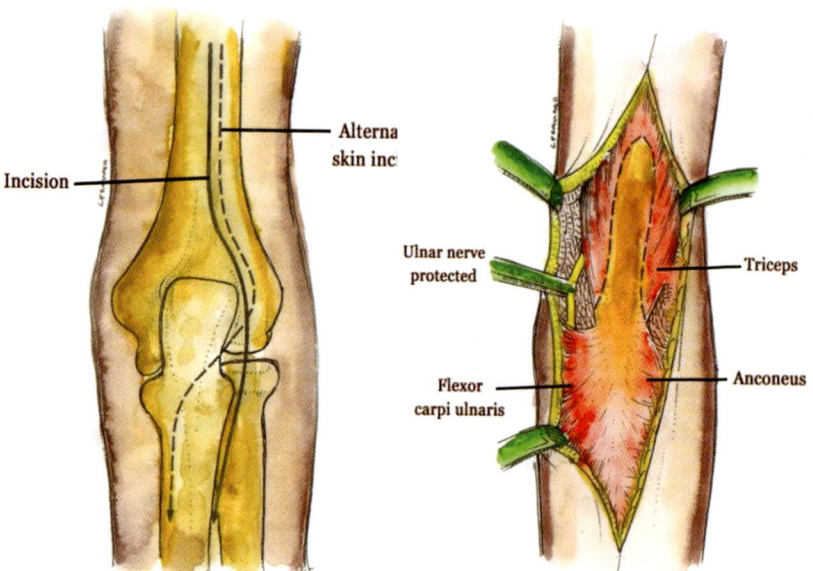

The apex of the tongue has fascia, the mid-portion fascia and muscle, and the base has the full thickness of the triceps muscle and tendon.

After reflecting the tongue, a longitudinal midline incision is made right up to the bone. Dissection to either side exposes the posterior surface of the lower end of the humerus and the joint.

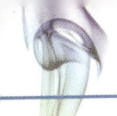

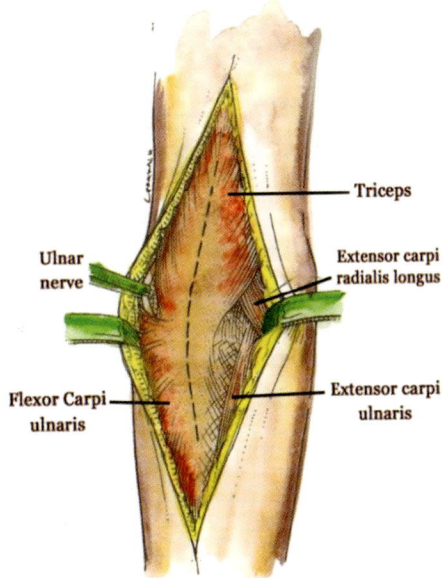

Ulnar nerve

Flexor Carpi ulnaris

Triceps

Extensor carpi radialis longus

Extensor carpi ulnaris

Indications

- Open reduction of unreduced elbow dislocations.
- Open reduction and internal fixation of supracondylar fractures in children and adults.
- Release of extension contracture of the elbow.
- Supracondylar osteotomy.
- Open reduction and internal fixation of comminuted intra-articular fractures. (Olecranon splitting exposures give a better exposure for these problems.)
- Total elbow arthroplasty.
- Excision arthroplasty.
- Resection of heterotrophic bone in this area.

Posterior Longitudinal Approach with or without Olecranon

Access

- Triceps tendon.
- The distal humerus and its articular surface.
- Elbow joint, the radial head and the olecranon.

Position: Same positions as for the posterior approach.

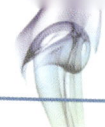

Incision: Straight midline incision over the olecranon, skirting lightly laterally just at the tip.

Approach: The triceps tendon is exposed in line of the incision.

The ulnar nerve is identified, dissected free and protected by a moist tape.

The olecranon is exposed by subperiosteal elevation of the flexor carpi ulnaris medially and of the anconeus laterally.

The lower humerus and elbow joint can now be exposed either by splitting the triceps tendon or olecranon osteotomy.

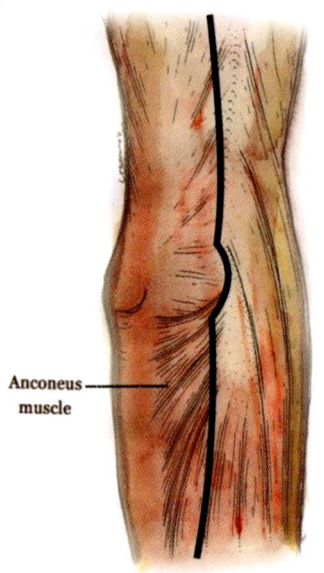

Anconeus muscle

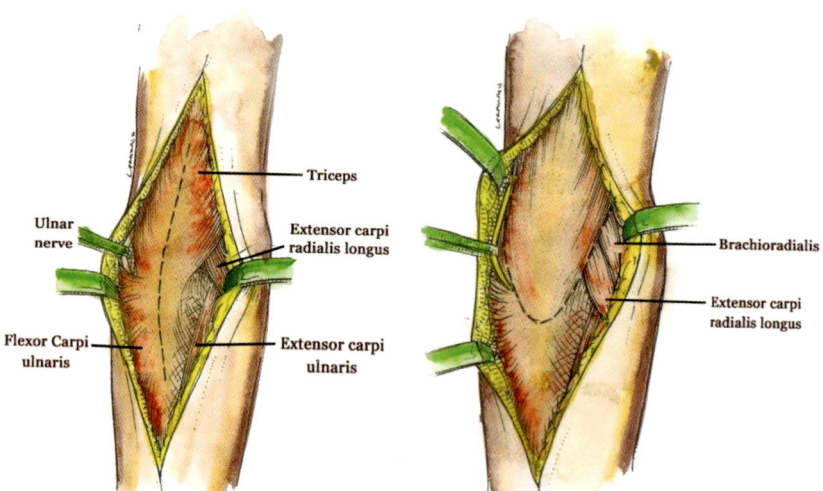

Triceps

Ulnar nerve

Extensor carpi radialis longus

Flexor Carpi ulnaris

Extensor carpi ulnaris

Brachioradialis

Extensor carpi radialis longus

For an olecranon osteotomy, it is divided either intra-articularly or extra-articularly.

Before the osteotomy, either a drill hole is made for cancellous screw insertion, or a pair of K-wires are inserted to be tension band wired later.

The extra-articular osteotomy is performed obliquely in a single plane with either a saw or a thin, sharp osteotome, the last part of subchondral bone being finally broken rather than cut. This will allow for a snap fit during reattachment.

The intra-articular osteotomy can be transverse or V shaped (chevronned) and is done by a sharp, thin osteotome to avoid loss of bone.

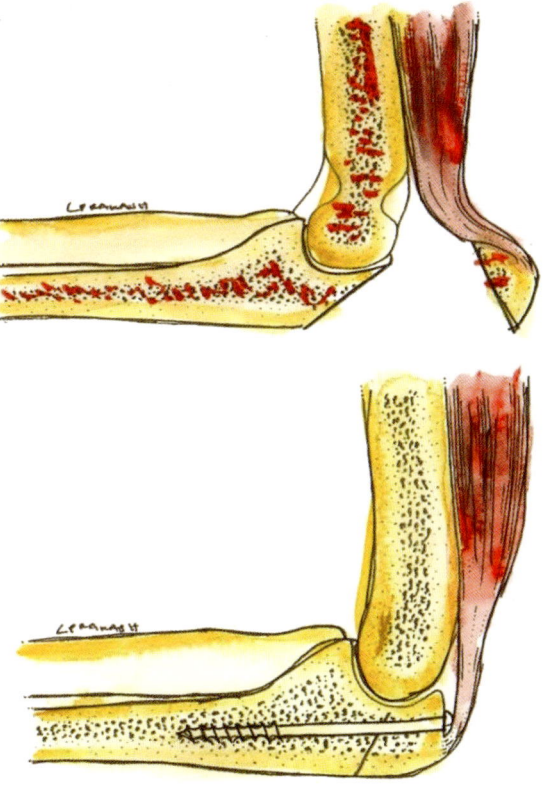

The osteotomized olecranon is deflected with the distal triceps tendon, which is cut to separate it from the anconeus and humeral shaft.

The ulnar nerve should be carefully protected.

During closure, restoration of the olecranon osteotomy should anatomic.

The ulnar nerve can be repositioned in its groove, but if it slips, it can be transposed anteriorly.

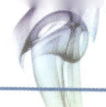

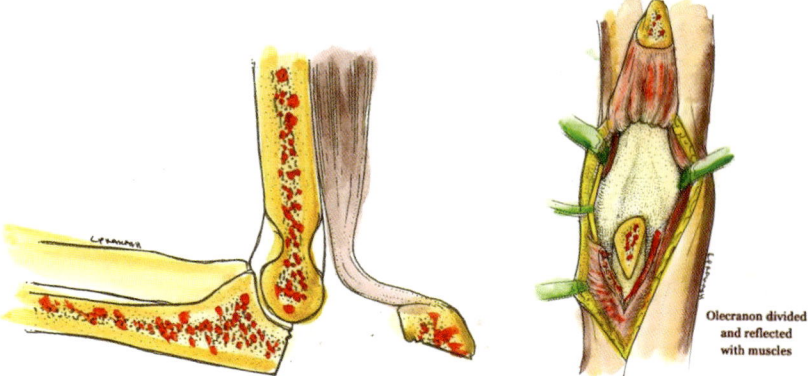

Olecranon divided
and reflected
with muscles

Indications

- Comminuted intra-articular fractures of the distal humerus.
- Delayed or non-unions needing fixations and grafts.
- Arthrodesis.
- Synovectomy.
- Removal of heterotrophic bone.

Posterior Transolecranon U Approach

Access: Distal humerus and its articular surface.

Position: Same as for other posterior approaches.

Incision: U shaped incision between the two humeral epicondyles, and a point about 2.5 cm below the tip of the olecranon.

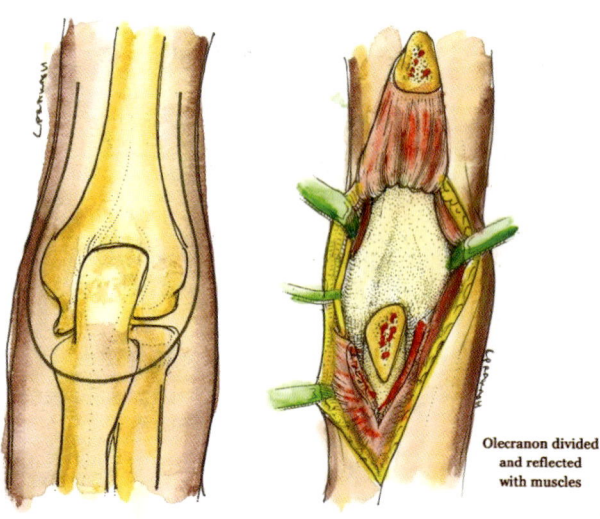

Olecranon divided
and reflected
with muscles

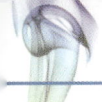

Approach: The tongue of the flap is retracted proximally and the olecranon is exposed.

The ulnar nerve is identified, exposed and retracted with a moist tape.

The olecranon is then osteotomized as previously described.

It is important to keep the subcutaneous tissue, triceps tendon and muscle as a single flap to avoid skin necrosis, probable by the U shaped incision.

During closure, restoration of the olecranon osteotomy should anatomic.

The ulnar nerve can be repositioned in its groove, but if it slips, it can be transposed anteriorly.

Indications
- Open reduction and internal fixation of comminuted intra-articular distal humeral fractures.
- Delayed or non-unions.
- Elbow arthroplasty.
- Olecranon resection.
- Arthrotomy, removal of loose bodies and synovectomy.

Lateral Approach

Access
- Lateral humeral epicondyle.
- Capitellum.
- Anterior and posterior compartments of elbow.
- Radial head, the radial collateral and annular ligaments

Position: The patient is supine on the operating table. The arm rests on an adjacent well-padded table, with the arm abducted and internally rotated. The elbow is flexed and its lateral aspect faces the surgeon.

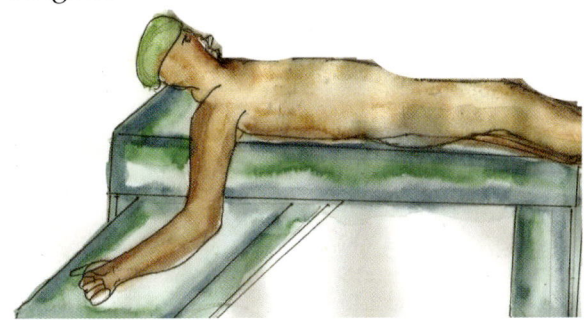

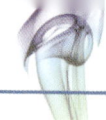

Incision: Beginning on the lateral supracondylar ridge, 2.5 cm above the elbow joint, the incision is brought over proximal forearm behind radial head, down to another 2.5 cm.

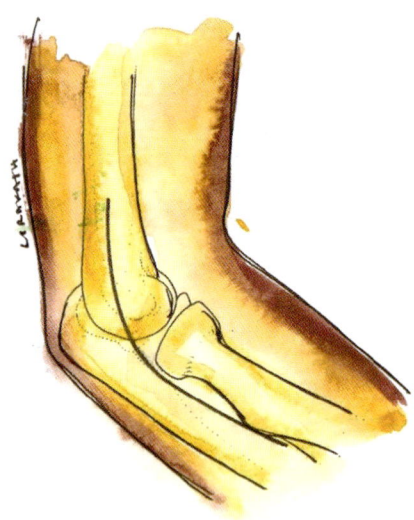

Approach: The deep fascia is incised in line with the incision.

The interval between the triceps muscle posteriorly and the brachioradialis and extensor carpi radialis longus muscles anteriorly is developed to expose the lateral humeral epicondyle, lateral joint capsule and radial collateral ligament.

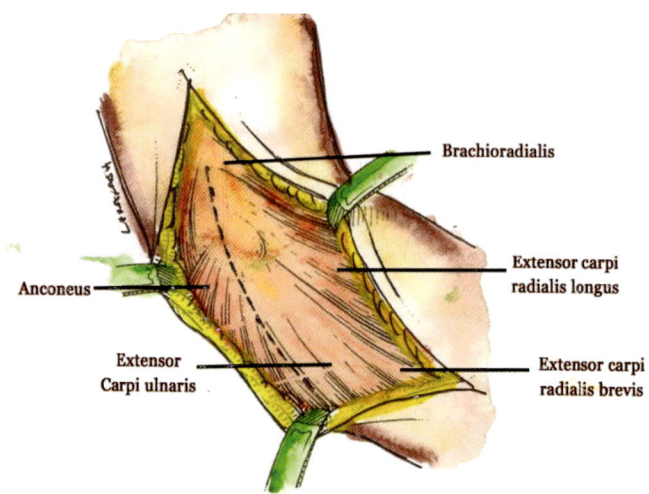

Brachioradialis

Extensor carpi radialis longus

Anconeus

Extensor Carpi ulnaris

Extensor carpi radialis brevis

The deep posterior interosseous branch of the radial nerve, lies close to the anterior capsule over the head the radius and is protected.

Distal exposure is between extensor carpi ulnaris and the anconeus.

Capsule and radial collateral ligament are incised over the lateral aspect of the head of the radius to expose the articular surface of the head and lower end of the lateral humeral epicondyle and the capitellum.

Subperiosteal reflection of the brachioradialis, extensor carpi, radialis longus, common extensor origins and triceps improves exposure.

Indications

- Surgery of fractures of the lateral humeral epicondyle.
- Fractures of capitellum and the head and neck of the radius.

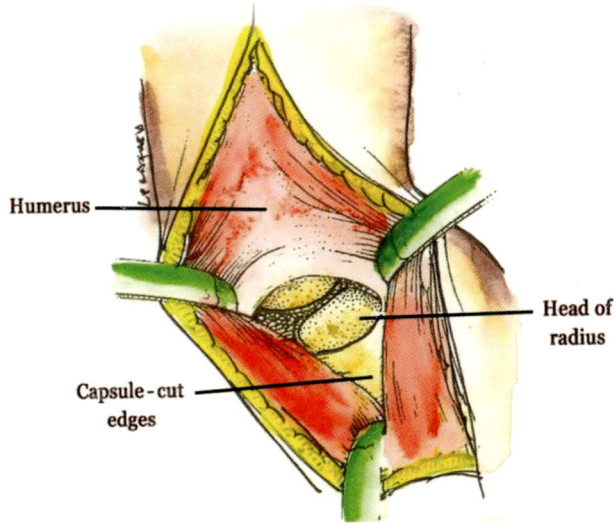

- Reduction of irreducible radial head dislocation.
- Arthrotomy for septic arthritis.
- Removal of loose bodies or foreign bodies.
- Tumours, heterotrophic bone and synovectomy.
- Tennis elbow and lateral epicondylitis.
- Flexion contracture of elbow.

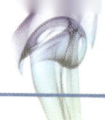

Posterolateral Approach

History

Emil Theodor Kocher: Emil Theodor Kocher (1841–1917, Berne) was the Swiss surgeon who won the 1909 Nobel prize for Physiology or Medicine for his work on the thyroid gland.

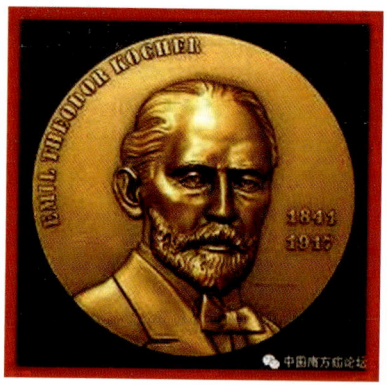
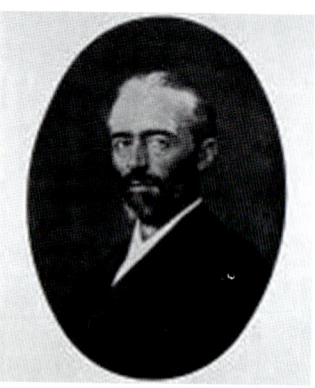

After qualifying in medicine at the University of Bern in 1865, Kocher studied in Berlin, London, Paris and Vienna, where he was a pupil of Theodor Billroth. In 1872, he became professor of clinical surgery at Bern, remaining head of the surgical clinic for 45 years.

There Kocher became the first surgeon to excise the thyroid gland in the treatment of goitre (1876). In 1883, he announced his discovery of a characteristic cretinoid pattern in patients after total excision of the thyroid gland; however, when a portion of the gland was left intact, there were only transitory signs of the pathological pattern.

His other surgical contributions include a method for reducing dislocations of the shoulder and techniques for surgery on hip, stomach, the lungs, the tongue, and the cranial nerves and for hernia. In surgical practice, he adopted the principles of complete asepsis introduced by Joseph Lister. He also devised many new surgical techniques, instruments, and appliances. The forceps and incision (in gallbladder surgery) that bear his name remain in general use.

He originally described the versatile posterolateral approach, which has many uses.

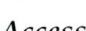

Access

- Lateral humeral epicondyle.
- Capitellum.
- Anterior and posterior compartments of the elbow.
- Radial head, radial collateral, and annular ligament.

Position: The patient is supine on the operating table. The arm is flexed and internally rotated. The elbow is flexed and held by the assistant on the opposite side. The posterior elbow faces the surgeon.

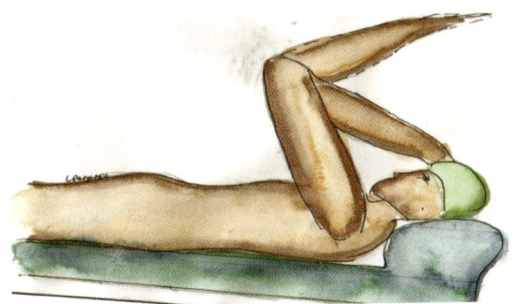

Incision: From the lateral aspect of the distal third of humerus 2.5 cm above the elbow it brought down to the elbow over the lateral epicondylar ridge.

After crossing the radial head, it is curved medially and posteriorly up to the posterior subcutaneous margin of the ulna.

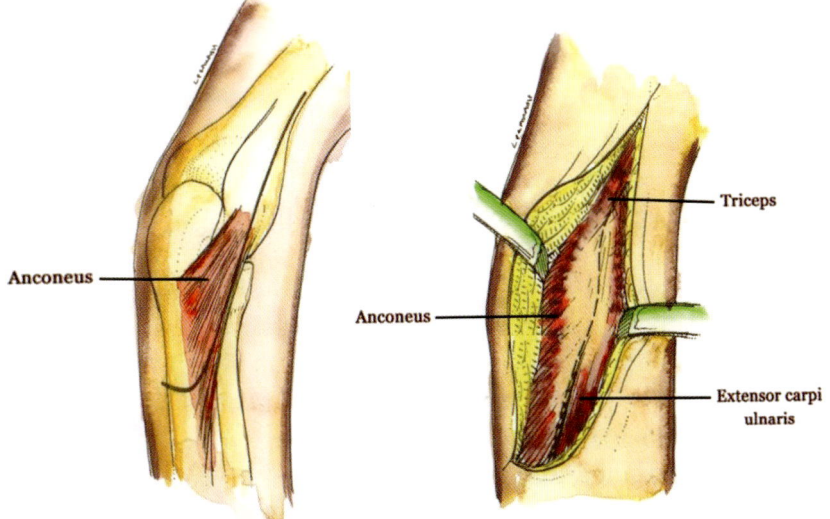

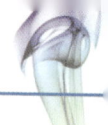

Approach: The deep fascia is incised in line with the incision.

The interval between triceps posteriorly and the brachio-radialis and extensor carpi radialis longus muscles anteriorly is developed to expose the lateral humeral epicondyle, lateral joint capsule and radial collateral ligament.

The dissection is then continued distally and the fibres of the anconeus and the extensor carpi ulnaris are separated.

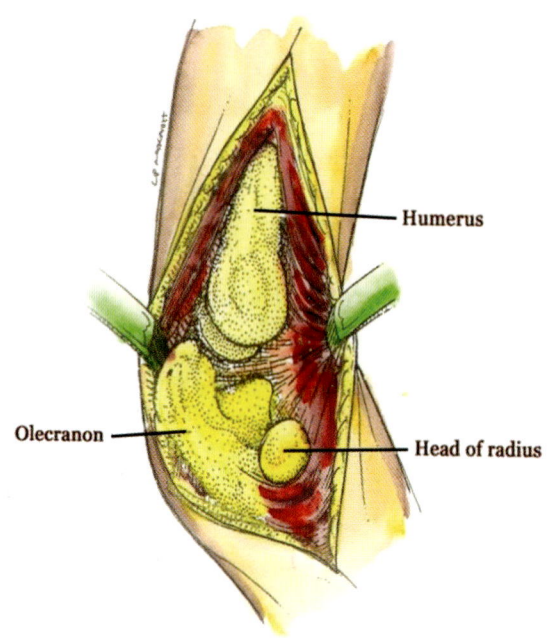

The fibres of supinator lying underneath are separated in their line.

The joint capsule is incised longitudinally to gain access to the joint.

Subperiosteal dissection of the brachioradialis, extensor carpi radialis longus, common extensor origin, anterior capsule, triceps, posterior capsule and anconeus will facilitate the exposure of the elbow, allowing its per operative lateral dislocation for wider exposure.

If the dissection is carried towards the medial humeral epicondyle, the ulnar nerve must be identified and protected.

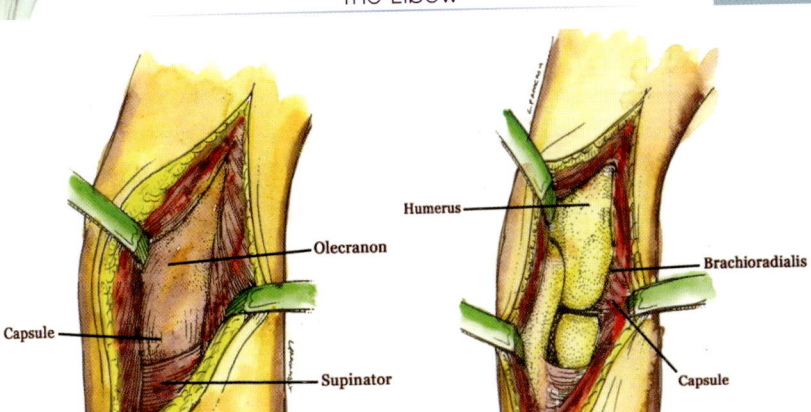

Indications

- Surgery of fractures of the lateral humeral epicondyle.
- Fractures of capitellum and the head and neck of the radius.
- Reduction of irreducible radial head dislocation.
- Arthrotomy for septic arthritis.
- Removal of loose bodies or foreign bodies.
- Tumours, heterotrophic bone and synovectomy.
- Tennis elbow and lateral epicondylitis.
- Flexion contracture of elbow.

Anterior Approach

Access

- Cubital fossa.
- Brachialis insertion.
- Coronoid process of the ulna.
- Anterior capsule of the elbow.

Position: Supine or mid-lateral, with the affected arm fully supinated and placed on a perpendicular side table, to allow its flexion extension.

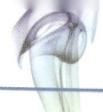

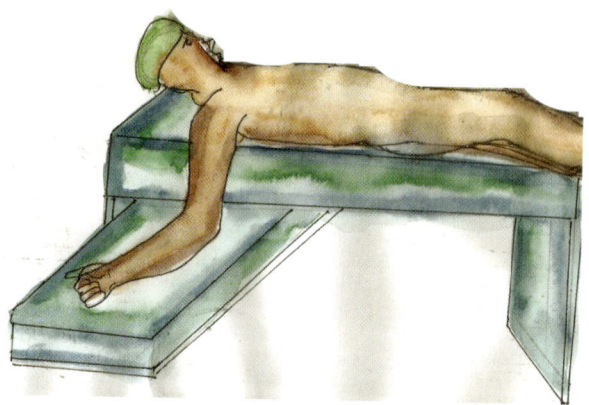

Incision: Beginning 2.5 cm above the elbow besides the medial edge of the biceps, the incision extends distally between the medial biceps and the lateral border of the pronator teres till the flexor crease.

It is then crossed obliquely, on the front of the elbow towards the medial edge of brachioradialis.

The incision can be extended up or down depending on the need.

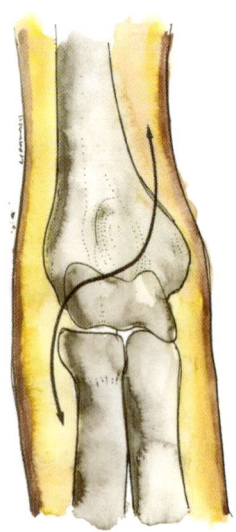

Approach: It may be necessary to coagulate or ligate the median antecubital and other small veins, but the cephalic and basilic veins are preserved.

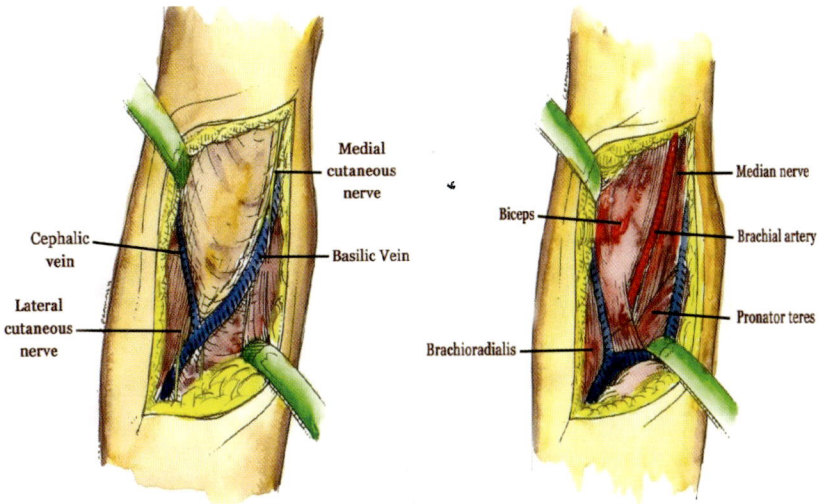

Dissection of the deep fascia exposes the contents of the fossa, which from medial to lateral are: median nerve, brachial artery and biceps tendon (MAD).

The insertion of brachialis is exposed by mobilizing the brachial artery and median nerve medially and the biceps tendon laterally.

The anterior capsule, the anterior portion of the distal humerus and the coronoid process are exposed by first mobilizing or splitting the brachialis and anterior joint capsule. The branches from the median nerve to the pronator teres must be protected.

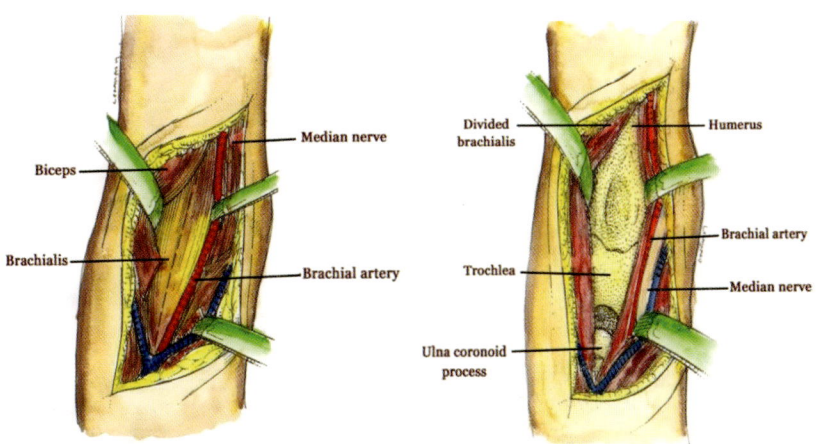

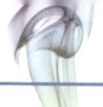

Indications
- Injuries to the biceps tendon.
- Biceps tendon transfers.
- Fracture—dislocations of the elbow associated with fractures of the coronoid process.
- Reconstruction of the elbow in cases of chronic instability.
- Flexion contracture release by lengthening biceps, brachialis, and anterior capsulectomy.
- Loose bodies in the anterior compartment of the elbow.
- Bronchial artery and median nerve exposure.

Medial Approach

Access
- Ulnar nerve at the elbow.
- Medial humeral epicondyle.
- Medial aspect of elbow joint, including the trochlea and the trochlear notch.

Position: Supine with the extremity placed on a side-table, with the shoulder abducted, externally rotated, and the elbow flexed.

Incision: A straight line centred over elbow extending 5 cm up and down, from medial supracondylar ridge, crossing medial epicondyle and over medial ulna.

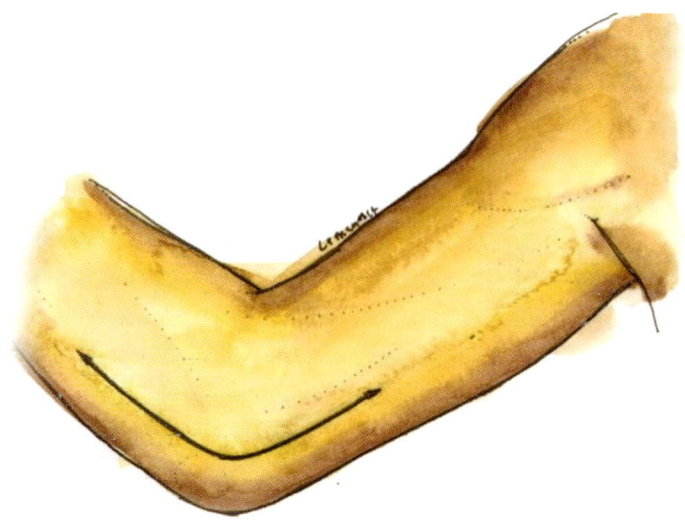

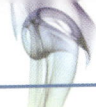

The posterior branch of the medial antebrachial cutaneous nerve is identified and protected.

In ulnar nerve surgeries, the skin incision is placed 1.25 cm anterior to the medial epicondyle to avoid nerve pressure between the operative scar and the medial humeral epicondyle.

The incision can be extended proximally or distally after locating the ulnar nerve and following it in both directions.

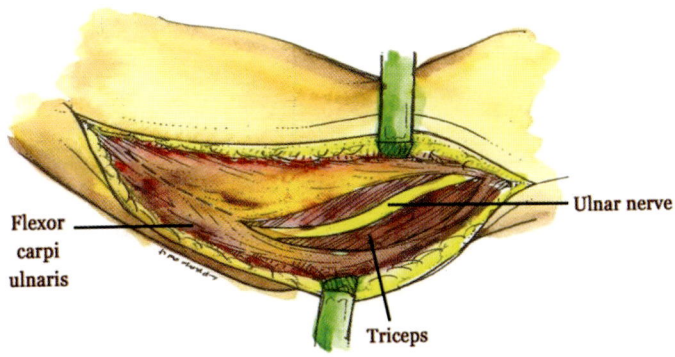

Flexor carpi ulnaris — Ulnar nerve — Triceps

Approach: Proximally, the ulnar nerve lies in the triceps groove, posterior to the medial epicondyle and distally between the two heads of the flexor carpi ulnaris.

For surgery of ulnar nerve entrapment, or anterior transposition, adequate decompression of the medial intermuscular septum proximally and the fascia of the flexor carpi ulnaris distally must be done.

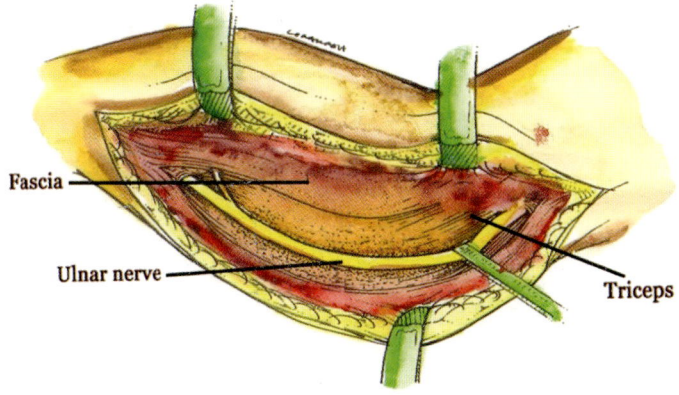

Fascia — Ulnar nerve — Triceps

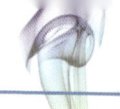

The ulnar nerve is retracted by a moist tape and its first supplying the elbow joint is sacrificed.

The second branch to the flexor carpi ulnaris must be protected.

At this stage, an additional osteotomy of the medial humeral epicondyle allows it to be deflected along with the flexor pronator origins as far as the coronoid process.

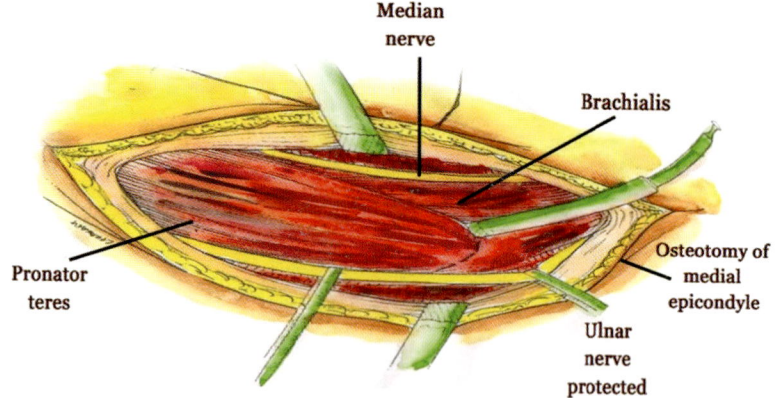

Then the median nerve is identified, lying on the brachialis belly, lateral to the pronator teres.

The capsule is incised longitudinally and spread anteriorly and posteriorly. For wider exposure, the periosteum is stripped with the capsule. The forearm is abducted to wedge open the elbow joint, hinging the lateral capsule and radial collateral ligament complex.

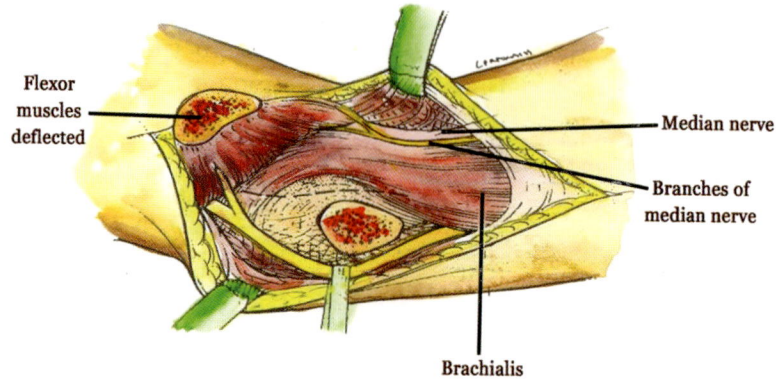

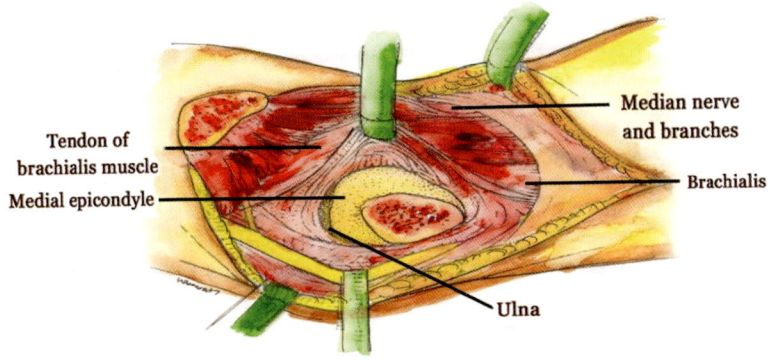

Labels: Tendon of brachialis muscle; Medial epicondyle; Median nerve and branches; Brachialis; Ulna

Indications

- Displaced medial epicondylar fractures and coronoid process.
- Decompression, transposition, repair or reconstruction of the ulnar nerve.
- Arthroplasties and reconstructive procedures for chronic elbow instability.
- Removal of heterotopic bone.
- Drainage of the elbow joint.
- Removal of loose or foreign bodies.
- Synovectomy.
- Anteromedial release for flexion contracture.
- Combined with an additional anterior incision, it is used for median nerve entrapment syndromes.

Posterior Approach to Olecranon and Proximal Ulna

Access

- Olecranon process.
- Proximal ulna.

Position: Supine with the shoulder adducted and the elbow flexed across the torso with the forearm supinated and supported by the assistant from the opposite side.

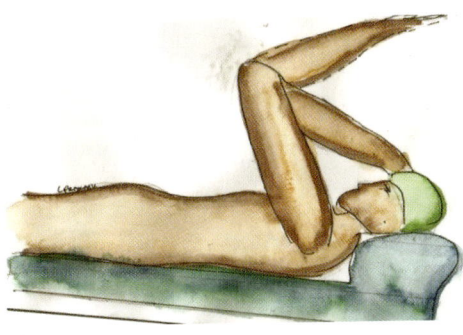

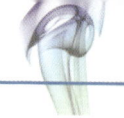

Incision: Midline incision just above the tip of the olecranon extending over the subcutaneous margin of the proximal ulna curving laterally to avoid crossing the bony prominence.

Approach: Below subcutaneous fat and deep fascia, the cleavage is developed between extensor carpi ulnaris medially, and anconeus and supinator laterally by subperiosteal dissection.

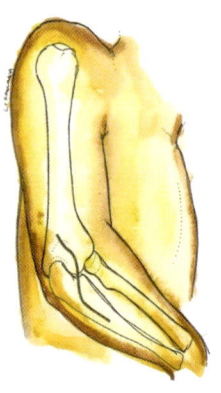

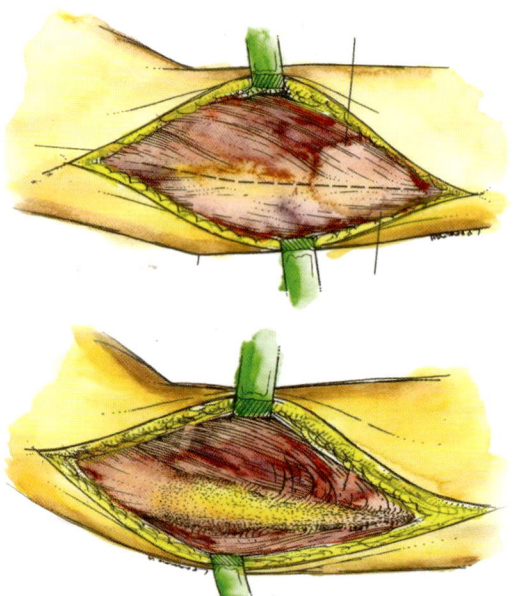

The muscle flap of flexor carpi ulnaris acts as an envelope protecting the ulnar nerve.

Proximally, the ulnar nerve lying medial to the olecranon coming from the cubital groove is identified and protected.

The posterior capsule is now exposed.

Indications
* Repair of olecranon.
* Proximal ulnar fractures.
* Excision of the olecranon.

The Forearm

RELEVANT ANATOMY OF THE FOREARM

Superficial Cutaneous Nerves

The posterior branch of the medial antebrachial cutaneous nerve in the proximal forearm and the dorsal sensory branch of the radial nerve in the distal forearm should always be protected to avoid painful neuromas.

The lateral antebrachial cutaneous nerve is an excellent donor for interfascicular nerve grafts for digital nerves, and complications from harvesting this nerve are rare.

The lateral antebrachial cutaneous nerve is a continuation of the musculocutaneous nerve emerging from behind the biceps, lateral to the tendon, and piercing the deep fascia at the level of the elbow.

Here it lies behind and between the cephalic and accessory cephalic veins dividing into anterior and posterior branches. The anterior branch continues along the radial half of the anterior forearm supplying the skin here.

Lying superficial to the radial artery at the wrist, it terminates by dividing

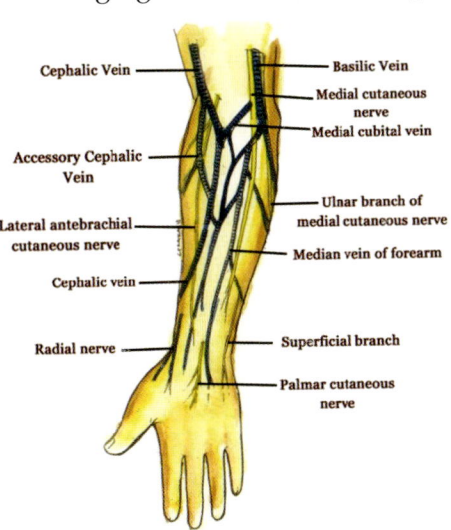

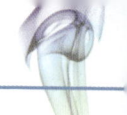

with the radial artery, supplying the thenar eminence and the dorsal surface of the carpus.

The posterior branch travels on the radial side of the forearm supplying the overlying skin.

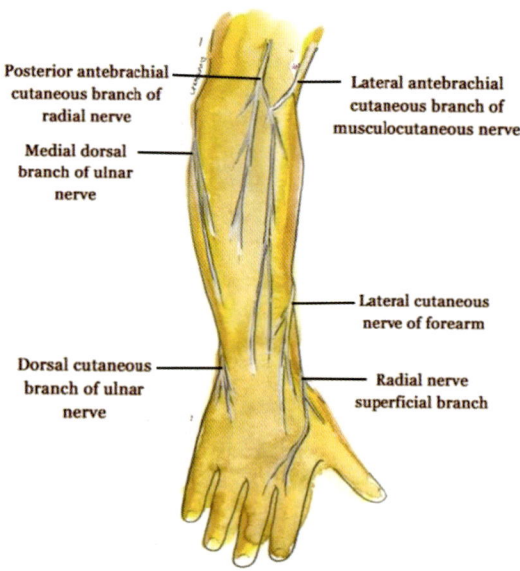

The medial antebrachial cutaneous nerve leaves near the medial side of the brachial artery and pierces the deep fascia at midarm with the basilic vein dividing into anterior and posterior branches.

The anterior branch continues besides the median vein on the ulnar side of the anterior forearm as far as the wrist, supplying overlying skin.

The posterior branch passes by the side of the basilic vein to the dorsoulnar aspect of the forearm, where it supplies the overlying skin.

The posterior antebrachial cutaneous nerve is one of the lateral group of radial nerve branches. Piercing the lateral head of the triceps, it penetrates the branchial fascia to run posteriorly to the lateral humeral epicondyle.

Then it courses down the middle of the posterior forearm as far as the wrist, supplying the overlying skin between the posterior branches of the lateral and medial antebrachial cutaneous nerves.

Deep Nerves and Vessels

Median nerve traverses the cubital fossa anterior to the brachialis and medial to the brachial artery.

Entering the forearm obliquely from medial to lateral over the ulnar artery and between the two heads of the pronator teres, it runs distally just lateral to the ulnar artery and superficial to the flexor digitorum profundus.

Entering between the two heads of the flexor digitorum superficialis and then deep to it, the nerve now surfaces from behind the superficial flexor, lateral to its tendons.

Moving anteriorly, it lies between the superficial flexor tendons to the index and middle fingers at the wrist.

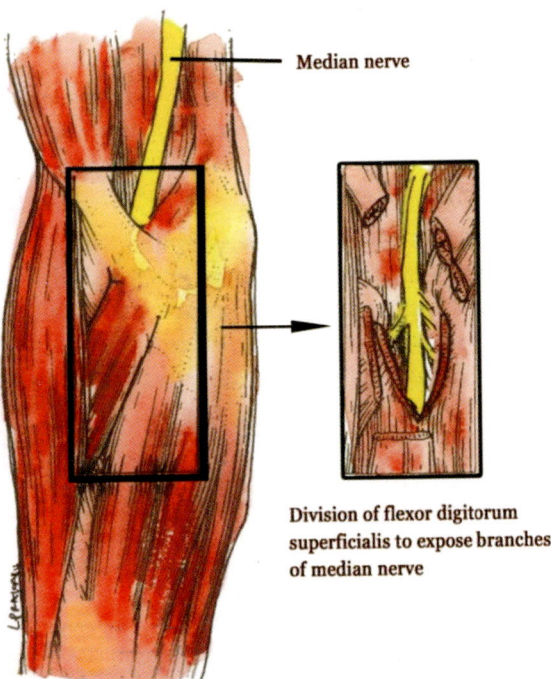

Median nerve

Division of flexor digitorum superficialis to expose branches of median nerve

The anterior interosseous nerve, its largest branch, arises about 5 cm distal to the medial epicondyle.

It runs obliquely from medial to lateral across the upper lateral portion of the flexor digitorum profundus and then descends on top of the interosseous membrane, with the anterior interosseous artery on its medial side.

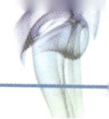

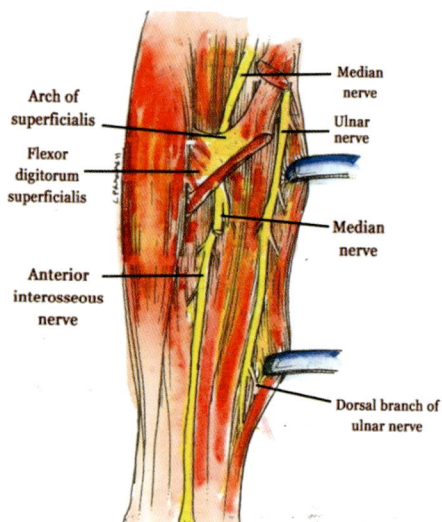

The palmar cutaneous nerve arises from the anterior surface of the median nerve above the wrist and pierces the deep fascia to become subcutaneous, dividing into radial and ulnar branches over the thenar eminence.

Ulnar nerve enters the forearm between the heads of the flexor carpi ulnaris, runs straight down the forearm to the wrist and is joined at the mid-forearm by the ulnar artery. The ulnar nerve and artery continue together to the wrist, where they surface just lateral to the flexor carpi ulnaris passing lateral to the pisiform bone.

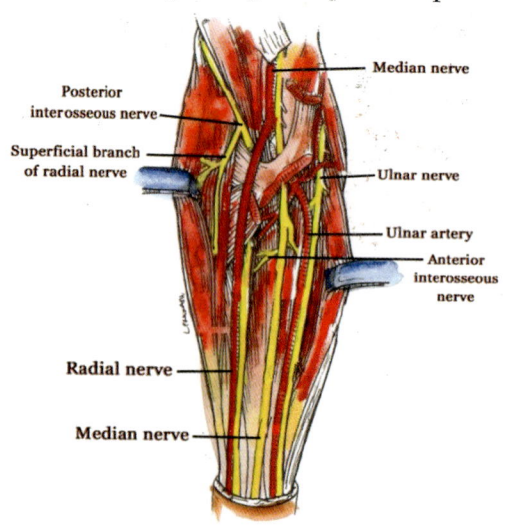

The branches to the flexor carpi ulnaris, flexor digitorum profundus, are given off here. The ulnar nerve has two cutaneous branches that arise distally in the forearm.

Radial nerve: A little below the tip of the lateral humeral condyles, the radial nerve divides into a deep motor branch, the posterior interosseous nerve, and a superficial sensory branch.

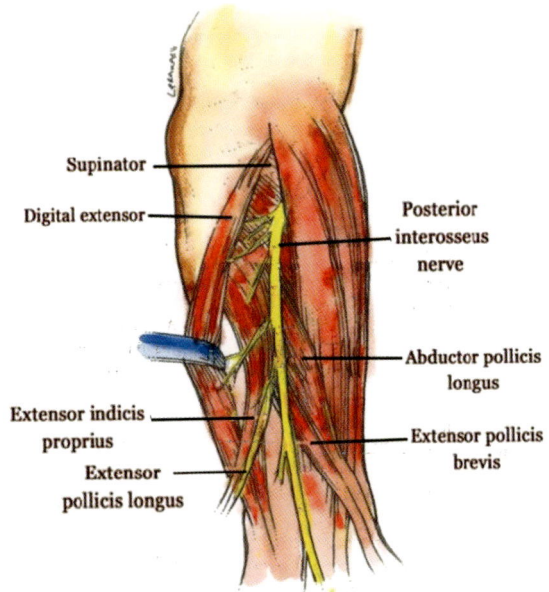

The posterior interosseous nerve is a purely motor nerve except for its distribution to the wrist joint, where it terminates.

After entering the forearm between the two heads of the supinator, its branches supply the superficial group of extensor muscles of the forearm; the extensor digitorum communis, the extensor digit minimi and the extensor carpi ulnaris. It also supplies the abductor pollicis longus, extensor pollicis brevis, extensor pollicis longus and extensor indicis.

The superficial branch of the radial nerve may give off a branch to the extensor carpi radialis brevis but is otherwise purely sensory.

Ulnar artery enters the forearm beneath the pronator teres and then accompanies the median nerve between the two heads of the flexor digitorum superficialis.

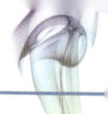

It continues distally lying under cover of the flexor carpi ulnaris, between it and the flexor digitorum profundus.

Accompanying the ulnar nerve up to the wrist, it gives off palmar and dorsal carpal branches. The ulnar artery gives off most at its branches under the flexor digitorum superficialis.

The common interosseous artery arises from the dorsolateral aspect of the ulnar artery, passes posterior to the median nerve and divides into the anterior and posterior interosseous arteries.

The anterior interosseous artery travels on the volar surface of the interoneous membrane, supplying the flexor digitorum profundus, the flexor pollicis longus, the radius and ulna.

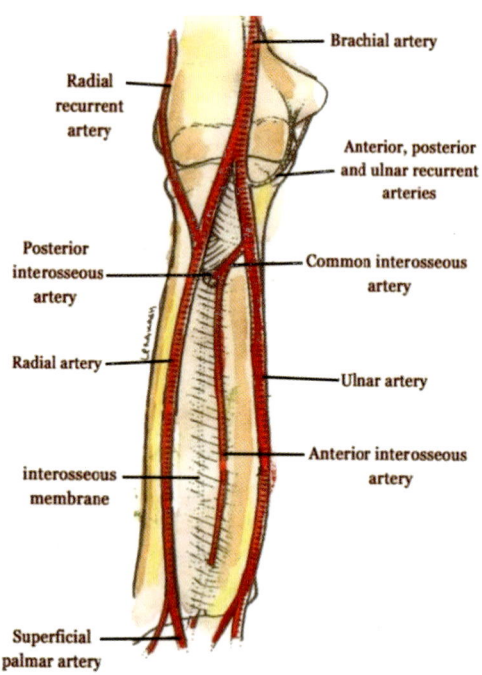

Proximally, it gives off the median artery and terminates by dividing into anterior and posterior branches at the superior border of the pronator quadratus muscle.

The posterior interosseous artery passes volar on the internosseous membrane, to emerge between the lower border at the supinator and the upper border of the abductor pollicis longus.

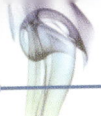

It then leaves the posterior interosseous nerve, remaining between the deep extensor muscles, supplying them and anastomosing with the posterior branch of the anterior interosseous artery at the distal portion of the interosseous membrane.

Radial artery: The radial artery runs laterally over the biceps tendon, the supinator and the pronator teres, coming to lie anterior to the flexor pollicis longus and later the pronator quadratus.

It is superficial in the wrist lying between the tendons of flexor carpi radialis and brachioradialis, where it is palpable.

Proximal to the wrist, the radial artery divides into the superficial and deep branches. The superficial branch continues subcutaneously, over the muscles of the thenar eminence, to the superficial palmar arch, while the deep branch passes deep to the tendons of the first dorsal compartment, across the anatomical snuff box, to the area between the thumb and index metacarpals.

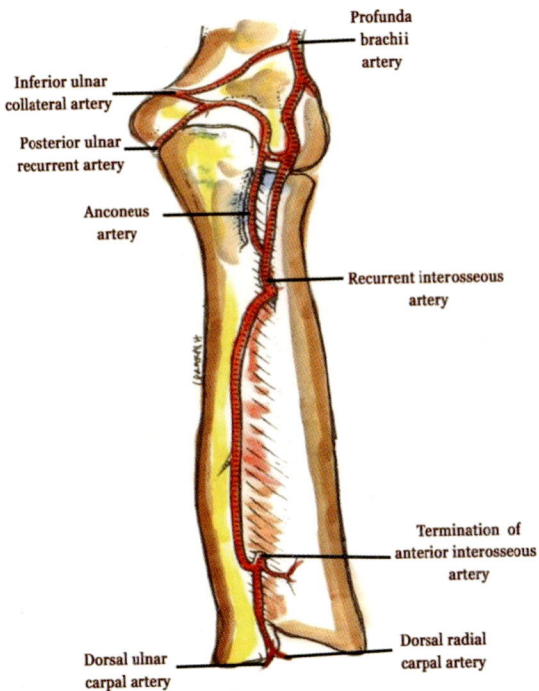

The first branch of the radial artery, the radial recurrent artery, is an important constituent of the collateral circulation around the elbow.

The Muscles and Tendons of Forearm

Anterior compartment: The muscles are arranged in three layers: superficial, intermediate and deep.

There are four superficial muscles (lateral to media): Pronator teres, flexor carpi radialis, palmaris longus, and flexor carpi ulnaris.

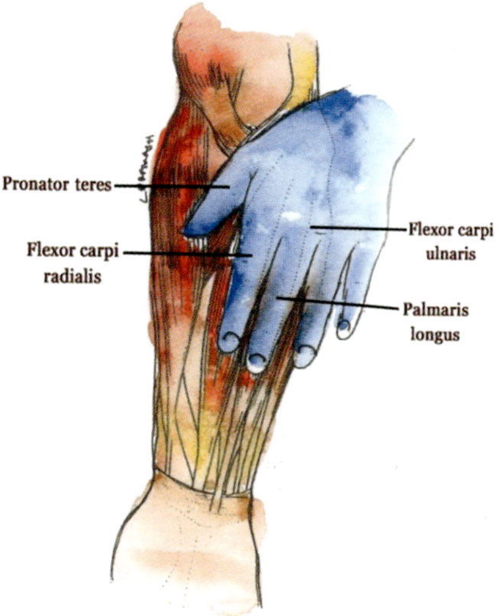

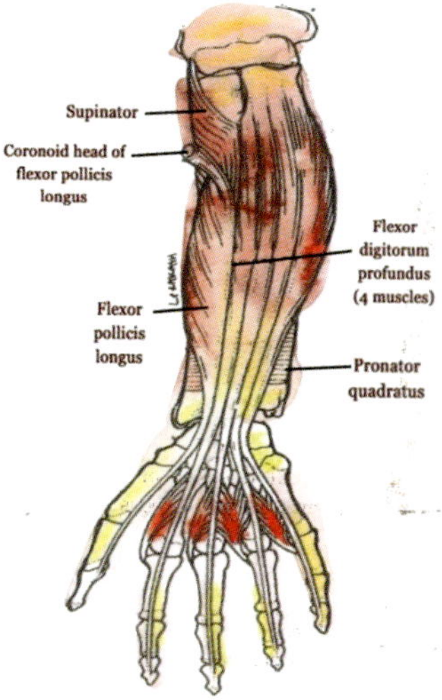

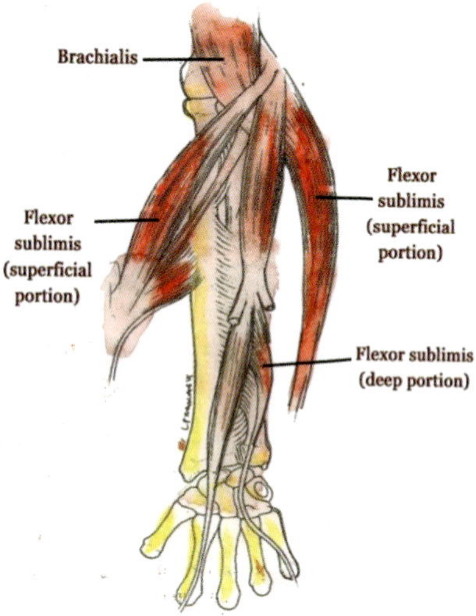

Pronator teres

Flexor carpi radialis

Flexor carpi ulnaris

Palmaris longus

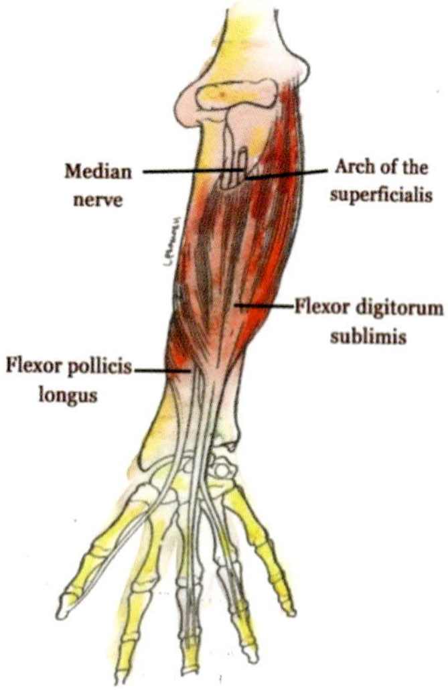

Median nerve

Arch of the superficialis

Flexor pollicis longus

Flexor digitorum sublimis

Supinator

Coronoid head of flexor pollicis longus

Flexor pollicis longus

Flexor digitorum profundus (4 muscles)

Flexor sublimis (superficial portion)

Pronator quadratus

Brachialis

Flexor sublimis (superficial portion)

Flexor sublimis (deep portion)

The single muscle of the intermediate group is the flexor digitorum superficialis and the deep group has flexor digitorum profundus and flexor pollicis longus.

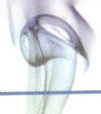

Posterior compartment contains three groups of muscles: The brachioradialis, extensor carpi radialis longus, and brevis, which form the 'mobile wad of three' as described by Henry in his "Extensile Exposures".

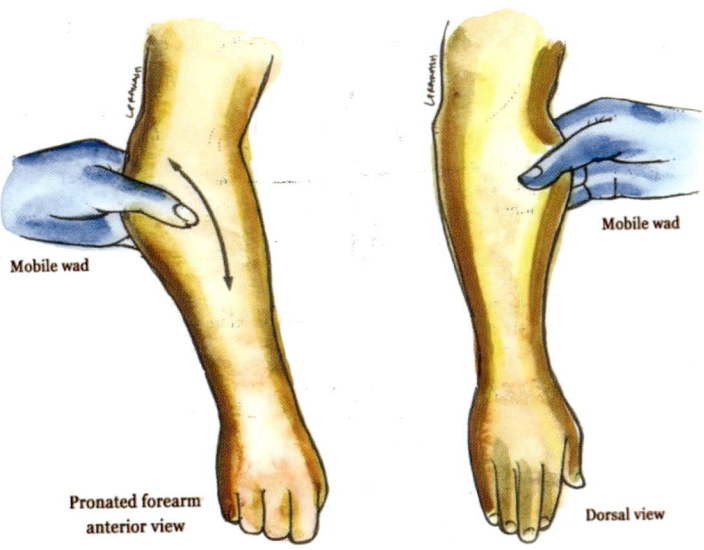

Mobile wad

Mobile wad

Pronated forearm
anterior view

Dorsal view

The superficial extensor muscle group consists of the extensor digitorum communis, extensor indicis, extensor digiti minimi, and the extensor carpi ulnaris.

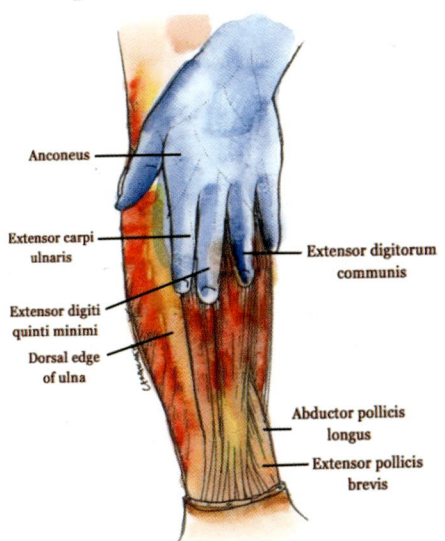

Anconeus

Extensor carpi
ulnaris

Extensor digiti
quinti minimi

Dorsal edge
of ulna

Extensor digitorum
communis

Abductor pollicis
longus

Extensor pollicis
brevis

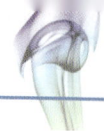

The deep extensor group consists of the supinator, abductor pollicis longus, extensor pollicis longus and brevis.

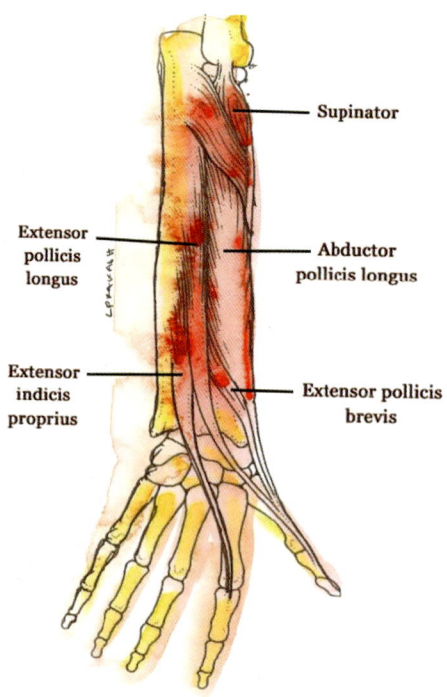

APPROACHES

- Proximal anterior for radius (Henry)
- Anterior distal (Henry)
- Posterolateral (Seed and Boyd)
- Posterolateral (Thompson)
- Combined posterior for radius and ulna

Proximal Anterior Approach for Radius

Access: Proximal and middle thirds of the radial shaft.

Distal radial nerve and deep posterior interosseous and superficial divisions.

Position: The patient is supine with the shoulder abducted and externally rotated. The upper extremity is placed on an adjacent arm table with the elbow extended and the forearm supinated.

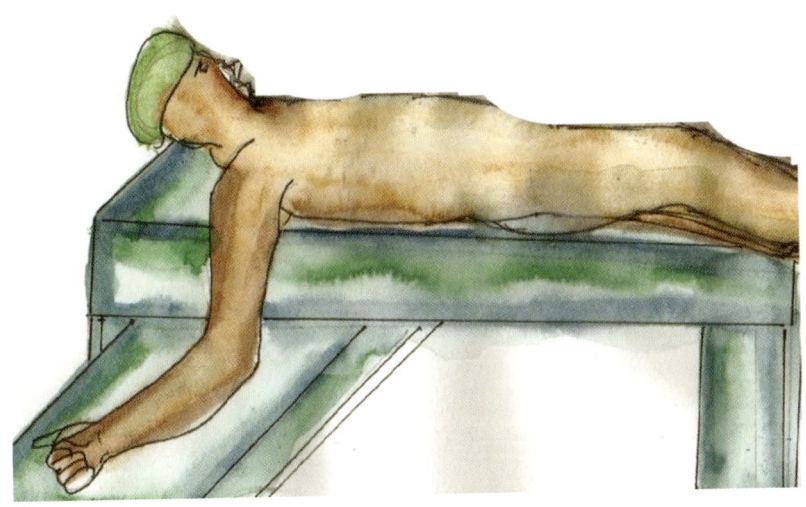

Incision: From the flexion crease of the elbow just lateral to the biceps tendon running parallel to the medial margin of the brachioradialis.

This can be extended both proximally and distally.

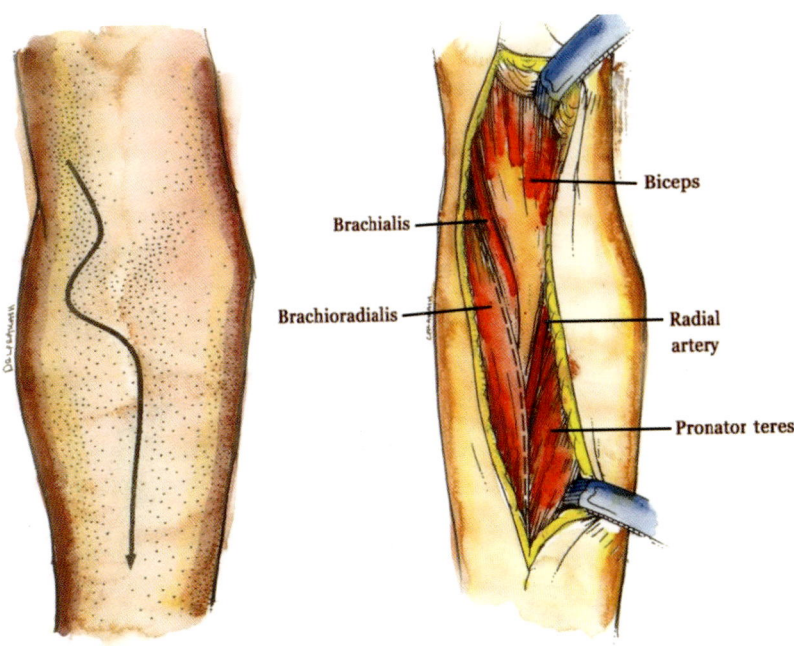

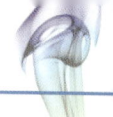

Approach: The brachioradialis and "mobile wad of three" are mobilized and retracted laterally, taking care to identify and protect the radial artery and the superficial branch of the radial nerve.

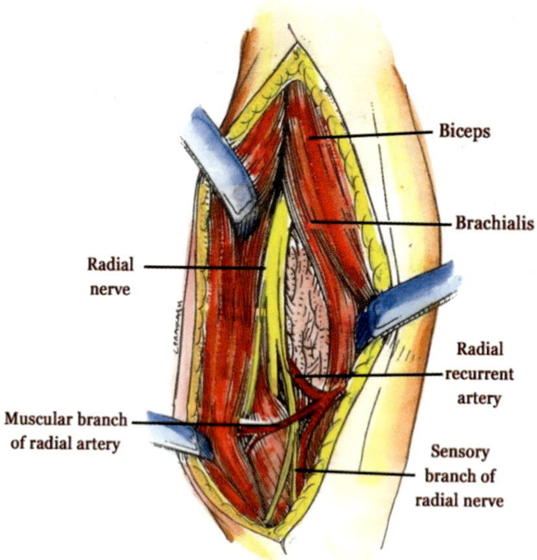

Biceps

Brachialis

Radial nerve

Radial recurrent artery

Muscular branch of radial artery

Sensory branch of radial nerve

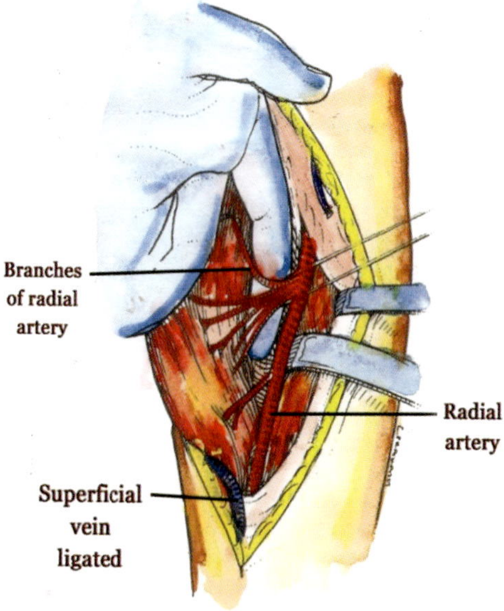

Branches of radial artery

Radial artery

Superficial vein ligated

The radial recurrent artery and veins are identified along with accessory branches, then ligated and divided. With elbow in flexion, the pronator teres and flexor carpi radialis are retracted to the medial side, and the brachioradialis and 'mobile wad' are retracted laterally, to expose the supinator.

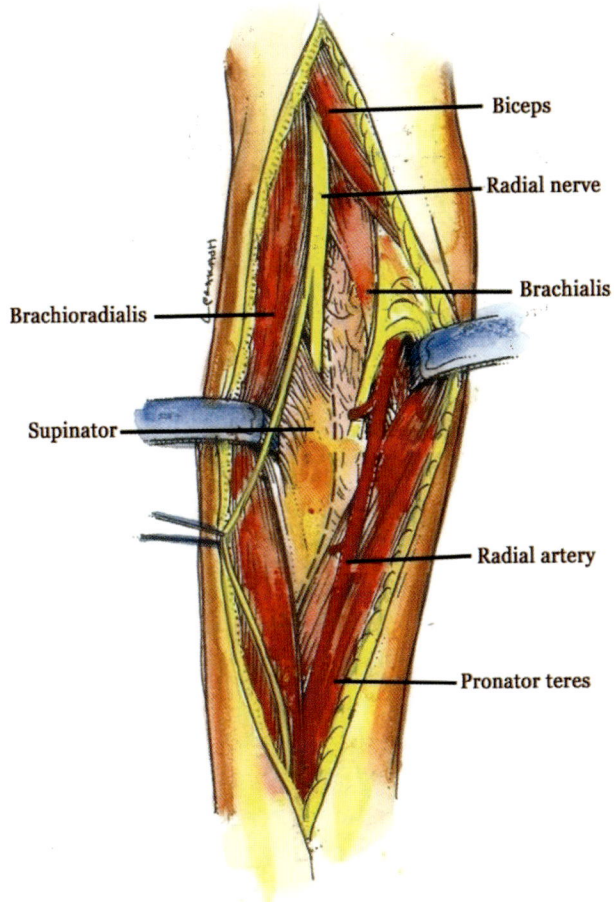

The periosteum is incised and the radial shaft is exposed by elevating the supinator subperiosteally, preserving the posterior interosseous nerve between its two heads.

The radial canal containing the posterior interosseous nerve can be released and explored, exposing the posterior interosseous nerve.

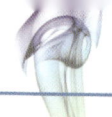

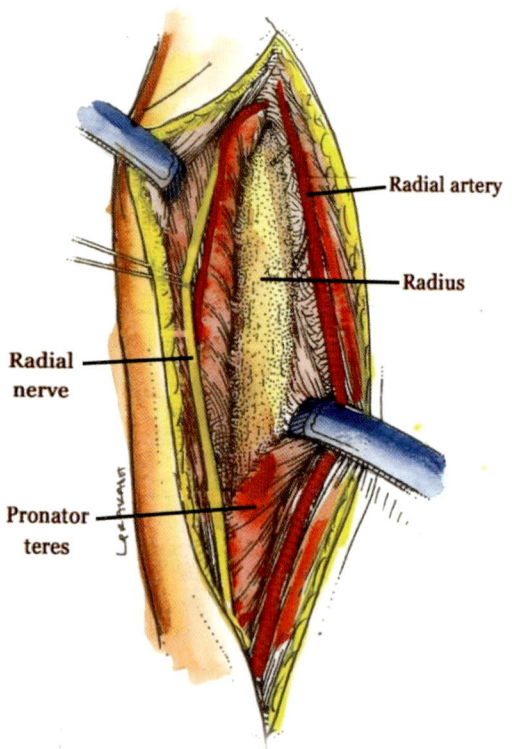

Indications: Decompression or repair the distal radial nerve and its deep posterior interosseus branch.

Fractures, deformities, delayed unions or non-unions in the proximal third of the radial shaft.

Combined with the anterior incision to the elbow, this may be used to approach the median nerve.

The incision may be further extended over the forearm to expose the median nerve or the radial artery for decompression, repair or reconstruction.

This versatile incision also provides access to the radial head, lateral elbow joint and capitellum.

Posterolateral Approach

Access

- Proximal third of the ulna.
- Proximal fourth of the radius.

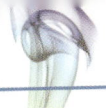

Position: Supine with the shoulder abducted and internally rotated, the upper extremity being supported on an arm table with the elbow flexed and the forearm pronated.

Incision: Beginning 2.5 cm above the elbow, lateral to the triceps tendon extending distally over the olecranon and subcutaneous border of the proximal ulna.

Approach: The clevage is developed between the insertion of anconeus and the flexor carpi ulnaris.

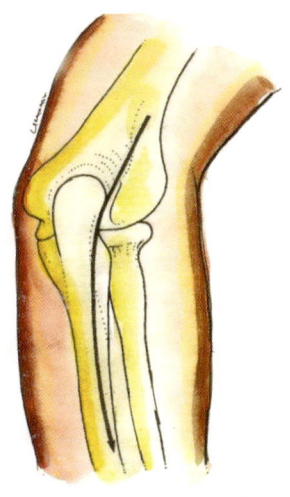

The anconeus is deflected laterally after erasing its ulnar insertion, exposing the proximal third of the ulna laterally and the supinator muscle.

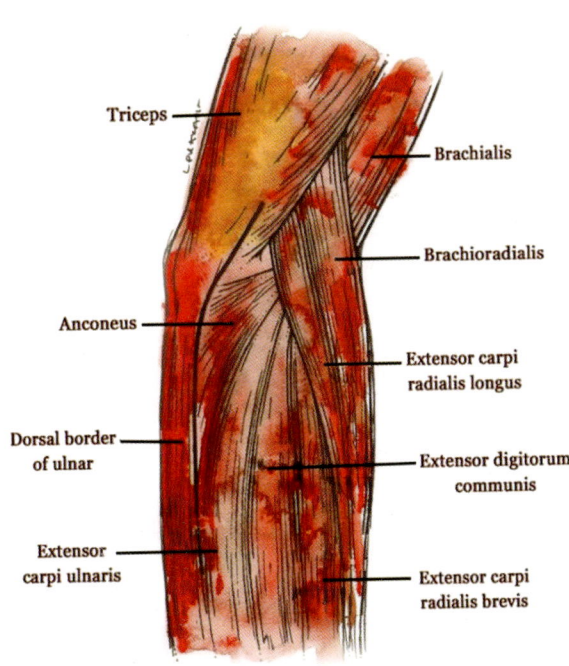

The supinator can be cut near its ulnar origin and dissected subperiosteally right up to the interosseous membrane.

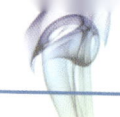

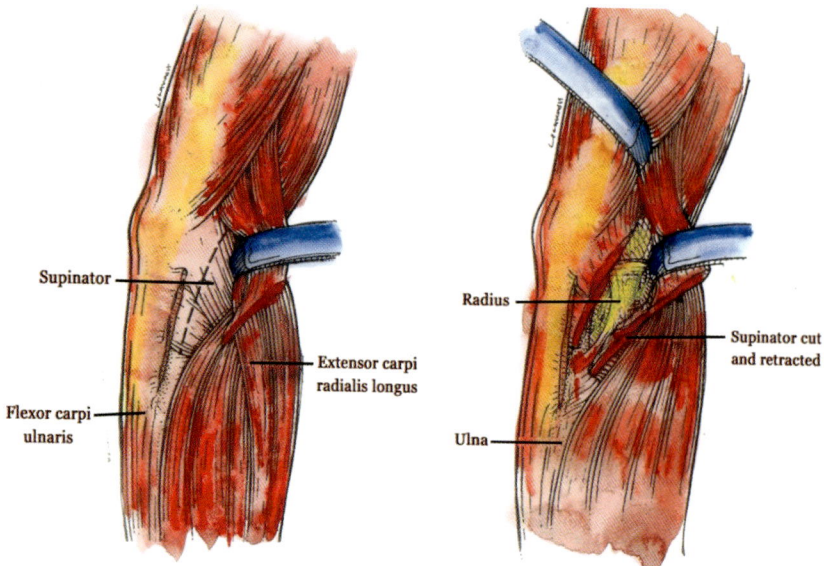

Supinator

Radius

Extensor carpi radialis longus

Supinator cut and retracted

Flexor carpi ulnaris

Ulna

Indications: Fractures of the proximal ulna associated with radial head dislocations.

Fractures, delayed unions and non-union of the proximal fourth of the ulna.

Fractures or dislocations of the radial head and neck with minimal risk of injury to the posterior interosseous nerve.

Posterolateral Approach

Access: Proximal two-thirds of the radius.

Position: Supine with the shoulder abducted and internally rotated. The limb is supported on an arm table. The elbow is flexed and the forearm pronated.

Incision: Straight incision over the proximal two-thirds of the radius on a line from the centre of the dorsum of the wrist to 1.25 cm anterior to the lateral humeral epicondyle.

The forearm is kept pronated.

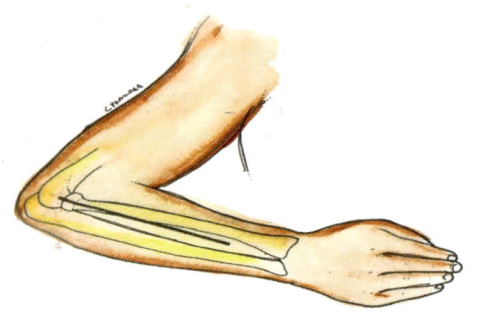

Approach: The plane is between extensor carpi radialis brevis and the extensor digitorum communis.

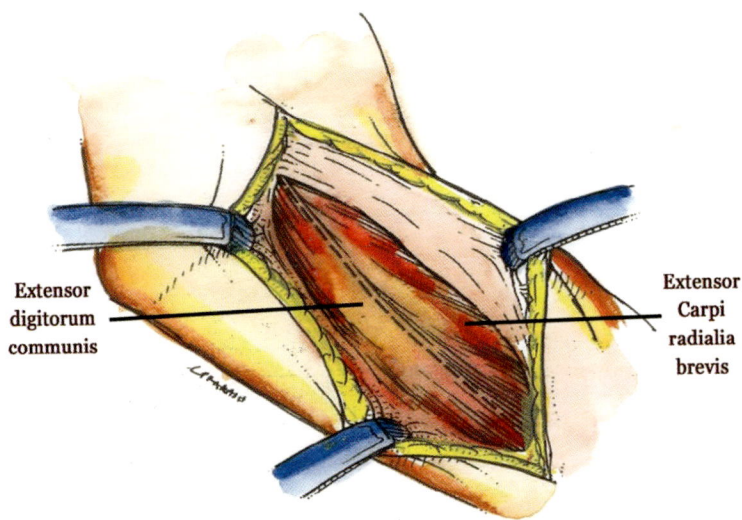

Extensor digitorum communis

Extensor Carpi radialia brevis

Separating these two exposes the supinator and the access can be improved by detaching the extensor digitorum origin from the lateral humeral epicondyle.

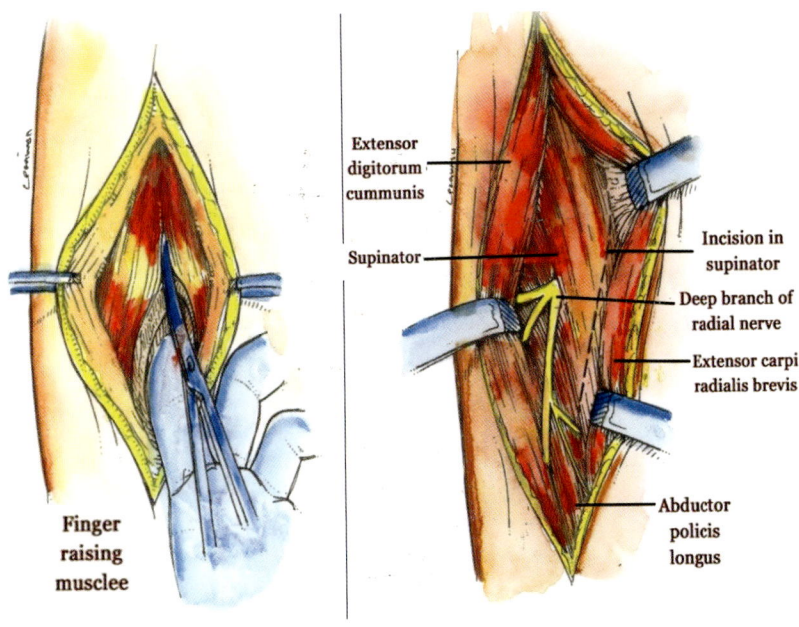

Finger raising musclee

Extensor digitorum cummunis

Supinator

Incision in supinator

Deep branch of radial nerve

Extensor carpi radialis brevis

Abductor policis longus

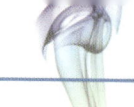

The insertion of the supinator to the radius is reflected medially, by subperiosteal dissection leaving the posterior interosseous nerve protected within its belly.

The posterior interosseous nerve can be identified as it emerges at the inferior part of the supinator.

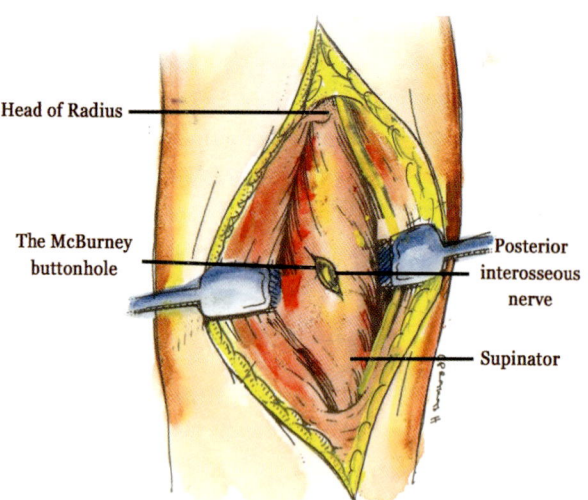

Head of Radius

The McBurney buttonhole

Posterior interosseous nerve

Supinator

The supinator and abductor pollicis longus are then gently retracted medially to expose the proximal two-thirds of the radius.

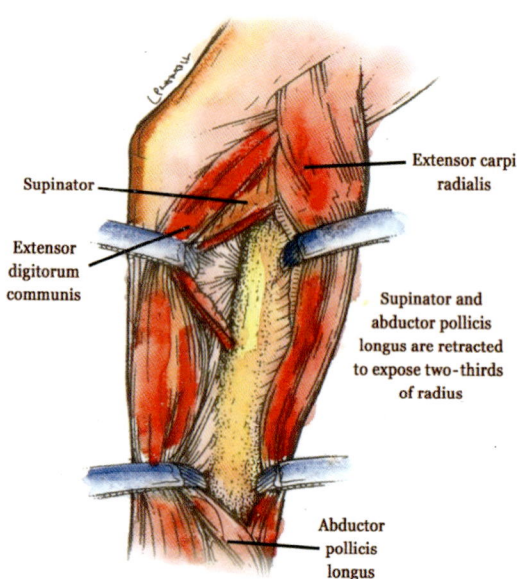

Supinator

Extensor digitorum communis

Extensor carpi radialis

Supinator and abductor pollicis longus are retracted to expose two-thirds of radius

Abductor pollicis longus

Indications
- Fractures, delayed or non-united fractures, in the proximal half of the radius.
- Tumours or infections in this area.
- Exploration of the posterior interosseous nerve.

Anterior Approach for Distal Radius

Access: Anterior surface of the distal half of the radius.

Position: The patient lies supine with the shoulder abducted and externally rotated. The upper extremity is placed on an adjacent arm table with the elbow extended and the forearm supinated.

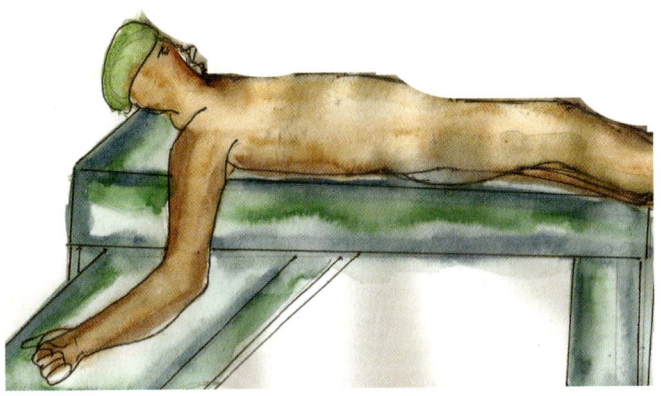

Incision: Beginning at the flexion crease of the wrist, the incision parallels the radial border of the flexor carpi radialis tendon for the distance required.

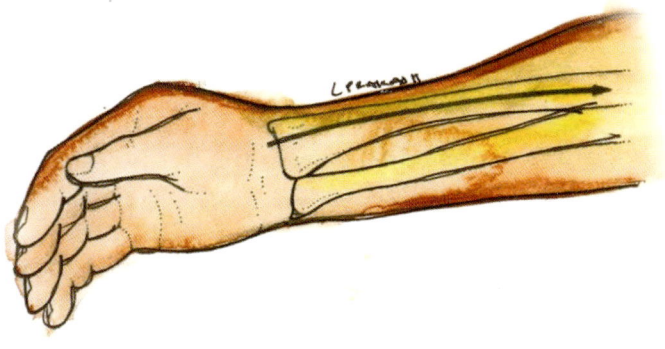

Approach: The radial artery is identified between the tendons of the brachioradialis and the flexor carpi radialis, protected and retracted medially.

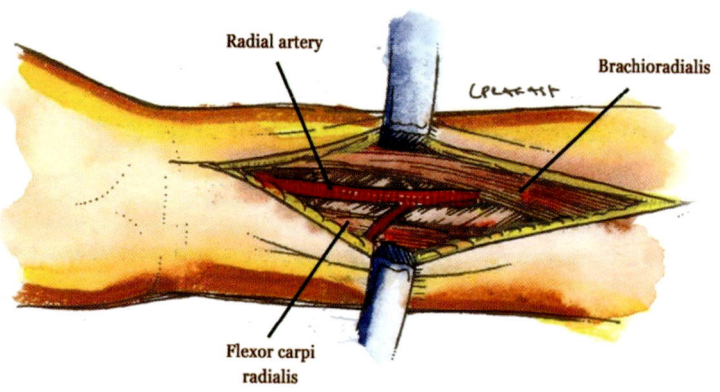

The sensory branch of the radial nerve is identified beneath the brachioradialis where it is protected and retracted laterally.

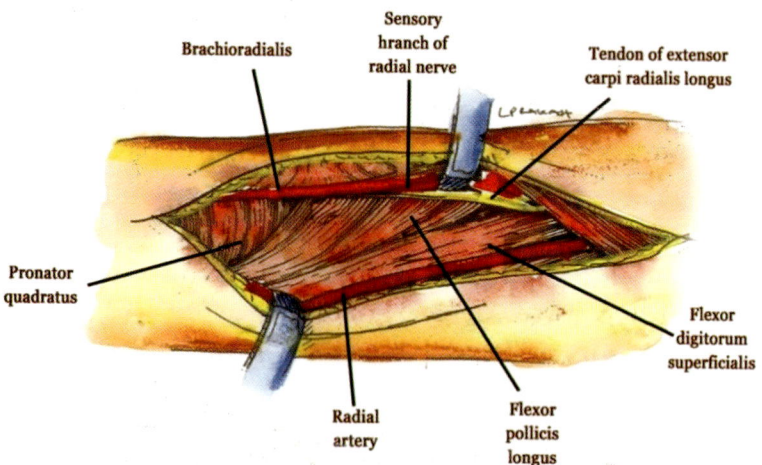

The forearm is pronated to expose the border of the radius lateral to the lateral edges of the flexor pollicis longus and the pronator quadratus.

The periosteum of the radius is incised in line with the pollicis longus and the pronator quadratus, reflecting these medially to expose the anterior border of the distal half of the radial shaft.

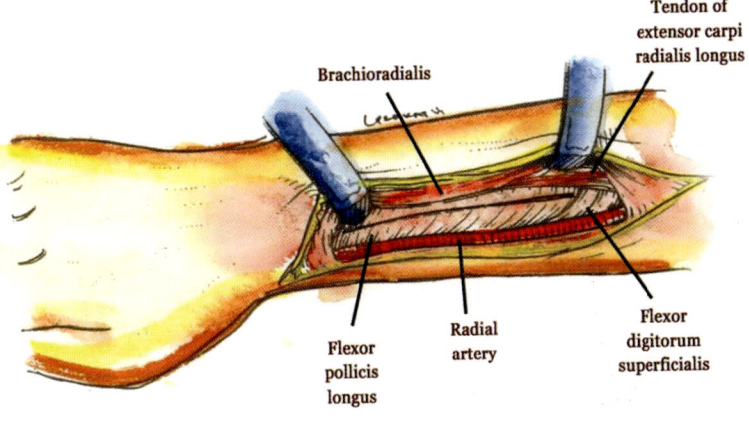

Tendon of
extensor carpi
radialis longus

Brachioradialis

Flexor
pollicis
longus

Radial
artery

Flexor
digitorum
superficialis

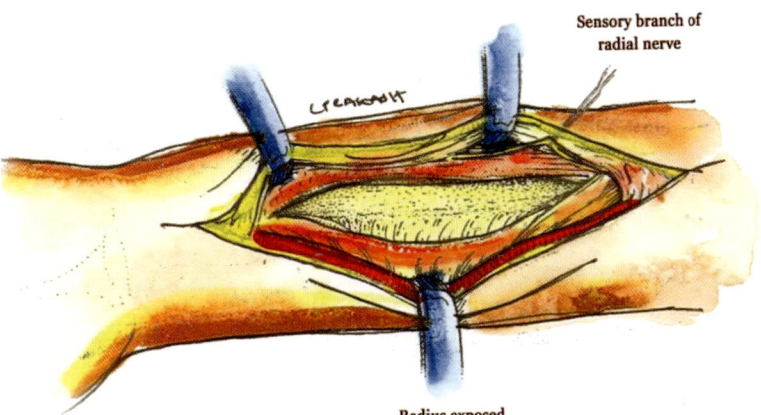

Sensory branch of
radial nerve

Radius exposed

Indications
- Fractures.
- Delayed and non-unions.
- Corrective osteotomy.
- Tumours or infections.

Combined Posterior Approach to the Radius and Ulna

Access (single incision)
- Proximal third of the ulnar shaft.
- Proximal two-thirds of the radial shaft.
- Access (double incision)
- Entire shaft of ulna.
- Proximal two-thirds of the radial shaft.

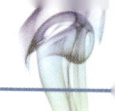

***Position*:** The patient is supine on the operating table. The arm is abducted and positioned on an adjacent table with the elbow flexed and the forearm supinated.

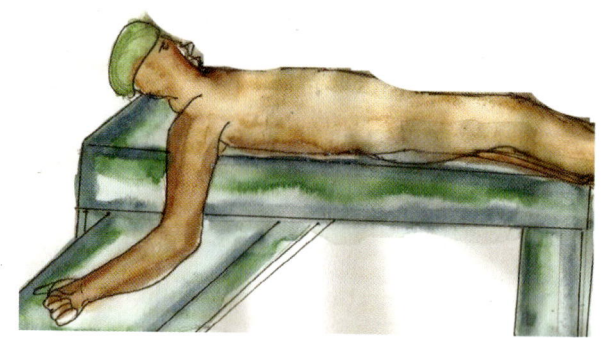

Incision

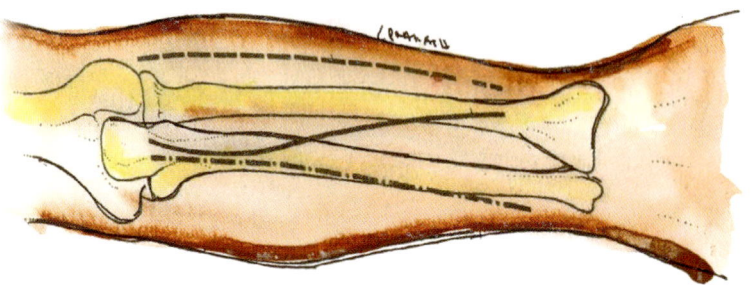

Single incision: Beginning at the elbow between the olecranon and the lateral epicondyle, curving over the proximal third of the ulna, and then back over the middle third of the radius.

Double incision: The ulnar incision is over its subcutaneous border from olecranon to ulnar styloid. The radial incision is standard Thompson posterolateral incision.

Approach

Single incision: A full thickness skin and subcutaneous fat flap is mobilized. The ulnar periosteum is incised along the subcutaneous margin of the bone and the extensor carpi ulnaris is separated laterally.

The upper two-thirds of the ulnar shaft is exposed between the extensor carpi radialis brevis and the extensor digitorum communis exposing the supinator and locating ulna below it.

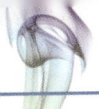

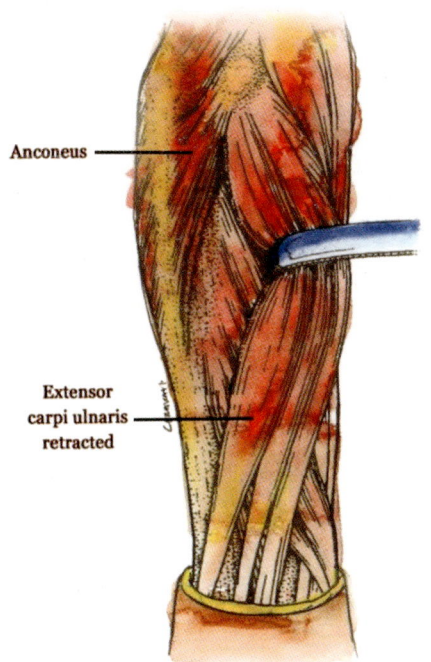

Anconeus

Extensor
carpi ulnaris
retracted

The deep posterior interosseous nerve is identified and visualized sufficiently to protect it.

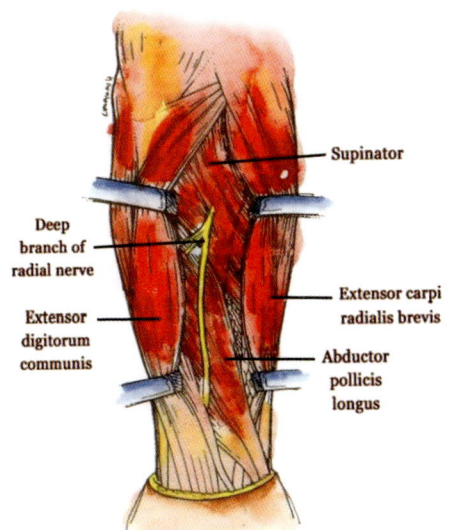

Supinator

Deep
branch of
radial nerve

Extensor
digitorum
communis

Extensor carpi
radialis brevis

Abductor
pollicis
longus

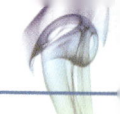

The supinator is divided longitudinally over the lateral aspect of the radius and retracted medially with the thumb muscles.

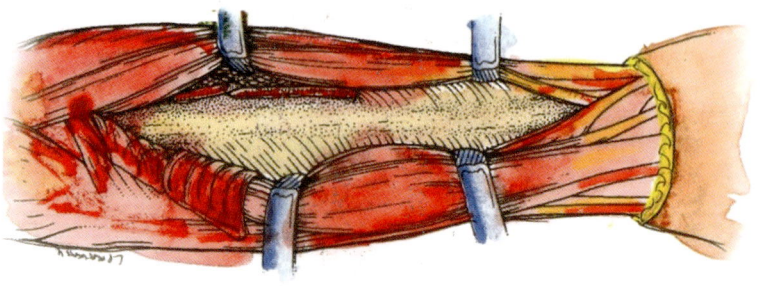

Double incision: The two separate incisions have sufficient skin space between them and should not be placed close together.

The ulna is palpated and the skin over the bone is incised.

The radius is approached by Thompson's approach.

Indications

- Fractures, delayed unions, non-unions and segmental bone loss.
- Corrective osteotomies.
- Benign or malignant tumours.
- Infections.

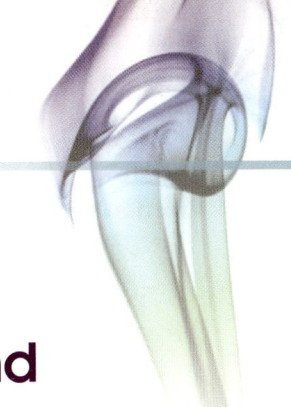

The Wrist and Hand

Hand surgery is a specialty, passionately coveted by both orthopaedic and plastic surgeons. A large number of bones, muscles, tendons, nerves and vessels crowd into a small irregular space, and share an intimate relationship.

More than with other parts of the body, here both the bone and soft tissue have to not only be treated together, but also probably by the same person. Unlike the lower limb where an orthopod would stabilize the bone, a vascular surgeon the vessels and the plastic surgeon the remaining soft tissues and skin, in the hand all these functions are done by a single person.

Thus the orthopaedic surgeon who deals with hand surgery should be as well versed with handling soft tissues, as should the plastic surgeon handling the bones be.

Similarly the exposures cannot be classified as simply as other areas, and the large varieties of incisions will depend on two aspects: The part to be exposed, and the extent of exposure required for that particular procedure.

Thus it can be logically inferred that a correct incision:
- Provides a large area to easily permit dissection
- Allows decent access to the area of lesions
- Will heal rapidly without scars limiting postoperative mobility
- Will reserve sensation and
- Avoid painful scars

On the contrary, incorrect incisions cause inadequate exposure, insufficient access, necrosis, contracture, anaesthetic areas and painful scars.

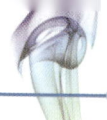

Flexion and extension of the fingers is a very important function, and scars that restrict this postoperatively are a disaster. In many cases, the patient seeks surgery for restriction of these movements due to scars.

The following are potentially damaging incisions, and should be avoided:

- Longitudinal incisions crossing flexion creases vertically in the palmar area.
- Incisions close and parallel to the web.
- Longitudinal anterolateral incisions causing damage to the neurovascular bundles.
- Incisions crossing thenar crease vertically in the hollow of the palm.
- Incisions on the palmar pulp.
- Circumferential/spiral incisions.
- Fish mouth opening of pulp leaves a painful scar.
- Incisions directly on the creases lead to maceration, delayed healing.

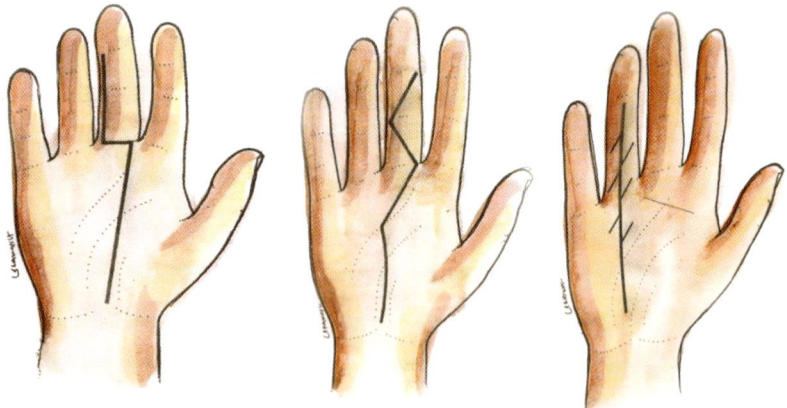

As a rule, incisions should not cross the flexion creases of the fingers, as subsequent contracture of the scar causes a flexion deformity (which could even have been the reason for surgery).

This can be avoided in the following ways:
A bayonet (or step incision) is used, in which the transverse incision over the flexor creases are joined proximally and distally

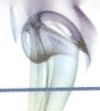
to horizontal ones. This may occasionally become a matter of necessity, because the pre-existing cut or scar would be transverse.

The incision is made in a zigzag shape, especially in the digits, so that it crosses the flexion creases at an outwards angle, to the end of the crease at the mid-lateral line.

A straight incision is made, but before closure is broken up by one or more Z plasties. Z plasties allow elongation of the incision, and their effect is cumulative.

Scars crossing the flexion creases in the palm result in a lesser incidence of flexion contracture and are often acceptable.

Scar contracture is a problem of the skin itself and not of the subcutaneous and deeper tissues. Once an incision has been made in the skin and properly developed, further incision into the deeper tissues can be made in any desired direction.

It is usually best to incorporate the earlier wound or scar into the new incision and this gives the opportunity to excise the scar, if it is hypertrophic.

If it is decided to ignore an old scar and plan a new elective incision, one must ensure that this will not compromise the blood supply distal to the old scar. Parallel wounds thus should not be too close together.

Complex tendon transfer operations needing access to many different parts of the hand, require multiple small incisions. The

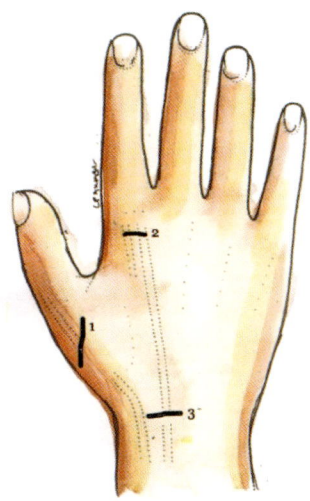

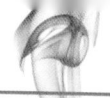

tendons can be detached or re-routed, through these small transverse incisions, causing the least possible scarring along the gliding surface of the tendon and an inconspicuous scar.

The cosmetic effect of scars is important. The hands and face are the only parts of the body which are normally exposed and as the hand is used in greeting or to give or receive something, a scar is noticeable.

Scars parallel to the creases of the skin are less likely to become hypertrophic. The finger creases have no subcutaneous fat, and skin and subcutaneous tissue are sutured together. Thus incisions should be parallel and near to a crease rather than over the crease.

SURGICAL APPROACHES

- Palmar fascia
  - Transverse incision
  - Longitudinal incision
  - Combinations of incisions
- Flexor tendons and median nerve
  - Carpal tunnel exposure
  - Extension above wrist
  - Flexor tendons in fingers and thumb
  - Mid-lateral incision
  - Zigzag incisions
- Extensor tendons
  - Carpus
  - Dorsal
  - Radial
  - Anterior

Palmar Fascia

The most common indication would be Dupuytren's contracture, which is an uncommon pathology in our parts of the world.

In the Western world, one of the most common disorders of the hand is Dupuytren's contracture.

The incision should, as far as possible, pass through the points of skin attachment, so that these thinnest parts of the skin flaps are at their edge and not in their base.

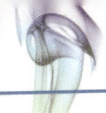

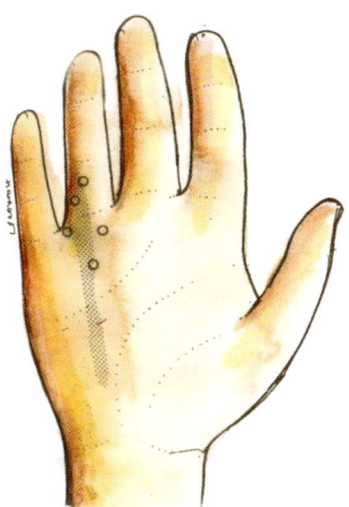

The pattern of disease will determine whether the incision is transverse, longitudinal, or a combination of both.

Transverse Incision

If the disease is confined mainly to the palm, a transverse incision on or around the distal palmar crease gives good access.

However, it may not always possible to approximate the skin edges for an intimate suture. McCash (1964) described a method by which the wound is left open to heal secondary intention.

After correction of the contracture, there may be a gap of up to 2 cm between the skin edges, even when there is no skin missing. Surprisingly, as the wound heals, the skin edges are drawn together to produce a linear scar over 4–6 weeks.

Alternatively, a transverse incision left open in the finger at the basal flexion crease can be deployed, but this gives only very limited access and is more suitable for open fasciotomy than for fasciectomy.

Longitudinal Incision

If the disease is distributed longitudinally from the palm into the finger, then an longitudinal incision gives the best exposure. However, this is modified to avoid a straight longitudinal scar in the finger. In the palm, scar contracture is seldom a problem and a gently tortuous incision is enough.

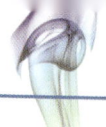

Straight incision with Z-plasties

A straight incision is made down the midline of the finger as far as the centre of the middle phalanx. The Z-plasties should not be made until the end of the procedure, to ensure that any thin skin is at the edge, rather than at the base, of any flap.

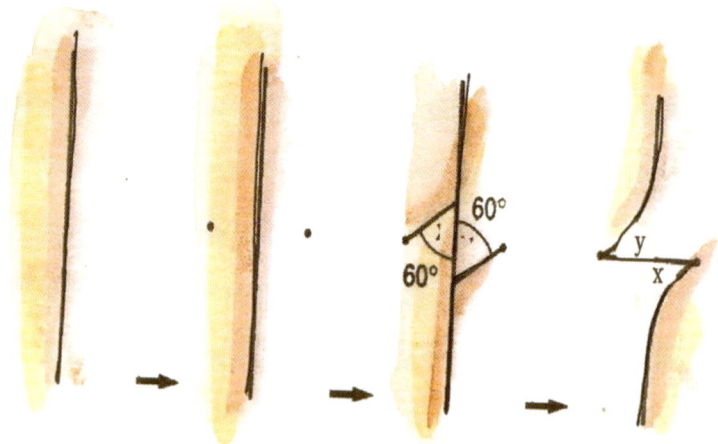

The skin should be handled gently with a fine skin hook and never with forceps.

Before closure, two spots are marked 7 mm on either side of the incision opposite each other preferably in the flexion creases. Parallel incisions are made, joining each spot to the previous incision at an angle of 60°.

It is best not to suture the transverse limb but to leave it open as this diminishes both tension and the risk of haematoma.

Zig-zag incision

The incision stays close to the longitudinal line of the disease; the sides should be about 1 cm long and the angle 90° or a little less. The parts of the incision which cross the flexion creases should coincide with one of the angles. There will also be angles in between these creases. Closure should be with stitches at the apices only, to allow free drainage of any blood.

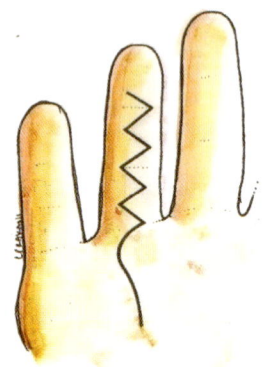

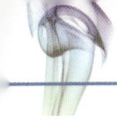

If the contracture is severe, it is preferable to use Z-plasties which actually lengthen the scar.

Combinations of Incisions

When more than one finger is involved, it is necessary to plan an incision combining both incisions described above.

The main concern is to preserve a blood supply to the distal skin flap between two longitudinal incisions. One solution is not to incise that part of skin, but to tunnel subcutaneously from the palmar incision to the base of the finger.

Alternatively, the longitudinal incisions for two fingers may join a transverse palmar incision. If this is done, the distal flap between them should be as broadly based as possible, and the transverse incision should not be sutured.

Any longitudinal incision made in the proximal part of the palm must not join the transverse palmar incision opposite the distal longitudinal incision, or a continuous longitudinal incision will result, which is very likely to cause a contracture.

Flexor Tendons and Median Nerve

A limited exposure for the release of a trigger finger or thumb can be obtained by a transverse incision placed over the proximal end of the fibrous flexor sheath, about 2 cm proximal to the basal flexor crease.

If there is more than one trigger finger, the skin incision can be extended to cover both.

Exposure of the Carpal Tunnel

The flexor retinaculum extends from the distal flexion crease of the wrist to the proximal end of the hollow in the centre of the palm.

It is attached at its four corners to the pisiform, the hamates, the tuberosity of the scaphoid and the ridge of the trapezium. The incision is longitudinal and lies between the medial and lateral margins of the retinaculum.

An incision here can endanger the palmar cutaneous branch of the median nerve resulting in painful hyperaesthesia in the palm.

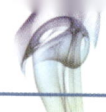

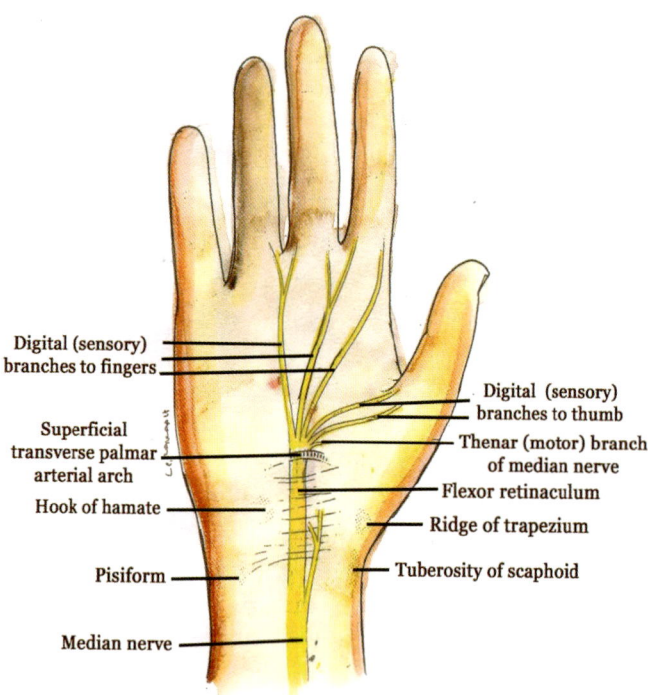

This branch usually arises from the radial side of the main median nerve, 3–6 cm above the wrist, and runs close to the tendon of flexor carpi radialis, so incisions in this area should be in the midline or slightly to the ulnar side.

Incision: The incision runs over the mid-point of the distal flexion crease of the wrist.

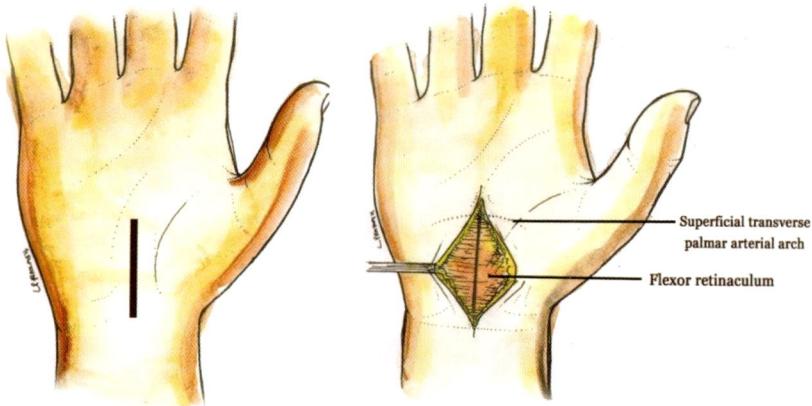

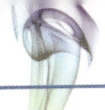
The incision must be in the midline or slightly to the ulnar side, in order to avoid the palmar cutaneous nerve. It should point roughly to the web between the middle and ring fingers.

Exposure: The incision is deepened to the insertion of the palmaris longus, until the flexor retinaculum.

The retinaculum is incised longitudinally, deepening the cut 1 mm at a time in the same place, until the carpal tunnel is entered.

This is enlarged to admit the curved end of a MacDonald's dissector, which is passed distally, keeping its tip as superficial in the tunnel as possible.

The cut is deepened down over the flexor retinaculum up to the dissector, which is now extracted and reintroduced the other way (going proximally).

The retinaculum is divided proximally till it thins out to become the deep fascia of the forearm.

Indications

- Decompression of the carpal tunnel.
- Extension above the wrist.

Approach: A step is added to the incision by incorporating a short transverse cut in the distal flexion crease of the wrist, and then continued proximally.

If there is a pre-existing transverse wound or scar, it is incorporated in the incision.

The approach is from the ulnar side of the midline, to avoid damage to the palmar cutaneous nerve and the long digital flexors lie.

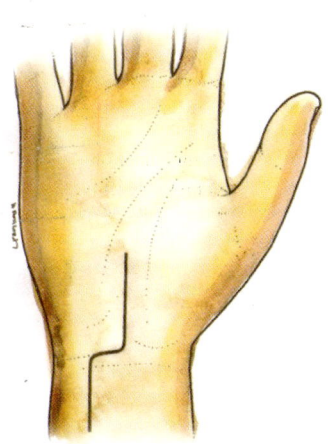

Indications

- Repair of cut nerves and tendons. Flexor tenosynovectomy (e.g. rheumatoid).
- Carpal tunnel syndrome following a Colles' fracture.
- Flexor tendon reconstructions, e.g. tendon graft to the thumb.
- Implantation of silastic joints.

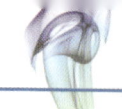

Flexor Tendons in the Fingers and Thumb

The flexion creases (three in each finger and two in each thumb) must be avoided, to prevent the development of a contracture.

It is also necessary to avoid injury to the digital nerves and vessels.

The anterior half of the finger is occupied by the flexor tendons in their sheath, covered by subcutaneous fat. The posterior half is occupied by the phalanx, over which lies the extensor tendon.

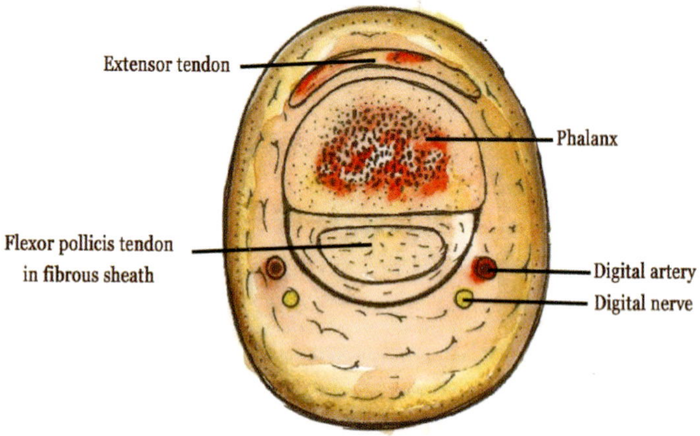

Extensor tendon

Phalanx

Flexor pollicis tendon
in fibrous sheath

Digital artery

Digital nerve

Dorsal

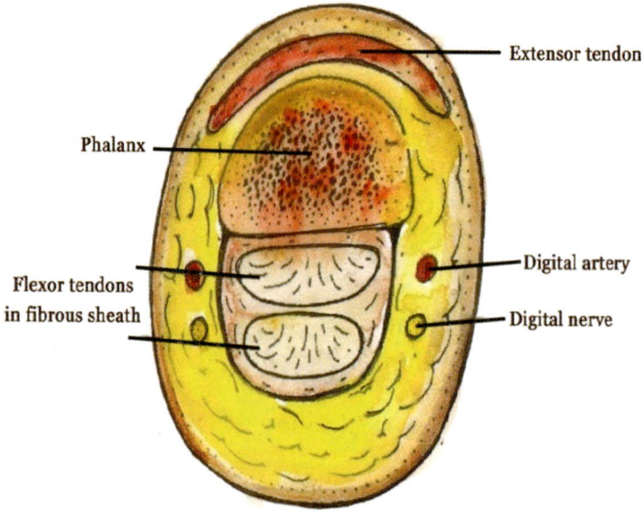

Extensor tendon

Phalanx

Flexor tendons
in fibrous sheath

Digital artery

Digital nerve

Palmar
finger

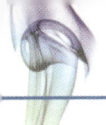

The digital arteries and nerves are anterior to the mid-lateral line, with the nerve lying in front of the artery.

In the thumb, the nerves and vessels are more anterior; and may lie partly in front of the flexor tendon sheath.

Approaches: There are two ways to avoid crossing of the flexor creases:

- A mid-lateral incision on the same side of the finger.
- Bruner zigzag incision, crossing the finger obliquely to the end of the next crease on the other side.

The advantages of the mid-lateral incision are two. It avoids scarring the anterior skin, and is easier to close with the finger flexed. However, a proper scar on the palmar surface does not cause problems.

The number of zigs depends on the length of the segment; the variability of this incision is one of its advantages.

1. Mid-lateral Incision

The advantages of the mid-lateral incision are two. It avoids scarring the anterior skin, and is easier to close with the finger flexed. However, a proper scar on the palmer surface does not cause problems.

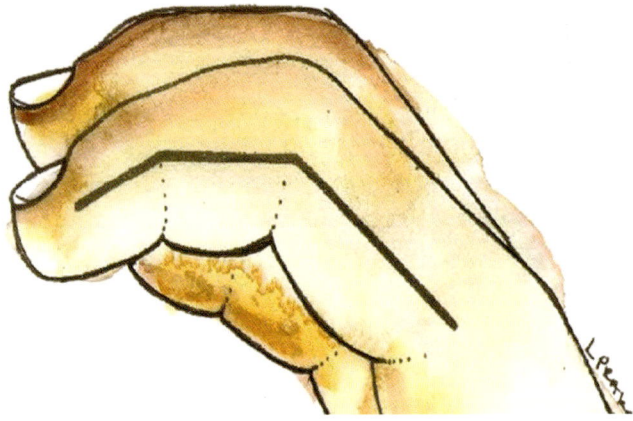

The ulnar side is preferable. On the index finger, the temptation to use the more accessible radial side should be resisted as this side of the finger should be left unscarred (as is so important in fine manipulations and key grip).

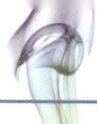

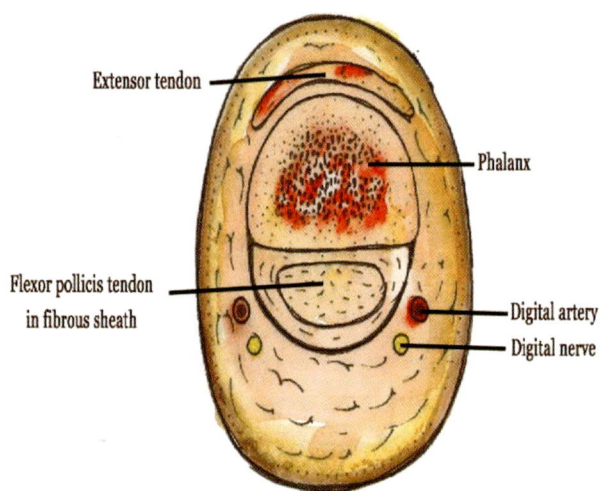

- Extensor tendon
- Phalanx
- Flexor pollicis tendon in fibrous sheath
- Digital artery
- Digital nerve

A line is drawn along the medial side of the finger between the ends of the flexion creases. Dissection is continued up to the side of the flexor tendon sheath, close to its attachment to the phalanx. Skin and fat are retracted anteriorly, using a small blunt hook, taking care to protect the digital nerve and artery.

The fibrous sheath is incised longitudinally to expose the flexor tendon. It may be necessary to incise the sheath transversely at one or both ends of the longitudinal incision in order to raise a flap of sheath to give a good view of the tendon.

2. Zigzag Incisions

The large zigzag incision gives good access to the flexor tendon sheath and to the digital nerve and artery.

Various other forms of zigzag incisions have also been described, all of which give better access to a narrower strip down the finger.

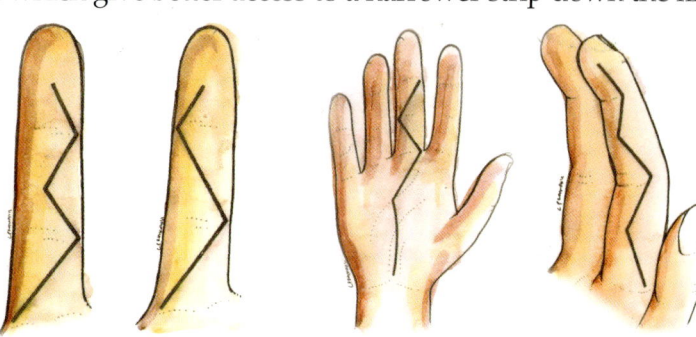

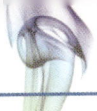

Indications
- Repair of cut flexor tendons.
- Tendon grafting.
- Flexor tenosynovectomy.
- Tumours involving the flexor tendons like pigmented villonodular synovitis.

Extensor Tendons

The skin on the back of the hand is lax and scarring is usually not a problem. Straight longitudinal incisions are adequate for most situations. In rheumatoids, where the skin is delicate, thick skin flaps are needed to protect vascularity.

The extensor retinaculum is not a single sheet of tissue across the tendons. It has six compartments containing varying tendons.

Approach: A straight longitudinal incision is made over the extensor tendon to be exposed.

The dissection is deepened to the retinaculum, and then bluntly separated off the fat. It is essential to keep the skin flap as thick as possible. Retraction must be very gentle, particularly in rheumatoid patients.

When it is necessary to expose more than one group of tendons, the sagittal septa which hold down the retinaculum must be divided so that the whole retinaculum can be lifted up as a flap.

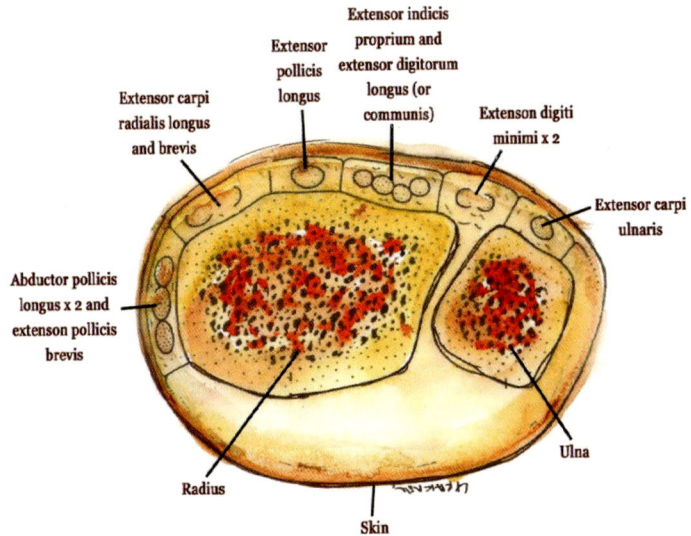

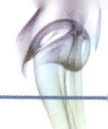

Starting from the radial side, the retinaculum is separated, leaving it attached on the ulnar side alone. Stripping can also be done from ulnar to radial, but in this case, there is risk of producing an ulnar slipping of the tendons postoperatively.

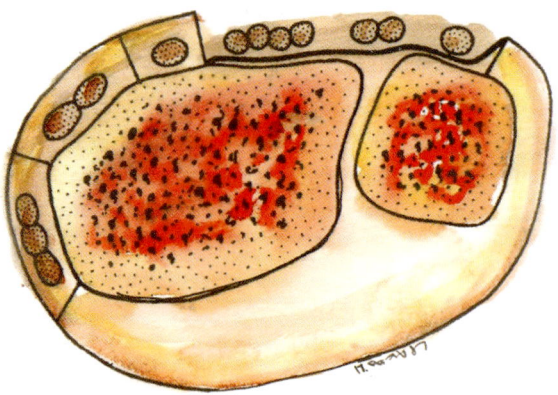

A small strip of retinaculum is cut in a step fashion which can later be made into a pulley to keep the extensor pollicis longus tendon in place on the ulnar side of Lister's tubercle.

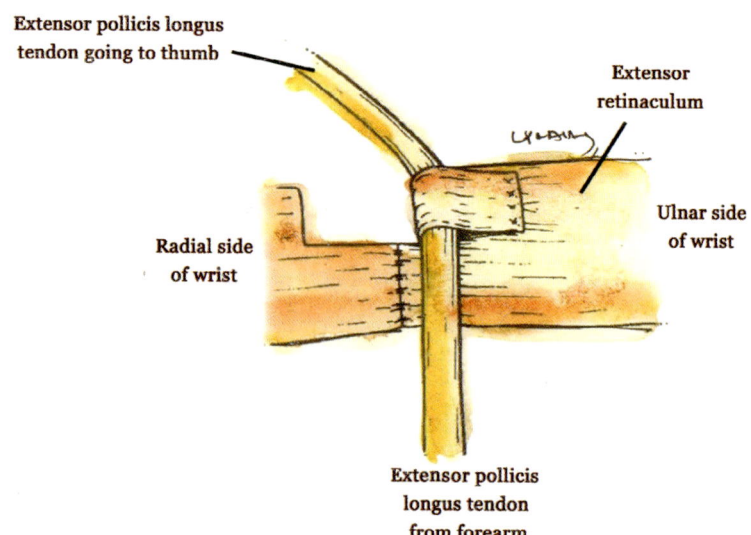

Extensor pollicis longus tendon going to thumb

Extensor retinaculum

Radial side of wrist

Ulnar side of wrist

Extensor pollicis longus tendon from forearm

Postoperatively, the retinaculum is not sutured to avoid constriction. In an case, release of the retinaculum is a part of the decompressive procedure.

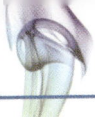
Indications

- Access to the extensor tendons.
- Tenosynovectomy for rheumatoid disease.
- Repair after trauma.
- Approaches to the carpal bones
- The approach chosen depends upon the area of the carpus to be exposed. Ulnar approaches are infrequently used, because access to the hamate, triquetral and pisiform is not often needed.
- The carpal bones are small, and it is easy to mistake one bone or joint for another. It is good practice to confirm the location after exposure, by pushing in a needle and confirm under a C-arm.

Dorsal Approach

Incision: The skin incision may be transverse or longitudinal.

If only limited access is required, as for a ganglion, a transverse incision leaves a less conspicuous scar.

If the whole length of the carpus is to be exposed, a longitudinal incision is necessary.

Thick skin flaps are essential, especially in rheumatoid patients who are very slow to heal.

Approach: Once through the skin, the approach is longitudinal between the extensor tendons.

The extensor retinaculum is divided longitudinally over the required area and retracted with blunt hooks, exposing the dorsal capsule of the wrist joint.

For a ganglion, the part of the capsule from which it arises must be excised together with the ganglion, to prevent recurrence.

The dorsal capsule is incised longitudinally over the part required, and then released by sharp dissection on either side from its attachments to the underlying bones.

The radiocarpal joint is identified by palpation before incising the capsule.

Indications

- Excision of dorsal wrist ganglion.
- Operations on the lunate.
- Ligamentous reconstructions.
- Partial or complete arthrodesis.

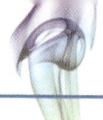

Radial Approach

Here there are two important structures to avoid:
1. The superficial radial nerve, which may be in one or two parts, running parallel by the radial side of the wrist.
2. The radial artery, with its accompanying veins coming from the front of the radius, to pass dorsally between the bases of the first and second metacarpals.

The artery is always preserved, and large hematomas may result from dividing its small branches whilst mobilizing the main artery.

These should be identified and coagulated at some distance from the main artery before they are cut.

Incision: The skin incision follows the line of the radial artery. The superficial nerve should not be damaged by the incision.

The nerve is retracted in either direction, and the anterior branches of the radial artery are coagulated and retracted dorsally.

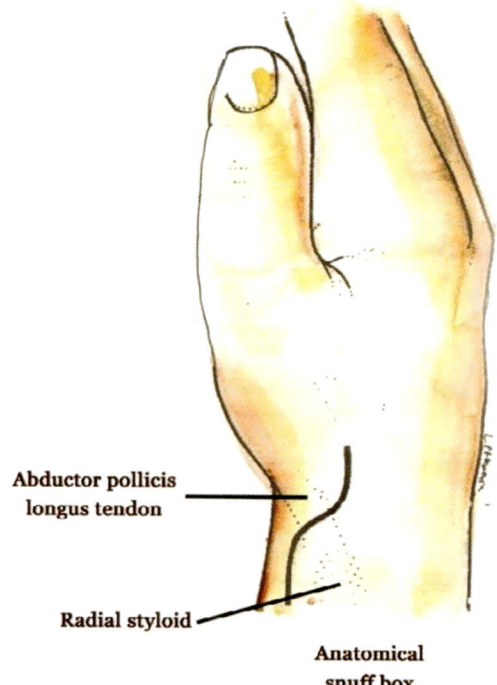

Abductor pollicis longus tendon

Radial styloid

Anatomical snuff box

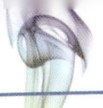

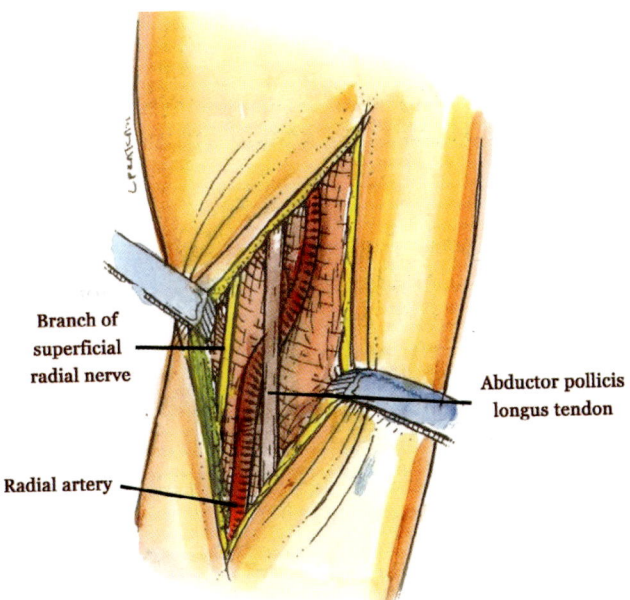

Branch of superficial radial nerve

Abductor pollicis longus tendon

Radial artery

Partial detachment of the abductor pollicis longus from its insertion on the base of the first metacarpal increases the exposure.

The capsule is incised longitudinally to reach the carpus.

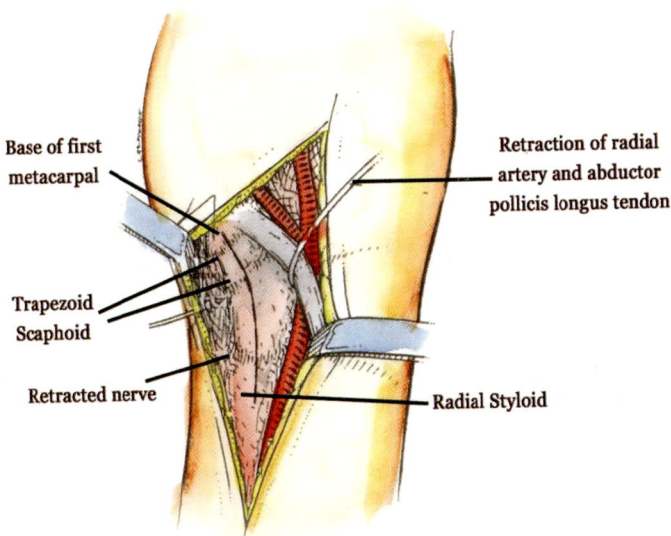

Base of first metacarpal

Retraction of radial artery and abductor pollicis longus tendon

Trapezoid
Scaphoid

Retracted nerve

Radial Styloid

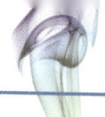

Indications
- Excision of trapezium.
- Arthrodesis or arthroplasty of trapeziometacarpal joint.
- Exposure of distal pole of scaphoid for internal fixation.

Anterior Approach

This is indicated only for open reduction of an anteriorly dislocated lunate or for reconstructions of the anterior ligaments.

An anterior approach more laterally gives access to the scaphoid, for bone grafting non-union.

Incision: The skin incision begins along the radial side of the distal inch of the flexor carpi radialis tendon and then continues across the wrist flexion crease, curving radially along the line of the radially abducted first metacarpal.

The radial side of the sheath of flexor carpi radialis is incised and the tendon is retracted to the ulnar side.

One or more small palmar branches of the radial artery may need to be ligated and divided.

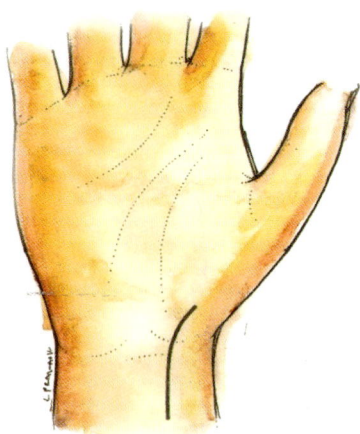

Going through the middle of the bed of the tendon exposes the scaphoid a little further towards the ulnar side, giving a better view of the proximal pole.

The anterior capsule of the wrist is divided in the line of the long axis of the scaphoid to expose the bone. The tuberosity protrudes anteriorly, while the waist and proximal pole are deeper.

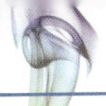

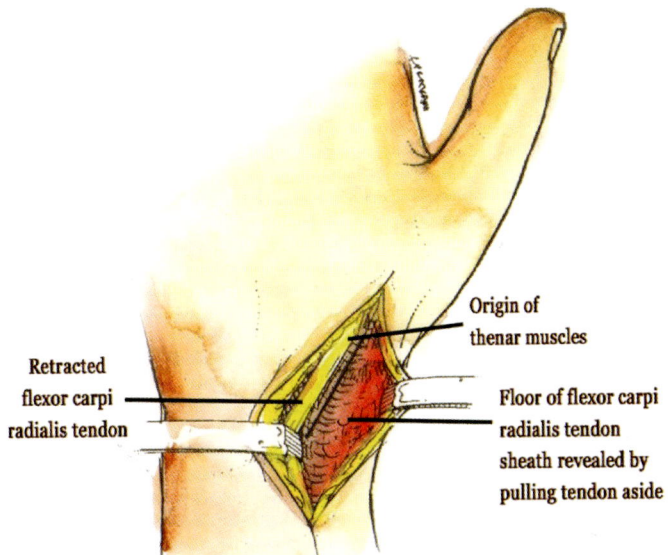

Origin of
thenar muscles

Retracted
flexor carpi
radialis tendon

Floor of flexor carpi
radialis tendon
sheath revealed by
pulling tendon aside

If a Herbert screw is to be inserted, the scaphotrapezial joint must be opened widely enough by splitting the origin of the thenar for about 1 cm in the line of their fibres and retracted to either side.

Indications: Fractures of scaphoid requiring bone grafting and/ or fixation with Herbert screw.

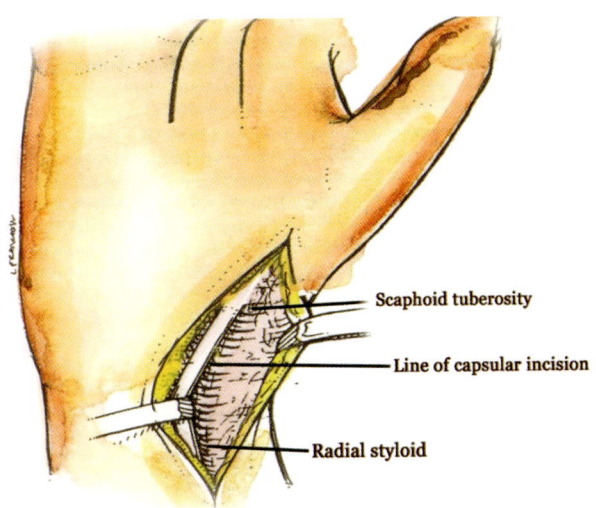

Scaphoid tuberosity

Line of capsular incision

Radial styloid

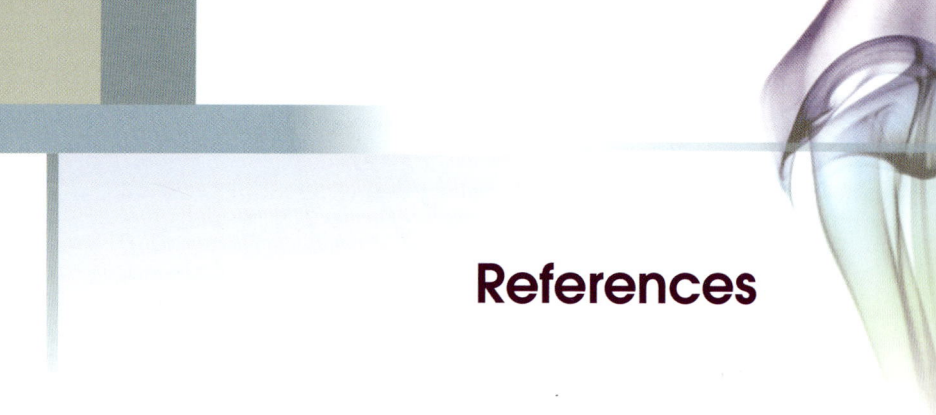

References

Abbott, LC and Carpenter, WF (1945) Surgical approaches to the knee joint. J Bone joint Surg., 27, 277.

Adams, JC (1948) Arthrodesis of the ankle joint. J Bone joint Surg., 303, 506.

Banks, SW and Laufman, H (1953) An Atlas of Surgical Exposures of the Extremities, WB Saunders, Philadelphia Harmon, PH (1945) A simplified surgical approach to the tibia.

Bonney, G, Birch, R and Marshall, RW (1990) A surgical approach to the cervico-thoracic spine. J Bone Joint Surg. 72B, 904-907.

Brackett, EG and Osgood, RB (1911) The popliteal incision for the removal of joint mice in the posterior capsule of the knee joint. Boston Med. Surg. J, 165, 975.

Brackett, EG (1912) Study of the different approaches to the hip joint. Boston Med. Surg., CLXVI, 235.

Gibson, A (1950) Posterior exposure of the hip joint. J. Bone joint Surg. 32B, 183.

Brackett, EG and Hall CL (1917) Osteochondritis dissecans. Am. I. Orthop. Surg., XV, 79.

Bruser, DM (1960) A direct lateral approach to the lateral compartment of the knee joint. J Bone Joint Surg., 423, 3, 8.

Campbell, WC (1949) Operative Orthopaedics, 2nd edn, Henry Kempton, London.

Campbell, WC (1956) Operative Orthopaedics, 3rd edn, CV Mosby, St Louis, p. 195.

Capener, N (1954) The evolution of lateral rachotomy. J Bone joint Surg., 368, 173-179.

Cauchoix, J and Binet, JP (1957) Anterior surgical approaches to the spine. Ann. R. Coll. Surg. Engl., 35, 237-243.

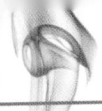

Charles, RW and Govender, S (1989) Anterior approach to the upper thoracic vertebrae. J Bone joint Surg., 71 B, 81-84.

Charnley, I (1979) Low Friction Arthroplasty of the Hip, Springer, Berlin.

Cloward, RB (1958) The anterior approach for removal of ruptured cervical disc.]. Neurosurg, 15, 602.

Colton, CL (1982) Watson-Jones Fractures and joint Injuries, Churchill Livingstone, Edinburgh, p. 1147.

Crenshaw, AH (1980) Surgical approaches in Campbell's Operative Orthopaedics (eds AS Edmonson and AH Crenshaw), CV. Mosby, St Louis.

Darrach, W (1945) Surgical approaches for surgery of the extremities. Am. J. Surg., 67, 237.

De And rade,]. R and MacNab, l. (1969) Anterior occipital fusion using an extra pharangeal exposure. 1. Bone joint Surg., 51A, 1621.

Devine, HB (1931) Exposure of the knee joint. Br. J. Surg., XIX, 306.

Erkes, F (1929) Weitere Erfahrungen mit Physiologischer Schnitt Fuhrung zue Eroffnung des Kniegelenks. Brunx Beitr. Klin. Chir., CXLVII, 221.

Evans, DL (1953) Recurrent instability of the ankle – a surgical treatment Proc. R. Soc. Med" 46, 343.

Fang, HSY and Ong , GB (1962) Direct approaches to the upper cervical spine. 1. Bone joint Surg., 44A, 1588.

Fang, HSY, Ong, GB and Hodgson, AR (1964) Anterior spinal fusion. The operative approach. Clin. Orthop., 35, 16.

Fiolle, J and Delmas, J (1921) In The Surgical Exposure of Deep Seated Blood-vessels (ed. C. G. Cumston), Heinemann, London, pp. 61-67.

for bone grafting and fibuiar transference. J. Bone joint Surg., 27, 496.

Fowler, AW (1959) A method of forefoot reconstruction. J. Bone joint Surg., 418, 507.

Gatellier, J. (1931) The juxta-peroneal route in the operative treatment of fracture of the malleolus with posterior marginal fragment. Surg. Gynecol. Obstet., 52, 67.

Gatellier, J and Chastang (1924) La voie d'acces juxta-retropéroniere dans le traitement sanglant des fractures malléolaires avec fragment marginal posterieur (technique opératoire). J. Chir, 24, 513.

Gibson, A. (1950) Posterior exposure of the hip joint. j. Bone joint Surg. 32B, 183.

Gillquist, J and Hagberg, G. (1976) A new modification of the technique of arthroscopy of the knee joint. Acta Chir. Scand., 142, 123-130.

Glasgow, M, Jackson, A and JamIeson, A. (1980) Instability of the ankle after injury to the lateral ligament. J. Bone joint Surg., 62B, 196.

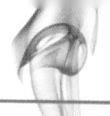

Gordes, W and Viernstein, Jr, K. (1980) Traitement de l'instabilité tibio-tarsienne par tenodése al' aide du court péronier lateral. Int. Orthop., 3, 293.

Grant, JCB. (1972) Grant's Atlas of Anatomy, Williams and Wilkins, Baltimore.

Hardinge, K. (1982) The direct lateral approach to the hip. 1. Bone joint Surg., 648, 17.

Harty, M and Joyce, JJ. (1963) Surgical approaches to the hip and femur. J. Bone Joint Surg., 45A, 175.

Helal , B. (1975) Metatarsal osteotomy for metatarsalgia. J. Bone Joint Surg., 578, 187.

Henderson , MS. (1921) Posterolateral Incision for the removal of loose bodies from the posterior compartment of the knee joint. Surg. Gynecol. Obstet., 33, 691.

Henry, AK (1924-25) Exposure of the humerus and femoral shaft. Br. J. Surg., 12, 84.

Henry, AK. (1957) Extensile Exposure, 2nd edn, E. & S. Livingstone, Edinburgh.

Henry, AK. (1966) Extensile Exposure, E. & S. Livingstone, Edinburgh.

Henry, AK. (1973) Extensile Exposure, Churchill Livingstone, Edinburgh, pp. 15-47.

Henry, AK. (1959) Extensile Exposure, 2nd edn, E. & S. Livingstone, Edinburgh, p. 305.

Hodgson, AR and Rau, ACM. (1969) Anterior approach to the spinal column. Recent Adv. Orthop., IX, 289.

Hollinshead. WH. (1932) Anatomy for Surgeons, volume. 3, Harper and Row, philadelphia.

Insall, J. (1971) A mid-line approach to the knee. J. Bone joint Surg., 53A, 1584 .

Jones, R. (1916) Disabilities of the knee joint. Br. Med. J., ll , 169.

Judet R., Judet, J. and Letournel, E. (1964) Fractures of the acetabulum: classification and surgical approaches for open reduction. J. Bone joint Surg., 46A, 1615.

Kaplan, EB. (1946) Posterior approach to the superoiateral region of the tibia. J. Bone joint Surg., 28, 805.

Kocher, T. (1903) Text book of Operative Surgery, 2nd edn (translated from 4th German edn), Adam & Charles Black, London.

Konig, F. and Schafer, P. (1929) Osteoplastic surgical exposure of the ankle joint. Zeit. chir, 215, 196 (Abstracted in 44th report of Progress in Orthopaedic Surgery, p. 17).

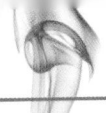

Langenbeck, B. von (1874) Ueber die Schussverletzungen des Huftgelenks Arch. Klin. Chir., 16, 263.

Louis, R. (1983) Surgery of the Spine, Springer, Berlin.

Ludloff, K. (1939) The open reduction of the congenital hip dislocation and anterior incision. Am. J. Orthop. Surg., 10, 438.

MacRae, R. (1987) Practical Orthopaedic Exposures, Churchill Livingstone, Edinburgh, pp. 24-50.

Marcy, GH. (1947) Posterolateral approach to the femur. J.Bone Joint Surg., 29, 676.

Marti, R, Reichen, A., Oberhammer, l. and Raaymakers, E. (1976) Talo-fibular tendon graft for recurrent instability of the ankle joint. In Injuries of the Ligaments and their Repair, Chapchal, Theime, Stuttgart, p. 219.

McConnell, JC. (1976) A dynamic transpatellar approach to the knee. South. Med. J., 69, 567.

McFarland, B. and Osborne, G. (1954) Approach to the hip. J. Bone joint Surg., 36B, 364.

Moore, AT. (1957) The self -locking metal hips prosthesis. J.Bone Joint Surg., 39A, 812.

Muller, ME, Allgower, M, Schneider, R. et al. (1979) Manual of Internal Fixation, Springer, Berlin.

Ollier, L. (1891) Traite des Resections et des Operations Conservatrices qu'on peut Practiquer sur Ie Systéme Osseux, Masson et Cle, Paris.

Payr, E. (1917) Einfaches und schonendes Verfahren zur beliebig Eroffnung des Kniegelenkes. Zentralbl . Chir., XLIV, 921.

Perry, J. (1977) Surgical approaches to the cervical Spine. In The Total Care of Spinal Injuries (eds E. 5. Pierce and VH Nickel), Little, Brown, Boston.

Putti , V. (1917) La mobilizazione chirurgica delle anchilosi del ginocchio Chit. Organi. Mov., 1, 1.

Querer Durchsagung der Patella. Dtsch. Med. Wohenschr., III, 389.

Romanes, C. J. (1976) Cunningham's Manual of Practical Anatomy, vol. 1, Oxford University Press, Oxford.

Ruedi, T., Hochstetter, AHC and Schlumpf, R. (1984) Surgical Approaches for Internal Fixation, Springer, Berlin.

Ruedi, T., von Hochstetter, A. and Schlumpf, R. (1984) Surgical Approaches for Internal Fixation, Springer, Berlin.

Sefton, GK, George, L, Fitton, JM and McMullen, H. (1979) Reconstruction of the anterior talo-fibular ligament for the treatment of the unstable ankle. Bone loint Surg., 61 B, 352.

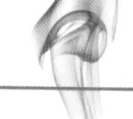

Smith-Petersen, MN. (1917) A new supra-articular approach to the hip joint. Am. I. Orthop. Surg., 15, 592.

Smith-Petersen, MN. (1949) Approach to and exposure of the hip joint for mold arthroplasty. J. Bone joint Surg., 31A, 40.

Somerville, EW. (1953) Open reduction in congenital dislocation of the hip. J. Bone joint Surg., 35B, 363.

Surgical approaches to the vertebral bodies in the cervical and lumbar regions. J. Bone Joint Surg., 39A, 631.

Textor, K. (1860) Resection des Kniegelenkes. Verh. Ges. Naturf . Arzte, xxxI, 177.

Thompson. JE. (1918) Anatomical methods of approach in operations on the long bones of the extremities. Ann. Surg., 68, 309.

Tillaux (reported by Gosselin) (1872) Rapports recherches; cliniques et experimentales sur les fractures malléolaires. Bull.Acad. Med. 5er.2 , 1,817.

Turner, PL and Webb, JK. (1987) A surgical approach to the upper thoracic spine. J. Bone Joint Surg., 678, 542-544.

Van den Brink, KD and Edmondson, AS. (1980) The spine. In Campbell's Operative Orthopaedics (eds AS Edmonson and AH Crenshaw), CV. Mosby, St Louis.

Von Langenbeck, B. (1878) Zur Resection des Kniegelenkes. Verh. Dtsch. Ges. Chir., VII, 34.

Von Volkman, R. (1977) Die Resection des Kniegelenkes mit Querer Durchsagung der Patella. Dtsch. Med. Wohenschr., III, 389.

Watkins, RG. (1983) Surgical Approaches to the Spine, Springer, New York.

Watson-Jones, R. (1936) Fractures of the neck of the femur. Br. J. Surg., 23. 7878.

White III, A. A. (1974) A precision posterior ankle fusion. Clin Orthop. 98, 239.

Wiltse, LL, Bateman, JG, Hutchinson, RH and Nelson, WE. (1963) Paraspinous muscle approach to the lumbar spine. J. Bone joint Surg., 50A, 919.